Psychiatry and Racial
Liberalism in Harlem, 1936–1968

Rochester Studies in Medical History

Senior Editor: Theodore M. Brown
Professor of History and Preventive Medicine
University of Rochester

Additional Titles of Interest

A complete list of titles in the Rochester Studies in Medical History series
may be found on our website, www.urpress.com.

Psychiatry and Racial Liberalism in Harlem, 1936–1968

DENNIS A. DOYLE

R UNIVERSITY OF ROCHESTER PRESS

The University of Rochester Press gratefully acknowledges the St. Louis College of Pharmacy for its generous support of this publication.

Copyright © 2016 by Dennis A. Doyle

First published 2016

University of Rochester Press
668 Mt. Hope Avenue, Rochester, NY 14620, USA
www.urpress.com
and Boydell & Brewer Limited
PO Box 9, Woodbridge, Suffolk IP12 3DF, UK
www.boydellandbrewer.com

Parts of chapter 6 were included in "Black Celebrities, Selfhood, and Psychiatry in the Civil Rights Era: The Wiltwyck School for Boys and the Floyd Patterson House," in *Social History of Medicine* 28 (May 2015): 330–50, and are reprinted with permission.

ISBN-13: 978-1-58046-492-5
ISSN: 1526-2715

Library of Congress Cataloging-in-Publication Data

Names: Doyle, Dennis A., author.
Title: Psychiatry and racial liberalism in Harlem, 1936–1968 / Dennis A. Doyle.
Other titles: Rochester studies in medical history ; v. 36. 1526-2715
Description: Rochester, NY : University of Rochester Press, 2016. | Series: Rochester studies in medical history, ISSN 1526-2715 ; v. 36 | Includes bibliographical references and index.
Identifiers: LCCN 2016022864 | ISBN 9781580464925 (hardcover : alk. paper)
Subjects: | MESH: Harlem Hospital (New York, N.Y.) | Psychiatry—history | African Americans—history | Community Mental Health Services—history | Hospitals, Psychiatric—history | Civil Rights—history | History, 20th Century | New York City
Classification: LCC RC451.5.N4 | NLM WM 11 AN7 | DDC 616.890089/96073—dc23
LC record available at https://lccn.loc.gov/2016022864

A catalogue record for this title is available from the British Library.

This publication is printed on acid-free paper.
Printed in the United States of America.

Contents

Acknowledgments

I have tried to acknowledge all the individuals and institutions that made this book possible. I hope I have not missed anyone.

First and foremost, I owe my deepest debt of gratitude to Nancy Tomes at Stony Brook University. She has supported this project, my career, and my family in countless ways. More than anyone else, she modeled how to think, research, and write like a historian of medicine. Her patience, sage advice, loyalty, and encouragement have always been invaluable resources to me.

This book also bears the imprint of so many other scholars. For starters, I need to thank the scholars and teachers who first taught me how to research and write history. During my undergraduate years at Eastern Connecticut State University, Evelyn Higginbotham, Barbara Tucker, David Frye, and Emil Pocock convinced me that I could become a historian. Pocock especially spent long hours reading as my honors thesis adviser, leading me through the research process and fine-tuning my writing. Without those mentors I would not have been ready to tackle graduate school.

The historians Ellen Dwyer, Andrea Friedman, Matthew Gambino, Ellen Herman, Kathleen Jones, Kraig Larkin, Mical Raz, Glenn Reynolds, Christopher Sellers, Martin Summers, Jason Morgan Ward, and the readers of the Yale University Working Group on the History of Psychiatry all read or commented on drafts that became book chapters. Their insights were much appreciated. At various conferences, a host of scholars and intellectuals—including but not limited to David Rosner, James Gilbert, Kirby Randolph, and Anne C. Rose—pushed me to clarify my thinking. Most important, the University of Rochester Press's two anonymous readers knew exactly what this project needed. Their recommendations enabled me to make some serious, much-needed revisions that improved the book.

Many thanks also go out to the archivists and libraries that granted me access to their collections. I am indebted to the Special Collections of the Milbank Memorial Library, Teachers College, Columbia University, the Rare Books and Manuscripts Library of Columbia University, the Beinecke Rare Books and Manuscripts Library of Yale University, the Schlesinger Library of the Radcliffe Institute for Advanced Study, the United States Library of Congress's Manuscript Division, and the Moving Images and Recorded Sound and Rare Book and Manuscript Divisions of the Schomburg Center for Research in Black Culture. I owe special thanks to the archivist Stephen Novak at the Archives and Special Collections of Columbia University Medical Center's Augustus C.

Long Health Sciences Library. My initial consult with Stephen shaped this project perhaps more than anything else. Not only did he suggest collections that proved absolutely invaluable, but he also actively supported this project even as it grew in unintended directions. A special word of thanks to Brooklyn College Library's administrative staff and student workers. As I researched their Special Collections, they created the friendliest, most relaxed work atmosphere I have ever encountered on an archival trip. That alone was worth the daily subway ride to Midwood.

I was fortunate to have my employers' support as I worked to complete this manuscript for publication. Thanks go to Alan Marcus, head of Mississippi State's Department of History. Not only did he give me my first full-time academic job, but he also encouraged me to publish even though my appointment was not tenure track. My current employer, the St. Louis College of Pharmacy (STL-COP), has done so much to bring this book to fruition. I must thank STL-COP's Research and Scholarly Activities Committee for providing me with three Faculty Research Incentive Grants that funded travel to archives in 2012, 2013, and 2014. My thanks also go out to Susan Mueller and the other participants in the Norton Summer Writer's Workshop for their good cheer as I worked on book chapters. So many colleagues and students have expressed interest in the project and encouraged me in a variety of ways—including Patrick Fontane, Brenda Walter, Eric Robinson, Elizabeth Rattine-Flaherty, Elizabeth Lemma, and Amy Suh. Most of all, I have benefited from the unwavering support of my Liberal Arts Department chair and fellow Stony Brook alum, Bob Zebroski. His mentorship, friendship, understanding, and cheerleading helped make this book a reality.

As I traveled to archives, several friends gave me a place to stay. My thanks go out to Andrew and Andrea Zercie, Mark and Monica Kehren, and Kraig Larkin for helping to lighten the financial burden of researching so far from home.

Of course I would be remiss if I did not thank this project's shepherd, Ted Brown. I am ever indebted to him for seeing the potential in my prospectus and early drafts. He continued to champion my work even when my manuscript took some unfortunate detours early on, and never lost faith in either me or the project. Owing to his patience, clear vision, honesty, and blunt criticism, I was able to transform the manuscript from a jargon-laden mess into a publishable monograph. I am so grateful.

I also thank my parents. My mother and father continually asked me about the book's progress, rooting for me to succeed. Their love and support humbles me still.

Last but not least, I must acknowledge that this book made it to press only because of my wife, Amy Gangloff, and my son, Miles. Amy knows how much she has sacrificed to ensure that I had the time and money to research and write. To his credit, Miles has put up with Daddy taking trips to faraway cities and spending precious time laboring away on his laptop. Without their love and understanding, none of this would have been possible.

Introduction

Across 110th Street

New York is the greatest city in the world—especially for my people.
Where else, in this grand and glorious land of ours, can I get on a
subway, sit in any part of the train I please, get off at any station above
110th Street, and know I'll be welcome?

—Dick Gregory, *From the Back of the Bus*

Located above Manhattan's 110th Street, Harlem had been the world's most famous predominantly black living space since the 1920s. On September 20, 1958, however, Martin Luther King Jr. did not receive the Harlem welcome the comedian Dick Gregory joked about. Instead, King, one of the rising stars of the civil-rights movement, encountered one of the truths about Harlem's postwar black community: it was not a like-minded monolith. The "Negro Capital of America" was home to a potent mix of generations, ideologies, languages, religions, cultures, classes, and mental states.[1] On that day, the civil-rights leader was at Blumstein's department store on 125th Street signing copies of *Stride toward Freedom*. While there, Izola Ware Curry, a black woman who lived nearby, stabbed King in the chest with a letter opener. After surviving a delicate surgery and a bout of pneumonia at Harlem Hospital, King told the press that he hoped "all thoughtful people will do all in their power to see that she gets the help she apparently needs."[2]

Following her arrest, Curry found herself on Bellevue Hospital's psychiatric ward. Based on the psychiatrist's recommendation, the court determined that forty-two-year-old Curry was "not of sound mind," committing her to Mattewan State Hospital that November.[3] Even before the court's ruling, Harlem's leading newspaper, the *New York Amsterdam News*, uncovered a history of behavioral problems. Relatives recalled her strange demeanor, ramblings, violent tendencies, and paranoid delusions about Communist conspiracies involving black ministers and the National Association for the Advancement of Colored People (NAACP). As far as her family knew, she had never seen a psychiatrist. Curry's nephew told the *Amsterdam News* that his aunt was "getting now what she should have had a long time ago—a psychiatric examination."[4]

How was it possible that Curry could have escaped medical notice in New York City, one of the postwar centers of psychiatric training, treatment, and innovation? Although other factors were involved, US medicine's longstanding mishandling and often outright neglect of African American health needs partly explains Curry's slip through the cracks. That history is marked by a lack of consistent access to quality care, exclusion from white institutions, substandard treatment by white professionals, segregated public facilities, and a reliance on the black community's own meager resources.[5] In 1958, Harlem Hospital, a public municipal hospital, was not equipped to deal with Curry's problems. It lacked inpatient psychiatric services and had no formal psychiatric department except for a small mental hygiene clinic. In Manhattan, inpatient mental health care was practically nonexistent above 110th Street. Since the 1940s, Harlem's outpatient care consisted mostly of underfunded clinics, social agencies with psychiatric consultants, and at least one child guidance center. Yet even those limited services were dwindling in number. The year Curry stabbed King, one of Central Harlem's busiest psychiatric providers—the Lafargue Mental Hygiene Clinic, run by volunteers in the basement of the St. Philip's Episcopal Church Parish House—closed its doors.[6]

By default, Bellevue's psychiatric ward was the primary mental health facility available to black Harlemites. To be sure, Bellevue was a place African Americans sought to avoid even more than white New Yorkers did. In Harlem, Bellevue had a reputation as both a den of racism and the first step along an inexorable path to a state mental institution—where Curry was eventually committed.

In 1962, less than four years after Izola Curry's commitment, the situation changed for black New Yorkers. The New York Department of Hospitals finally equipped Harlem Hospital with its own formal psychiatric division, Ward 9-K. Dr. Elizabeth B. Davis, a black Harlem native, was in charge. Ward 9-K featured brand-new in-patient services, emergency care, and pioneering community-health programs for African Americans living "across 110th Street."[7] The new psychiatric ward even employed young, socially conscious clinicians set on promoting racial justice through mental health care.

What accounts for Ward 9-K's development in 1962? Was it chiefly inspired by Dr. King and the civil-rights movement of the 1950s and early 1960s? Had racial liberals—citizens convinced that equal access to government resources would best reduce racial disparities—suddenly become a political majority? Was this new urban policy, then, the result of a sweeping liberalization of American attitudes toward race? Unfortunately, none of those potential explanations are adequate. As we shall see, Ward 9-K's origin extends back much further than King's appearance on the national scene. Neither does some alleged across-the-board shift in American values account for why Harlem Hospital was able to open a psychiatric department in 1962. Instead, this book contends that the facility was the product of racial liberalism's partial institutionalization within New York City's social-welfare apparatus—a historical process spanning more than three decades.

Racial Liberalism and Psychiatry:
Psychological Equality of the Races

The movement to make New York's municipal government more receptive to the mental health needs of Harlem's black population did not arise out of some sea change in white American attitudes toward African Americans. A wholesale liberalization of America's racial beliefs never happened, and certainly not before Harlem Hospital's psychiatric department opened in 1962. Consequently, racial liberals never comprised a large segment of the population. Despite their small numbers, they did manage to chip away at institutional racism in midcentury New York. Clusters of racial liberals, working as civil servants with access to local power, helped expand the range of mental health services that the courts, public schools, and even Harlem Hospital offered African Americans.

My narrative traces the work of the individuals who helped improve black Harlem's access to publicly funded mental health care between 1936 and 1968. Networking across disciplinary lines, racial liberals in the fields of psychiatry, social work, education, and juvenile justice became a small but powerful presence within New York's mechanisms of urban policy and social services. At various times they clustered within the juvenile courts, the correctional system, the public schools, and Harlem Hospital. The people working in these pockets of racial liberalism included Judge Justine Wise Polier, the Harlem school psychiatrist Max Winsor, Columbia faculty member Viola Bernard, the Department of Hospitals' chief Ray E. Trussell, and Harlem Hospital's first director of psychiatry, Elizabeth B. Davis. Wherever they gained a foothold within New York's system of mental health care, these public employees and administrators altered the culture of their workplaces, changing the way race mattered in American psychiatry.

Racial liberalism impacted the operation of racial assumptions in mid-twentieth-century America by transforming how social service and health professionals understood the relationship between race and human psychology. As psychodynamic thinking infiltrated the fields of health care, education, jurisprudence, and corrections, racial liberals mapped their assumptions and politics onto this process, shaping how the public sector delivered psychiatric care within the African American community. The racial liberals featured in this book injected New York City's public schools, courts, medical schools, and the Department of Hospitals with the faith that whites and blacks were endowed with the same emotional makeup and potential.[8] They expected their colleagues, students, and employees to assume that African Americans were innately capable of benefiting from modern psychiatry. Once this belief in the psychological equality of the races had been institutionalized within New York's systems of health, education, and law, African American mental health became a policy goal worthy of public investment. Racial liberals initiated inclusive new programs that included the Children's Court diagnostic and treatment clinics, two major wartime experiments with child-guidance services in Harlem public schools, and the creation of Harlem Hospital's Psychiatric Division.

Yet as we will see, these well-meaning attempts to combat institutional racism at the municipal level were problematic. At crucial moments, political resistance, mixed results, controversy, and the contradictions nearly inherent in a color-blind, race neutral, universalist[9] approach to medicine hindered these publicly funded psychiatric interventions within Harlem life. Nevertheless, the story of racial liberalism and psychiatry's intersection in midcentury Harlem offers new insight into the complex historical relationship between race and health disparities.

Racial Liberalism in the Long Civil-Rights Era, 1936–68

This is a story of institutional change in the civil-rights era. More to the point, it is a study of how public institutions concerned with citizens' psychological well-being became more racially inclusive over the course of those decades. For the events of this narrative cannot be neatly bracketed between the 1950s and early 1960s—the decades most associated with the United States civil-rights movement. Some of the activists and public servants who helped make Ward 9-K possible had been combating institutional racism in New York's mental health care system as far back as the 1930s. And that is precisely when and where this story begins.

The timing and location of the antiracist actions this book documents were neither anomalous nor unprecedented. More than a decade ago, Jacqueline Dowd Hall and other leading students of the African American experience expanded the scope of the civil-rights movement's narrative, identifying the Great Depression rather than the early years of the Cold War as its more likely starting point. In this revised timeline, the "long civil-rights era" ran from the 1930s well into the 1980s and included much more than the war against Jim Crow and disenfranchisement in the South.[10] Especially before the Cold War began, activists in the NAACP, the Urban League, the National Negro Congress, and other civil-rights organizations pursued racial fairness in the distribution of wealth and public resources. From the 1930s through the 1950s, New York City was at the forefront of the black community's struggle for economic justice. Local African American activists pushed for an end to racial discrimination and inequity in unions, employment, policing, housing, and education.[11] It should come as no surprise, then, that Manhattan also became an early battleground in the fight against institutional racism and racialism in mental health care.

When this process of institutional change began, racialism—the premise that biological race determines an individual's personal capabilities—still pervaded the United States.[12] Ever since "race" emerged as a social category in the colonial era, it has been intimately involved in shaping how Americans understand the way the world works. Since race is socially constructed, its meaning and operation does not remain fixed for long. Each extended moment in race's career as an American social category possessed its own historically specific complex of institutions, practices, and meanings.[13] Culturally rooted in both racialism and white supremacy—the racist assumption that whites are innately superior to people of color—institutional racism pervaded mid-twentieth-century America. As a state-supported form of discrimination against people of color, institutional racism systematically generated inequalities in wealth, social condition, and access to opportunity and resources.[14]

Within New York City's systems of health, justice, and education, racial liberals led the challenge against institutional racism in the civil-rights era. Even though the histories of racial liberalism and the civil-rights movement often intersected, they were still distinct campaigns.[15] Although the black freedom struggle was itself not one single unchanging entity, it largely remained a creature of civil society.[16] Racial liberalism, however, was a more state-bound phenomenon, operating at all levels of government. Between the 1930s and the 1960s, its proponents believed that racial inequality would recede once African Americans enjoyed equal access to the expanding public sector. This book's use of the term "racial liberalism" relies on the historian Robert Self's definition of its political orientation. According to Self, racial liberals were dedicated to opening up "racially equal opportunity in social and political life" and promoting "some state intervention to achieve an equal playing field."[17] In my study, the historical actors are largely public employees themselves. As institutional insiders, they saw their fellow citizens enmeshed within a complex web of governmental institutions and social services, each with its own rules, bureaucracies, and resources. In their estimation, health disparities in Harlem resulted and persisted because the African American community was chronically underserved by multiple strands of that web.[18] These institutional insiders sought ways to expand the scope and power of their respective institutions and transform them into tools of racial justice and social engineering. Not surprisingly, equal inclusion of individual African Americans within the expanding public sector became a racial liberal's primary solution to racial disparities.[19]

Public institutions, however, did not become more racially inclusive merely by including more African Americans. Indeed, one of the primary outcomes of both racial liberalism and the civil-rights movement was that the public sector had become the leading employer of African Americans by the 1970s.[20] A variety of antidiscriminatory legislation and judicial decisions enacted between 1942 and 1988 reduced explicit barriers to African American participation in education, military service, social services, housing, financing, and health care.[21] All this is well known. Nevertheless, historians have not adequately explored the internal changes public institutions underwent so that they could start including African Americans as employees, clients, or patients. Dislodging institutional racism in mental health care involved more than the formal removal of a color bar. It required an adjustment in how African Americans should be treated once they were formally included. Even after World War II, places such as the prestigious New York Psychiatric Institute, run by Dr. Nolan D. C. Lewis, still operated on the racialist premise that African Americans were incapable of benefiting from modern psychiatry. Given that racialism and institutional racism persisted in other arenas of American life in that era, what explains their decline within the institutions this book examines?

Liberal Consensus on Race?

This book seeks to determine just how antiracist the United States needed to be before racial liberals could challenge institutional racism's hold over mental health care policy. How did America's public institutions become more racially inclusive during the civil-rights era? Eventually, racial liberalism became institutionalized within the expanding public sector. This included health-care facilities and social-welfare services. In New York City's midcentury system of mental health care, new policies rooted in notions of "racial fairness" and "universal standards" of care began to replace ones grounded in "racial exceptionalism" and "exclusion." When governmental institutions became more racially inclusive, did this happen because the racial sensibilities of most American citizens had become more progressive, more liberal?[22]

This book does not support the largely discredited thesis of "liberal consensus." Over the last twenty years, civil-rights historians have generally abandoned an older narrative in which the public—especially in the North—became more liberal and antiracist in the 1950s and governmental institutions simply followed the will of the people. Historians have determined that no such "liberal consensus" on racial equality existed in the civil-rights era.[23] Racial discrimination in public policy did not decrease because of some alleged nationwide shift in white attitudes. Instead, scholars typically explain institutional racism's decline within the public sector as the product of complex political pressures, grassroots black activism, and the Cold War competition for allies in postcolonial Africa, Asia, and the Global South.[24]

My work seeks to modify this historiography, reinserting cultural change as a cause for the liberal assault on racial disparities within social policy. I am not trying to revive the myth of a postwar liberal consensus on race. As recent literature indicates, most white citizens did not suddenly become enlightened in the civil-rights era. As well, I am not contesting Daniel Martinez HoSang's argument that postwar liberalism's "conceptual grammar" of race-neutral equality became part of the dominant political discourse even though white racial sensibilities had not changed all that much. According to HoSang and others, postwar white Americans tended to pay mere lip service to a color-blind ethics of fairness. And most of them only adopted that language of race neutrality as a way to preserve rather than eliminate racial inequalities. A wholesale change of hearts and minds this was not.[25]

Racial Liberalism: Institutional
Pockets within the Public Sector

Even though a major cultural shift in American racial attitudes did not occur between the 1930s and 1960s, policymakers and public servants in New York still managed to make mental health care more available to Harlem's black residents. Cultures never shape values, lives, and imaginations whole cloth.[26]

Especially in complex modern societies, individual institutions can develop their own workplace cultures. They can take on a life of their own, somewhat isolated from mainstream values. This is likely to happen in offices staffed and run by nonelected experts wielding professional knowledge and bureaucratic power. Historical actors within these institutional pockets could even develop far-reaching policies informed by their workplace's own expectations rather than the values of the culture at large.[27]

That is the way racial liberals challenged racism within mental health care. Working within small but powerful pockets of the public sector, they institutionalized their shared conviction that blacks and whites were psychological equals. But these racial liberals supplanted institutional racism in only a partial way. Small groups of psychiatrists, juvenile court judges, and social workers did not change the culture as a whole. They did not convince the average white citizen that blacks could benefit from psychiatry just as much as whites. Instead, these civil servants typically mounted their antiracist challenges within the confines of one municipal department's institutional culture. Combating institutional racism in this piecemeal way, these professionals within health care, education, and law disseminated their shared egalitarian racial sensibilities only within their specific bureaucratic niches. In those public workplaces where racial liberals had successfully installed their race-neutral understanding of psychiatry's usefulness, racist patterns and policies of exclusion began to decline.

Public Investment in Emotional Health

Racial liberalism was perhaps most effective in dislodging racialism and institutional racism from institutions seeking to help citizens exercise self-control. As urban social services expanded between the 1890s and 1920s, authorities worked to produce Americans who could be expected to regulate their own emotional states, habits, and conduct. Concentrating their efforts within education, medicine, correctional facilities, probation, parole, case work, and child guidance, urban policymakers chose to invest in the maturation, management, and rehabilitation of emotionally stable adults. These efforts often entailed an unprecedented level of government intrusion in a citizen's personal life.[28] If we understand power as a relationship rather than as something that one possesses and wields over someone else, the aim of such direct interventions was—ironically enough—the creation of a more indirect form of power. In this modern relationship between states and citizens, authority was not exercised *over* citizens per se. Instead, such power was generated when states governed *through* the psyches of individuals well-adjusted enough to police themselves. In societies pursuing such a diffuse model of power, governments no longer relied exclusively on purely punitive or even destructive shows of authority. Instead such authorities could afford to govern at a distance to some extent. They promoted order and security by helping citizens to regulate their own affect and conduct in accordance with the norms of that era.[29]

As modern governments began to manage personal life, psychiatry expanded its authority. A medical specialty formerly confined to asylums and the care of the severely mentally ill, psychiatry became a tool used in the prevention of juvenile delinquency, crime, and poverty. Entering the 1930s, psychiatric experts actively worked to help individuals acquire and maintain the emotional stability expected of productive, law-abiding citizens. When the long civil-rights era began, psychodynamic theory was fast becoming the dominant framework through which many civil servants imagined the self. A psychological understanding of personhood quickly become a kind of institutional "common sense" in courts, clinics, prisons, schools, and other agencies interested in shaping human behavior.[30] Employees within those services came to think of psychological space as a deep, complex world driven by innate and subconscious needs, impulses, and the residue of childhood experience. They no longer understood the self as the product of individual will alone. Instead they deemed it a work in progress shaped largely by forces beyond a person's conscious awareness. As policymakers came to regard crime, delinquency, and even poverty as symptoms of emotional illness, they called on psychiatry to help prevent these social ills.[31]

In Depression-era Manhattan, health professionals and their allies in corrections, juvenile justice, and education identified the citizenry's emotional stability as a goal worthy of public expenditure.[32] Psychiatrists and other experts armed with psychodynamic theory often operated as gatekeepers. They determined which citizens deserved to have more local resources invested in their psychological development, identifying who did and did not possess the innate capacity for emotional stability and self-control.[33] In Harlem, African Americans were disproportionately the targets of police brutality and arrest quotas. Yet very few resources—including psychiatry—had been dedicated to help Harlem prevent crime. Before policymakers could even consider using precious resources to promote the emotional development of African Americans, they first had to assume that the black psyche was capable of handling what psychiatry had to offer.

Making Color-Blind Psychiatry an Institutional Expectation

According to historians of race and medicine, race played a role in determining whose psychological potential was deemed worthy of public investment.[34] In the early twentieth century, racialism heavily influenced mental health policy. For racialists, the psyches of black and whites were innately different and unequal.[35] The black personality was primitive, less evolved, with less potential for development. Evolution had not equipped African Americans with whatever allowed whites to achieve emotional stability and self-control in adulthood. Racialists posited that even black adults remained arrested at the emotional level of children or adolescents. Since African Americans could not be expected to adequately regulate their feelings and impulses, psychiatrists helped to deny the use of public resources to support the maturation, rehabilitation, and management of the black psyche.[36] Although racialists often stated their psychiatric theories in race-neutral terms, they assumed that psychological normalcy and self-control were properties inherent to whiteness. In practice, these psychiatric norms really only applied to whites, with African Americans figuring as nature's inferior exception.[37]

In contrast, racial liberals assumed that blacks and whites were psychological equals. To the judges, psychiatrists, social workers, and educators fighting institutional racism in New York's mental health care system, the human self was a space where biological race did not intrude. Well before these cosmopolitan New York civil servants even began reading psychodynamic theory, most of them were already convinced that biological race did not determine one's personal capabilities. Many of these individuals came from backgrounds—including organized labor, the Ethical Culture movement, and Reform Judaism—that had given them a sense of social justice. They were people already inclined to believe that citizens deserved equal access to any opportunities they were able to use. Although psychiatry had long been saddled with the intellectual baggage of racialism, these individuals had not. So when they trained their attention on mental health care, these select New Yorkers helped change how race mattered within psychiatry. Collectively, they generated an institutional shift in perception that was as simple as it was historically necessary. By mapping their egalitarian racial sensibilities onto contemporary psychodynamic theory, they simply took it for granted that no fundamental differences existed between the psyches of blacks and whites, making it nearly impossible for them to even consider psychiatric racialism a valid point of view.[38]

Beginning in 1936, Justice Polier and other racial liberals within New York's system of courts, corrections, and education referred to their race-neutral understanding of psychiatry as the "psychiatric point of view."[39] The adherents of this view did not conceive of black psychological development as a racial exception to modern psychiatry's whites-only standards. They rejected racialism. For them, there was no reason to make racial exceptions. Rather, they understood psychiatry's benefits in race-neutral terms. Both races contained the same emotional makeup, the same human potential for psychological stability. Racial liberals expected the black psyche to operate, develop, and break down in accordance with the ostensibly universal patterns articulated in psychiatric texts. In other words, they transformed psychiatry from a profession colored by racialism into one whose theories and practices were to be understood as color-blind or universal in intent and application.[40]

This reimagining of the black psyche made it possible for African Americans to receive greater access to psychiatric services.[41] Far fewer black Harlem residents would have been included within New York's mental health care system had civil servants and policymakers continued to assume that blacks were biologically incapable of making full use of psychiatric care. When tracing major shifts in the way race worked within the twentieth-century United States, most historians have underestimated the ways in which an emerging race-neutral understanding of human psychology helped pry open new opportunities for African Americans.[42] Certainly institutional racism did not decline because most white

Americans suddenly changed their assumptions about what blacks could do, think, or feel. Even though a small social-justice-minded portion of Manhattan did assume that blacks and whites were psychological equals, that in itself was not enough to enact change either. What made the difference was that the New Yorkers who shared this relatively rare sensibility were able to gain access to governmental power and authority far in excess of their small numbers. Within the public institutions in which they worked, these individuals managed to install their antiracist assumptions as new policymaking expectations. Once color-blind psychiatry became an accepted expectation within key pockets of Manhattan's systems of health, justice, corrections, and education, African American access to municipal mental health services increased. What follows is the story of the men and women who created those institutional pockets and struggled to reduce racial disparities in mental health care. I explore the historical circumstances that enabled those racial liberals to gain a foothold within New York's social services, affording them a chance to craft inclusive public policies and ostensibly race-neutral standards of care.

Color-Blind Psychiatry: Its Expansion and Limitations

The first three chapters document how changing ideas about race, mental health, and human selfhood affected the relationship between public policy, medical care, and African American lives. Chapter 1 offers a snapshot of both mental health care in central Harlem and the psychiatric profession's understanding of the black psyche prior to 1936—the year that Justine Wise Polier and the Domestic Relations Court began tackling institutional racism in mental health care. That chapter not only examines racialism and racial disparities in mental health delivery in Harlem, but it also documents the presence of clinicians—such as Bellevue's Lauretta Bender—who expressed some ambivalence regarding racialism and scientific racism's validity.

Chapter 2 examines the first efforts to combat racial inequalities in the public sector's delivery of mental health care. Judge Polier led these early efforts from within the Domestic Relations Court between 1936 and 1942. The daughter of two leading Jewish American activists, Polier was New York City's first female judge. After her family's political ally, Mayor Fiorello La Guardia, appointed her to the bench in 1936, she became a fierce advocate for both racial justice and a psychological understanding of juvenile delinquency. She expected that her court's staff would consider the emotional needs of African American children in a race-neutral way. Holding an expansionist view of the court's power to pursue social justice, she used her authority to cultivate court personnel and outside allies who shared this new institutional expectation. Mobilizing her new allies—including the mental hygiene pioneer Dr. Marion E. Kenworthy and the publishing magnate Marshall Field III—she persuaded court authorities to open an interracial treatment clinic in 1937. In adjudicating the cases of black Harlemites, Polier regularly attempted to apply psychodynamic concepts without taking race into consideration. Although Polier's court recognized the psychological needs of African American children, New York's childcare agencies retained the right to discriminate on the basis of race before 1942, frustrating the judge's efforts to secure psychiatric care for them.

Chapter 3 examines the development of the Harlem Special Child Guidance Service Unit (the Harlem Unit), a Board of Education initiative that ran between 1940 and 1942. The brainchild of the school psychiatrist Dr. Max Winsor, the program extended psychiatry into select Harlem public schools through the auspices of the New York City Board of Education's Bureau of Child Guidance (BCG). Winsor proposed that the public schools could prevent juvenile delinquency in Harlem if the BCG concentrated its resources in the neighborhoods with the highest youth arrest rates. Polier, who had befriended Winsor when he was a reform-school clinician in 1937, championed his proposal, securing La Guardia's approval. Polier hoped the program could help prevent more young people from stepping foot inside her courtroom. She also imagined that it could provide additional information on the psychological needs of the children who appeared before her court. Enlisting the cohort that had created the Domestic Relations Court's treatment clinic, Polier recruited personnel for Winsor's Harlem Special Child Guidance Service Unit. The program lasted two years, concentrating psychiatric care, teacher training, and counseling services within three Harlem junior highs and one kindergarten.

At the same time, Polier and some of her fellow civil servants in the BCG and the juvenile courts—including the gifted young Harlem Unit psychiatrist Dr. Viola Bernard—took administrative control of an interracial reform school, the Wiltwyck School for Boys. Racial liberals hoped that the reformatory would eventually enable at least some troubled African American youth to see a child psychiatrist.

Chapter 4 examines the wartime circumstances that compelled some of these activists to consider the mental health disparities facing Harlem's adult population. Given their positions within the courts and schools, Polier, Winsor, Bernard, and the BCG director Carolyn Zachary were narrowly concerned with the mental health disparities facing the African Americans they served: children. But in 1942, these four—as well as several of the judges, psychiatrists, BCG staff, and philanthropists that had shared that narrow focus on children's needs— joined a new civil-rights organization, the City-Wide Citizens Committee for Harlem (CWCCH). Between 1942 and 1947, these civil servants, acting as private citizens, successfully inserted their mental health agenda within Harlem's civil-rights movement. Polier and her longtime collaborators won CWCCH support for both their new Harlem Project (a 1943–45 expansion of the Harlem Special Child Guidance Service Unit) and their bid to keep the Domestic Relations Court's treatment clinic open. Both campaigns were designed to help prevent juvenile delinquency in Harlem. Exposure to the civil-rights movement compelled these child-welfare experts to consider the mental health needs of black adults. This collaboration with the CWCCH prompted Bernard and others to articulate an expanded mental health agenda for Harlem, one that went beyond the needs of children. It included the recruitment of black psychiatrists and a proposal to create a psychiatric division for Harlem Hospital.

Chapter 5 examines the impact antiracist New York psychiatrists had on postwar public discourse. When writing about black patients for medical journals and public reports, they outright rejected racial stereotypes while at the same reinforcing popular gender stereotypes. Racialists had long seen African Americans as exceptions to normative white gender conventions. In print, antiracist psychiatrists such as Dr. Bernard revealed their expectation that black men and women would be as psychologically different from each other as white men and women were supposed to be. A good bit of the chapter examines the Wiltwyck School for Boys' efforts to promote its alleged therapeutic benefits for young African American men. It pays particular attention to Bernard's role as adviser on *The Quiet One,* a 1948 film about the reform school. Representations of the black male psyche became a matter of real debate within postwar Manhattan psychiatry. Not all of New York's antiracist psychiatrists believed that the racial liberals in Polier's courtroom, the BCG, and Wiltwyck really understood African Americans. Dr. Fredric Wertham and his colleagues in the short-lived Lafargue Mental Hygiene Clinic—an independent Harlem facility named in honor of Karl Marx's son-in-law—doubted whether forced encounters with psychiatry in correctional institutions served the best interests of black male youth. Lafargue clinicians criticized Bernard and *The Quiet One* for blaming juvenile delinquency on gender dynamics and black families rather than on structural factors. Yet despite their ideological differences over the best way to publicly discuss the black psyche, Bernard and the Lafargue staff tended to agree on one thing: published work claiming that psychological differences existed between the races no longer deserved a place in the psychiatric literature.

The last two chapters cover the creation and early operation of Harlem Hospital's new psychiatric department. Chapter 6 looks at the roles racial liberals played in the founding of Harlem Hospital's psychiatric wing. It examines how well-placed individuals within Columbia University and the New York Department of Hospitals created Ward 9-K and staffed it with clinicians committed to racial justice, including Drs. Elizabeth Davis and June Jackson Christmas. As the 1950s began, Cold War conditions made it difficult for New York's public schools and children's court to continue taking an active role in the struggle against psychiatric racism. In the meantime, Columbia University and Wiltwyck sheltered clinicians and activists who still believed that New York's public sector had a responsibility to provide Harlem with more psychiatric care. While the Wiltwyck School's Board of Directors sought aftercare facilities for clients returning home to Harlem, Bernard's community psychiatry program at Columbia pushed for a locally based model of care. In 1961 Mayor Robert Wagner appointed Bernard's sympathetic colleague Dr. Ray E. Trussell as the Commissioner of Hospitals. In forging an alliance between Columbia and Harlem Hospital, Trussell enabled the seventy-five-year-old hospital to open a full psychiatric division in 1962, satisfying both Wiltwyck and Bernard's plans for Harlem.

Chapter 7 concludes with an assessment of the first six years of color-blind psychiatry's presence within Harlem Hospital's new psychiatric department. The chapter probes its uneven impact on Harlem. On the one hand, the new division's first director, Dr. Elizabeth Davis, frequently consulted with local social organizations to gauge the Harlem community's mental health needs. As well, local residents participated as lay workers and hospital liaisons, helping the clinician Dr. June Jackson Christmas's pioneering psychiatric rehabilitation program to succeed. Yet a disconnect still existed between the hospital and the local population. In seeking to assess central Harlem's health needs in a race-neutral way, Davis and her staff instead investigated the psychological impact of class within Harlem. But without an unpacking of the demeaning racial assumptions embedded in their ostensibly color-blind analysis, these otherwise well-intentioned clinicians ended up perpetuating the historical overdiagnosis of psychosis among African Americans. Perhaps most emblematic of color-blind psychiatry's pitfalls was a 1965 Harlem Hospital program that offered sterilizations as a treatment for postpartum psychosis. In response to the program, Dr. Davis' administration faced criticism from Black Power leaders.[43]

The conclusion considers the complicated legacy of both color-blind psychiatry and the efforts to increase African American access to psychiatric care. It examines the problems inherent to a one-size-fits-all approach to humanity, paying particular attention to the ways in which the neglect of race still allowed for other social categories to reinforce racism. Racial liberals had identified the mental health issues that seemed to be most endemic to black communities. Racism had helped generate those health gaps. Race-blind solutions generally did not attend to the ways that racism had structured life chances within central Harlem. Even as they ignored race, well-meaning city officials and mental health professionals often found themselves relying on racially loaded concepts of gender, class, culture, and selfhood. Consequently, they tended to blame individual African Americans and their families for Harlem's mental health disparities. In failing to pay attention to the historical relationship between race and place, color-blind policies and practices did sometimes reinforce and even create new health disparities in black communities—a legacy that continued into the so-called postracial age.

It is my hope that this book will help readers discover just how much the history of medicine broadens our understanding of the civil-rights era's transformations. Given that the emergence of the black body as an equal bearer of political rights historically converged with new claims to health care as a right, the history of medicine is best suited for an analysis of that intersection.[44] In particular, the history of psychiatric care in Harlem illuminates the role racial liberalism played in changing the American experience of race, health, and selfhood. While this story demonstrates how changing assumptions about African Americans and mental health relates to changes in racial policies and practices, it also reveals that the racial liberals' limited influence on urban social policy cannot serve as evidence that America had entered some postracial phase. As we shall see, refracting this critical moment in US history through the lens of medical history not only alters our vision of race in the past, but of its continuing operation in the present as well.

Chapter One

Before Racial Liberalism

Depression-Era Harlem and Psychiatry, 1936

In 1935 and 1936, Benjamin Malzberg, a prominent psychiatric statistician, published two intriguing findings concerning mental illness in New York. First, he found that the black rate of admission to state mental hospitals exceeded the white rate by a ratio of 2.3 to 1. Malzberg's statistical findings inspired others to seek explanations for this racial disparity, making similar comparisons with their own institutions. Initially, Malzberg speculated that the higher admission rates for African Americans demonstrated that their race was more susceptible to mental illness—especially severe psychosis. Such racial determinism was not unique. Since the antebellum era, psychiatrists and politicians tended to interpret black rates of disease as evidence of racial inferiority, no matter if such rates were higher or lower than white rates.[1]

In 1936 Malzberg published his second finding: the majority of New York's mental patients had been born out of state, in the South mostly. In light of this new data, he recanted his earlier theory. He now let this second finding explain the first. He concluded that the "excess of the Negro rate in New York state must therefore be ascribed not so much to racial characteristics, as to the economic and other social difficulties to which a migratory population is subject." He argued that so many blacks had been committed because urban life had been too stressful for rural migrants from the slower-paced South.[2]

Although some critics were pleased that he abandoned racialist thinking, others were none too thrilled with his cultural mismatch argument. One critic was Dr. Ernest Y. Williams, an African American professor of psychiatry and neurology at Howard University. Williams did not doubt that black Southerners were overrepresented in the New York's mental hospitals. What he disagreed with was Malzberg's explanation of this racial disparity. Williams argued that the high rate of institutionalized blacks could best be interpreted as proof that uptown Manhattan, where most of the state's African Americans lived, lacked local psychiatric alternatives to the old asylums. Afflicted whites were less likely to end up in state hospitals because they had other mental health care options available to them. With most local care off-limits to African Americans, state hospitals were the primary placement option for mentally disturbed blacks.[3] Owing to institutional racism within both the private and public sectors, the symbolic capital of black America had very little access to city-based psychiatric care in 1936. As we shall see, much of the care they did receive was delivered within punitive contexts, producing an antagonistic relationship between black citizens and psychiatry.

This chapter reconstructs the relationship between Harlem and psychiatry in 1936. That was the year racial liberals first began to promote psychiatry's expansion in Harlem. Examining 1936 gives the reader an overview of the racial disparities those activists were about to encounter and seek to ameliorate. Employing a two-pronged strategy, this chapter excavates the common racial assumptions and practices of the white New Yorkers administering psychiatric care to African Americans that year. First, it offers a snapshot of US psychiatry's engagement with race. Second, it compares Manhattan's psychiatric culture of race with these national patterns, relying primarily on the private papers and published work of Bellevue Psychopathic's renowned child psychiatrist, Dr. Lauretta Bender. Her records shed light on the racial climate at Bellevue—the site of many if not most black encounters with psychiatry in 1936 New York.

This analysis of Harlem's mental health care in 1936 reveals that practitioners were confused about how they should think about, diagnose, and treat the black psyche. Racialist beliefs in the black psyche's exceptionality still informed the theory and practice of many white clinicians. Yet even before racial liberals intervened, biological determinism faced some contestation. As Bender's writings show, not all psychiatrists were sure how race should matter in the clinic. Given black urban population growth and the introduction of antiracist ideas, what white psychiatrists thought about African Americans was in flux. Although psychiatry was becoming more open to progressive racial thought in the midthirties, racialism and institutional racism still actively informed psychiatry's engagement with African Americans.

African Americans and Central Harlem in 1936

At the close of the 1930s, Claude McKay, the renowned Jamaican American poet and novelist of the Harlem Renaissance, published a book entitled *Harlem: Negro Metropolis*. Racializing Harlem in this way was fairly common during the Great Depression. In the popular imagination at least, Harlem was the most famous black-identified living space in the United States. Nevertheless, Harlem's demography in 1936 was not entirely black. White Americans were still the majority in some sections of uptown Manhattan. What McKay and other locals had in mind when they referred to Harlem was just one section of that region: central Harlem. Central Harlem lies between 110th Street and 155th Street from south to north, and the Harlem River and St. Nicholas Avenue from east to west.[4]

Owing to rampant discrimination in the housing market, central Harlem was one of the few places open to black home seekers.[5] Consequently, it became a disproportionately black space. In 1930, over 6.5 million whites lived in New York City, whereas only 327,706 African Americans lived there. Of those black New Yorkers, 68.6 percent lived in the borough of Manhattan, and 91 percent of those black Manhattanites lived in Harlem.[6] These figures included not only homeowners but also renters, the primary occupants of Harlem's brownstones. Given that not all of Harlem was hospitable to prospective black residents, African Americans clustered into smaller, overwhelmingly black neighborhoods—mostly in the center and the west. By 1930 much of this clustering occurred between 126th and 146th streets. There, 96 percent of residents were black.[7]

African Americans of all socioeconomic classes lived and worked in Harlem. Most black Harlemites worked in domestic servitude or unskilled manual labor. Harlem also contained the black middle class and elites. They tended to cluster in the posh Sugar Hill neighborhood between 145th and 155th streets.[8] Harlem's black community was culturally heterogeneous as well. Central Harlem's sidewalks, stoops, and renowned 125th Street soapboxes must have produced a uniquely polyphonic soundscape, ringing out with the mingled sounds of native New Yorkers, Southern migrants, and African and Caribbean immigrants.[9] Each group brought their own traditions, including a wide range of Protestant Christian churches, from Baptist to Episcopal, and even local cults led by dynamic figures such as Father Divine.[10] Entering the 1930s, Harlem remained a global symbol of black artistic achievement. Still, Harlem's entertainment district was no longer the hub of black-white interaction it had been in the Harlem Renaissance of the 1920s to the early 1930s.[11] After the 1935 Harlem Riot, the Cotton Club and other interracial after-hours spots closed. Nevertheless, Harlem still nourished new talents in art, big-band jazz, and literature, perhaps most notably the young novelist Richard Wright.[12]

The Great Depression hit Harlem's black community hard. Even before the 1930s, a racially segmented labor market left blacks with the lowest average income of any racial group in New York. They also paid some of the highest rents in the city—the unfortunate result of artificial housing scarcity triggered and consolidated by racial covenants, blockbusting, racial steering, vigilantism, and redlining.[13] As the economic crisis enveloped Manhattan, African Americans were the "last hired, first fired," leaving over half of Harlem's black labor force unemployed and struggling to pay rent. Black Harlemites did whatever they could to make ends meet. They turned to stingy home relief, held multiple low-paying jobs, relied on neighbors, or joined the underground economy.[14]

The Harlem Riot of 1935

As the Harlem Riot of 1935 demonstrated, blacks faced even more than economic dislocations entering 1936. Harlem's predominantly black neighborhoods were also riddled with declining schools, poor health care, police brutality, and inequality within the criminal justice system.[15] These problems were nothing new. From 1931 to 1935, a wide range of civic organizations, churches, political groups, and consumers' movements—including the National Association for the Advancement of Colored People and the "Don't Buy Where You Can't Work" campaign—actively worked to draw attention to the racial inequalities plaguing central Harlem. Before March 19, 1935, Mayor La Guardia's administration had done little to address the black community's long list of grievances. The events of that day proved too destructive for La Guardia to ignore.[16]

Beginning that afternoon and ending the next day, crowds looted and destroyed white-owned stores on 125th street, Harlem's busiest thoroughfare. The immediate trigger for the uprising was a rumor that New York police had beaten a Harlem teenager. After police contained the destruction, La Guardia appointed a committee to investigate the cause of the riot and propose ways to prevent another one. The Mayor's Commission on Conditions in Harlem concluded that black frustration over racism had caused the Harlem Riot. African Americans had not been fully included within the social services offered by either the city or the New Deal. The committee recommended that La Guardia end his administration's political neglect of Harlem.[17] In response to this pressure, La Guardia made public housing available to black Harlemites for the first time, authorized Harlem Hospital to hire black nurses, and appointed African Americans to high-profile positions on the courts and in his administration. He eventually increased the resources available to Harlem's public schools. Nevertheless, New Yorkers continued to suffer racially disproportionate rates of unemployment, poverty, arrests, and mortality throughout 1936 and beyond.[18]

African Americans, State Hospitals, and the Lack of Local Options

In the interwar period, Africans Americans held a racially disproportionate share of beds in state mental institutions. As the Great Depression wore on, their presence on America's mental hospital wards increased. Nationwide, starting as early as 1910, annual rates of state institutionalization among blacks outstripped the general black population's growth. In 1933, the US Department of Commerce reported that the black rate of admission had not only increased by 10 percent over the last decade, but also exceeded the native-born white majority's rate of admission to state mental hospitals and asylums.[19]

This influx of black New Yorkers in state mental hospitals had multiple causes. As both Malzberg and Williams noted, Southern migration played a role. The Great Black Migration of the early twentieth century was triggered by the desire to escape Jim Crow's racial restrictions. It was also driven by the expectation that northern cities offered more opportunity and freedom. This movement caused a dramatic demographic shift within the urban North. Between 1910 and 1930, New York City's black population tripled, whereas the white population rose by only 41 percent. Given that formal medical care was still largely unavailable to African Americans below the Mason-Dixon Line, transplanted black Southerners accounted for most first-time admissions to New York's mental hospitals. Of the

US-born blacks admitted to the state's mental hospitals for the first time between 1929 and 1931, 90.7 percent had arrived in the Great Black Migration.[20] As well, the decline in official policies of racial exclusion and segregation also helped the number of blacks within New York's state hospital system to swell.

Nonetheless, those factors do not fully explain the racial imbalance in public mental hospitals. As Ernest Y. Williams suggested, the dearth of local private options for black adults also contributed to those historically high rates of black institutionalization.[21] Private facilities were not a realistic option for most black New Yorkers. Even for wealthier Harlem families who could afford private care, racial discrimination was an obstacle. Many private-care facilities, including the New York Neurological Institute, maintained policies of racial exclusion well into the 1940s. Some families did care for the severely mentally ill at home, sometimes relying on a combination of "medical, religious, and occult" understandings of madness transported from the rural South. But this home option became less viable during the Great Depression.[22] The costs of caring for a mentally ill relative had become too prohibitive.[23]

Harlem's black families also had little access to private psychotherapy. Psychoanalysis was still relatively new in the 1930s. Psychotherapists understood the human psyche to be deep and multilayered, composed of both conscious thought and a subconscious level of mental activity. This inner self was complex and psychodynamic. Through a series of timed stages, the psychodynamic self would develop in response to pressures generated by both internal (innate instincts and drives) and external forces (parents and siblings). For psychoanalysts and others influenced by Sigmund Freud, most emotional problems originated on the subconscious level, the result of a failure to adequately complete some childhood stage. The analyst probed the patient's subconscious through expensive, long-term private sessions, teasing out the specific internal conflict responsible for the patient's arrested development.

Manhattan's notoriously high fees were not the only reason few African Americans were able to see a psychoanalyst. There were no private black psychiatrists anywhere in the United States. Few whites were willing to take a black analysand.[24] Even when a clinician might have recommended that a black Harlemite seek private therapy, white psychoanalysts rejected blacks for fear of losing their white clients. When they accepted blacks, they often charged them higher fees.[25] These black clients were from the upper and middle classes, people who had been introduced to Freudian ideas about human subjectivity through both the mainstream and African American media.[26]

Nevertheless, most mentally ill African Americans were not diagnosed with the diseases psychoanalysts treated. Of the black adults that received some psychiatric care in the 1930s,[27] most had been diagnosed with psychoses: personality disturbances that allegedly prevented the afflicted from adjusting to everyday life. Analysts generally rejected such cases. They considered their talk therapy ineffective for anyone with severe psychoses such as dementia praecox or manic-depression. Instead, private psychoanalysts worked with patients who were neurotic—an interior state that analysts had normalized as within the range of mental health. In the modern psychiatric languages of psychodynamics, psycho-biology, and mental hygiene, neurotics were considered emotionally ill or mal-adjusted, to be sure. Yet psychiatrists imagined neurotics as individuals who had not lost touch with reality. They were still adjusted enough to function normally in the outside world. They could hold a job, socialize, and obey the law. On the other hand, psychotics were unable to apprehend reality. They could not control their emotions and behavior when interacting with others. Institutionalization was often recommended for psychotics. With psychosis disproportionately diag-nosed among African Americans, commitment to a state mental hospital was a likely outcome, helping account for the overrepresentation of black patients in the nation's old asylums.

The Black Psyche: Not Quite the Same

Institutional racism helps explains the historical overdiagnosis of psycho-sis among African Americans. According to the anthropologist Emily Martin, "medical categories working in combination with cultural categories define race in relation to human capacity in historically specific ways."[28] A racialist mode of thinking still informed the typical white psychiatrist's perception of a black patient's emotional makeup. Owing to cultural predispositions extending back to the nineteenth century, interwar psychiatrists still tended to assume that the interior worlds of black and whites contained innately different potentials, that they were "almost the same but not quite."[29]

Psychiatrists did not invent the proposition that race determined an indi-vidual's temperament. That claim was as old as the race concept itself.[30] White psychiatrists were prepared to regard black patients as racially exceptional, encountering them through a racial lens informed by fairly widespread racialist assumptions about black character.[31] Yet when it came time to make a specific diagnosis, racialists often experienced difficulty determining whether a black patient even had a mental illness.[32] At Boston Psychpathic Hospital in the 1920s, clinicians there often held blacks and whites to different standards as to what was psychologically normal or abnormal.[33] Typically, they seemed to think that even normal African Americans were naturally prone to affect and behaviors that whites would have been diagnosed as psychotic for exhibiting.[34] According to Emily Martin, blacks were thought "impulsive, volatile, and prone to extreme emotional outbursts, while at the same time (and paradoxically) lacking human emotion and feeling."[35] In 1917 the psychiatrist E. M. Green expected that an African American's "normal emotions [could] become exaggerated with slight cause," making it hard for him and other white clinicians to determine if a black patient even had a mental disease.[36]

Given that racialists regarded the black race as almost psychotic by nature, they rarely diagnosed African Americans as neurotic. In the early decades of the twentieth century, psychiatrists expected that blacks' unique emotional makeup left them more prone to severe mental illness—psychoses, mania, and dementia praecox. It also made them less susceptible to stress-related disorders and conditions associated with the more sensitive, neurologically complex white race: neuroses, anxiety, depression, alcoholism, and suicide.[37] In 1914 the psychiatrist Mary O'Malley asserted that "the colored do not react in any pathological sense to mental stress."[38] Not all interwar clinicians went that far. Yet most assumed that African Americans were endowed with a higher tolerance for stress, naturalizing neuroses and anxiety as white emotional states.[39] In 1921, the clinician William Bevis claimed that "sadness and depression have little part in [the Negro's] psychological make-up." Despite the fact that black Southerners possessed their own terminology for sadness and deep depression, psychiatrists rarely diagnosed neuroses and melancholia among blacks, prompting the psychiatrists Nolan D. C. Lewis and L. D. Hubbard in 1932 to refer matter-of-factly to the "low rate of depression among the negro as a race."[40]

For these psychiatrists, the black race's allegedly psychotic tendencies explained the disproportionate African American presence in state hospitals. Since psychotherapists did not treat psychotics, racialists expected that African Americans were more likely to see the inside of padded cells then to end up on an analyst's couch. In 1936 this racialist presumption still prevailed within psychiatry. As psychiatric authority expanded into city hospitals, schools, courts, prisons, and reformatories, racialism traveled along with it.

Failure of the Public Sector:
Harlem Hospital and the Public School System

The racial determinism that generated such high rates of black institutionalization and kept black neurotics out of private offices also helped justify Harlem's lack of mental health services. Harlem itself contained almost nothing in the way of locally based inpatient or outpatient care. Entering 1936, the mental hygiene movement had not yet come to Harlem. Mental hygienists took psychiatry out of the asylums, using modern psychiatric principles to treat the mild, everyday troubles of ordinary people. Initially, mental hygienists hoped that early treatment of minor emotional problems could prevent more severe mental illness, eventually stemming the need for long-term hospitalization. Since the 1920s, mental hygiene clinics opened across the country as local outpatient alternatives to both state mental hospitals and private care.[41] By 1928, the United States contained over 470 mental hygiene clinics, several in Manhattan.[42] In the 1930s some private citizens even petitioned La Guardia for a Harlem mental hygiene clinic, but to no avail.[43]

Harlem did have a local public hospital: Harlem Hospital.[44] But it did not have its own psychiatric department. Psychiatric units were becoming common features in interwar urban hospitals. That a hospital serving one of the world's most densely populated spaces lacked such a unit was a glaring sign of racial inequality. Even its nursing staff was untrained in basic psychiatric principles or methods.[45] Not until the end of World War II did the city provide Harlem

Hospital with an outpatient mental hygiene clinic, supervised by the black psychiatrist Dr. Harold Ellis. In the 1930s, Harlem residents did have limited access to three other uptown Manhattan hospitals: Community Hospital, St. Luke's on Columbia University's campus, and the charitable Sydenham Hospital.[46] None of them offered substantial inpatient or even outpatient psychiatry.

Whereas some New Yorkers first experienced psychiatry through mental hygiene in the public schools, black children generally did not have this chance. The child-guidance movement had not yet arrived in Harlem. Child guidance was an offshoot of mental hygiene.[47] Between the 1920s and 1940s, its experts helped psychologize childrearing. Initially, they were concerned with identifying and treating the emotional problems that caused juvenile delinquency.[48] In practice, child guidance was administered by an interdisciplinary team of psychiatrists, psychologists, and a new kind of mental health professional: the psychiatric social worker. Once this team had identified the various factors that allegedly caused a child to misbehave, it relied on a variety of services to help promote his or her healthy emotional growth.[49]

The New York City Board of Education first introduced child guidance into some of its schools in 1932. To administer this care, it created the Bureau of Child Guidance (BCG). According to a BCG report, its units provided diagnostic and treatment services, testing, counseling, teacher training, and referrals, all in an effort to "develop healthy personalities in children as the foundation for wholesome adult personalities."[50] Yet for the first four years of its existence, the BCG did not provide Harlem's forty public schools with those services.[51] Rather than a benign oversight, the Board of Education's neglect of Harlem reflected a nationwide pattern of institutional racism within crime prevention.[52] Owing to what the historian Khalil Gibran Muhammad refers to as "racial criminalization: the stigmatization of crime as 'black,'" white reformers and policymakers assumed that "black criminality" was natural and something government could not prevent. Since white crime was individualized and considered preventable, white ethnic neighborhoods received the bulk of crime prevention programs. In contrast, commentators attributed black crime to either an inborn racial disposition or some deficiency within black culture.[53]

It was only in the aftermath of the 1935 Harlem Riot—under pressure from several political commissions criticizing the lack of crime prevention measures in Harlem—that the Board finally authorized a Harlem child guidance unit. Its creation in June 1936 was little more than a political gesture, timed to demonstrate that LaGuardia was doing something to combat violent crime and juvenile delinquency in Harlem. As late as 1938, that single Harlem unit—at P.S. 124 on East 128th Street—still did not have a child guidance team assigned to it.[54]

Psychiatry for African Americans in Punitive Contexts

Despite these barriers, some of Harlem's school-age black children were exposed to psychiatry—but only once they were arrested and charged with juvenile delinquency. Those children were arraigned in the Children's Court, a division of the city's Domestic Relations Court. Given the American criminal justice system's institutional culture of "racial criminalization," children's courts tended to handle white and black children differently.[55] Comparing the fates of black and white New Yorkers, Khalil Muhammad found that African Americans were "twice as likely to be arraigned in Children's Court, [and] more likely to be found guilty."[56] Once the verdict was reached, judges typically did not place young black delinquents with a local agency or on probation. New York City's child welfare system lacked caregiving agencies of its own. Traditionally the city did contract with local private providers. They provided some of the court's charges with quality rehabilitative services. Statistically, however, white delinquents tended to be the only beneficiaries of this privatized, tax-supported care.[57] Black children were usually sentenced to upstate public reformatories known as the New York State training schools. The reason for this institutional racism was simple. Before 1942, Manhattan's private institutions retained the right to racially discriminate. Many refused to take the court's black charges. Consequently, a majority of the state training schools' inmates were African Americans with Harlem addresses.[58]

In contrast with many of the whites-only private schools, the state training schools were slow to incorporate psychiatry into their institutional setup. Case in point was the Warwick State Training School for Boys. Most of Harlem's black male delinquents between twelve and sixteen years of age had been sent to that facility. In 1932 the Warwick Training School contracted Columbia Presbyterian Medical Center to provide medical care. The care included a Psychiatric Clinic Unit.[59] Since this public reform school had been open only since May 1, 1929, it represented the first attempt on the school's part to render psychiatric services.

In everyday practice, Herbert D. Williams, Warwick's superintendent since 1935, neglected the clinic's therapeutic possibilities. Despite the Columbia-trained staff's progressive intentions, Williams only used the clinic to screen new students for psychosis. In accordance with the New York State Charity Law, Warwick denied entrance to any new arrivals diagnosed as psychotic, forcing courts to reassign them to state mental hospitals.[60] Once the clinic cleared new arrivals, those inmates never saw the head psychiatrist again. This failure to provide black teens with modern rehabilitative services can be seen as the product of what the historian Martin Summers identified as a "larger intellectual formation in which blackness was associated with excess, violence, and criminality, further legitimizing the classification and control of black bodies within sites that were more carceral than curative well into the twentieth century."[61] Most of the school's young men probably never knew the clinic's actual purpose. To them the clinic team must have seemed to be the mysterious proctors of seemingly pointless tests. Or even worse, perhaps they appeared to be conspiratorial adults invested in keeping them locked away from their family and friends. Either way, it was unlikely that black adolescents left Warwick convinced that psychiatry was a helping profession.

Incarceration in a reform school afforded Harlem's so-called delinquents a negative introduction to psychiatry, and other African Americans made their first contact with psychiatry in the adult criminal justice system. Unsurprisingly, the "racial criminalization" of African Americans produced racially disparate outcomes for black adults. Owing to race-based dragnets, police brutality, and other systematic harassment, two predominantly black sections of Harlem possessed the highest arrest and conviction rates for a variety of crimes in the 1930s.[62] Since blacks in custody were far more likely to have their cases go to trial, they stood a good chance of meeting the court psychiatrist. Starting in 1932, New York's Court of General Sessions provided every convicted male felon awaiting sentencing with a psychiatric exam.[63]

Some prisoners received more than personality assessments at the court clinic. Between 1935 and 1943, the court clinic's director, Bellevue psychiatrist Walter Bromberg, allowed a few prisoners to undergo psychotherapy at the clinic. Bromberg hoped that psychiatry could become a standard part of rehabilitation. He claimed that the court's clinic psychiatrist could educate the prisoners about the "mental hygiene idea" during these limited sessions. He hoped that exposure to mental hygiene principles (also called the "psychiatric point of view" by contemporaries) might encourage prisoners to understand their "criminal activity as evidence of psychological and personality distortion." If they could gain some such insight into the deeper personal reasons for their past misconduct, these convicts could be motivated to change their behavior.[64]

Although there is no hard evidence black convicts internalized this mental hygiene idea, some at least attempted to manipulate psychiatrists. A court clinician's report from the 1930s revealed that an eighteen-year-old black prisoner "facing his fourth charge and therefore a very long sentence . . . had been advised by fellow prisoners to pretend that he was crazy." The young man received a pretrial psychiatric exam, standard practice when the defendant's mental competence was disputed. The clinician found the teen sane and the inmate confessed to his deception. This case suggests that some African Americans saw the psychiatrist as a weak link in the criminal justice system's otherwise punitive world of armed police, unforgiving judges, brutal jailers, and vicious inmates. The psychiatrist appeared to be a soft adversary that citizens could exploit as they sought to avoid incarceration.[65]

Bellevue Psychopathic and Black Harlem

Outside of corrections and state institutions, the majority of black Harlemites who experienced psychiatry in 1936 did so at Bellevue Psychopathic Hospital. Bellevue was one of the nation's oldest hospital complexes. It was also one of the only New York hospitals that offered psychiatric care to blacks. As a public hospital, Bellevue received patients who were to pay. With few private facilities willing to take neglected and delinquent black children, the Children's Court sent a disproportionate number of those cases to Bellevue for both psychiatric and custodial care. Between 1932 and 1937, black children were 18 percent of the children's ward.[66]

For several reasons, black Harlemites did their best to avoid to Bellevue. According to the Brooklyn-bred writer Ralph G. Martin, Dr. Menas S. Gregory's psychiatric division had an "unenviable reputation in Harlem."[67] Understaffed and overcrowded, the all-white staff's dismissive and often hostile treatment of black patients was well-known above 110th Street. Even after Mayor La Guardia's administration had forced the hospital to hire its first black staff members in 1938, it still retained a racist reputation.[68] Second, Bellevue was too far from Harlem. It was located downtown on First Avenue between Twenty-Sixth and Thirtieth Streets, making the trip long and logistically difficult for those who lived across 110th Street—especially if one had to travel on the IRT subway or in a cab with a loved one who was experiencing a frightening episode. Third, Bellevue was also the first stop for many Harlemites on their equally unwanted path to a state mental hospital.[69]

Not surprisingly, few African Americans *chose* to enter Bellevue Psychopathic. As one writer put it as late as 1946: "Negroes have to be carried in there; few walk in."[70] Of those who had to be carried into Bellevue, loved ones or an authority figure generally did the carrying. An adult was often accompanied at admission by either a spouse or a close family member. Since Bellevue had such a poor reputation in Harlem, the choice to admit a family member was often made out of sheer desperation. Families typically sought Bellevue's help only when an afflicted loved one became too destructive or disruptive. Lena, a twenty-five-year-old immigrant from the British West Indies, was admitted by her sister on April 6, 1934. The sister decided that enough was enough when Lena arrived at her house and "started smashing the windows." Likewise, Arnette's husband had brought her down from Harlem on December 8, 1932, after "she had been screaming for several hours."[71]

The police also admitted black adults that had allegedly disturbed the peace or simply frightened white officers.[72] Between 1931 and 1933, the police brought in several black Harlemites whose public behavior, the officers claimed, became bizarre and unmanageable after smoking marijuana.[73] In deciding whether an intoxicated state merited hospitalization, racialist assumptions must have been part of this calculus. In run-ins with whites under the influence, a simple citation for disorderly conduct was common. Hospitalization in a mental ward could be potentially embarrassing. The police may have been sensitive to this fact when dealing with whites. Yet given Western culture's long association of blackness with madness,[74] the officers might not have felt that same need to shield blacks from the stigma of mental illness.[75]

Parents and city authorities also admitted black children with behavioral and learning problems into Bellevue Hospital. Some parents brought their children in when they found their behavior inexplicable and beyond correction. Others brought them in with school referrals, usually for classroom misconduct.[76] Harlem schools also referred children with learning difficulties. For example, a mother brought her preschooler to the mental hygiene clinic "because of retardation in speech."[77] In the 1930s, the Children's Court also referred cases of neglected and delinquent black children with mental illness.[78] With such a wide range of troubled children from all age groups, the children's ward was often terrifying for the youngest and most vulnerable.[79]

In 1936, a black Harlemite's typical experience with psychiatry was still rather coercive and custodial, much in the older state asylum model.[80] Few chose to see a psychiatrist. Such a meeting was either forced on them or chosen for them. Since local mental health options were so limited, psychiatry was something African Americans tended to encounter only if they had become ensnared within the criminal justice system. Psychiatry facilitated or even replaced prosecution, sentencing, and punishment. Even outside of jails and courthouses, the black experience with mental health professionals still featured involuntary confinement, estrangement from family and neighborhood, and exposure to people with frightening and dangerous emotional states and dispositions. As long as African Americans were overdiagnosed with mental illnesses for which there was little hope of recovery or prevention, authorities were chiefly interested in warehousing them. At this time, policymakers still did not think that the promotion or restoration of black mental health warranted public investment.

Early Twentieth-Century Psychiatry and Racialism

Once an African American entered Bellevue Psychopathic, how did his or her race matter on the wards? As the historian Jonathan Metzl noted, "racial tensions are structured into clinical interactions long before doctors or patients enter examination rooms."[81] In one sense, white psychiatrists internalized their culture's assumptions about race, gender, and class. They then diagnosed and treated patients through a perceptual lens mediated by those biases.[82] These clinical interactions, outcomes, and policies were influenced by more than personal prejudice. Early twentieth-century psychiatry's institutional culture possessed its own particular way of framing the way clinicians imagined how, when, and why race would matter. Besides the tendency to overdiagnose African Americans with psychoses, how and why did the racial identity of black patients matter to most white clinicians in the interwar period?

Summarizing psychiatry's relationship with race in the early twentieth century, Gerald Grob, dean of the history of US psychiatry, writes: "While race clearly shaped patterns of care and treatment, it never became a distinctive element in psychiatric thought."[83] If one narrowly defines race as a category of inherited physiognomic traits, Grob is correct. Psychiatry never explicitly included racial categories within their basic concepts of personhood, child development, disease causation, or pathology. Early twentieth-century medical schools and textbooks, with their emphasis on "teaching the general properties of all sick bodies" and minds, rarely taught students how race mattered.[84] Entering the 1930s, psychiatrists consistently claimed that the same general psychic forces governed both black and white psyches. As well, the psychiatric literature indicated that blacks and whites developed mental illnesses in the same way, with no specific diseases identified as afflicting only African Americans.[85]

Race, however, refers to more than just inherited skin-color variations. Race is not something that naturally inheres in the human body. Rather, it is just one way of seeing and creating meaning out of human bodies.[86] Humans have not always perceived population diversity through the lens of race. According to most scholars of race, the belief that humanity divides neatly into biologically distinct breeds distinguished by skin-color differences dates only as far back as the age of European colonization and transatlantic slavery. What is more, it was not just the human body that came to be seen and evaluated through this racial lens. In the United States, the logic of race, working in concert with other social categories (including gender, class, sexuality, and citizenship), informed how Americans made sense of the world around them. Over time, citizens began associating living spaces, jobs, behaviors, attitudes, customs, and other aspects of the culture with specific races. For something to have become racialized meant that it had acquired the same value Americans assigned a particular race. By the twentieth century, the United States had become so thoroughly racialized that skin color did not always have to be explicitly invoked for some assumption, practice, or policy to do the work of race.[87]

The cultural history of race explains how so many modern psychiatrists could believe in universal psychological forces and yet expect them to operate within black bodies and white bodies in slightly different ways. A closer look at interwar psychiatry's literature reveals that racialized assumptions lurked behind its apparently race-neutral language. As the historian Nayan Shah has shown, "modernity . . . promotes ideas of universality on the one hand, and on the other hand, obsessively objectifies difference."[88] Modern psychiatry's general principles and diagnostic categories were expressed in putatively universal terms. Still, American clinicians tended to "read them through a set of clearly racial assumptions" about normal and abnormal psychology.[89] When writing about black patients, racialist psychiatrists made sure to note the patient's skin color. By contrast, psychiatrists wrote about white patients without any reference to racial identity. Through this selective deployment of race neutrality, many psychiatric writers equated human normality with whiteness. Although they constructed their profession's various principles and theories with this imagined white subject in mind, racialists expressed those ideas in print without mention of skin color. Owing to this disingenuous race neutrality, race's influence on psychiatric thought was often imperceptible, giving outsiders the false impression that psychiatry's truths applied to all races.[90]

Yet within the professional literature, psychiatry revealed its racial scaffolding when clinicians published their encounters with the "Negro patient." In the late nineteenth and early twentieth centuries, with few blacks in Northern asylums, the profession had marginalized the black psyche as a Southern problem.[91] Following the Great Black Migration of the 1890s—1920s, the "Negro patient" became a figure of national concern. By 1931, George van Dearborn, a white neuropsychiatrist in the Bronx with several popular books on psychology, declared that someone ought to write "an elementary text book on negro psychiatry."[92] Dearborn's comment was an admission that what psychiatry taught about the human psyche was only meant to describe the interior life of white patients.

In 1936 many clinicians still considered the black psyche a racial exception to existing psychological precepts. In 1933, one critic observed that most of the writers in American psychiatric journals "generally have a preconceived notion (conscious or unconscious), that some races are inferior to others."[93] For the most part, psychiatrists writing about black patients expressed these racist sensibilities in their analyses of black psychological capacities.[94] Chiefly, they expected black patients to possess a unique and inferior "racial character makeup."[95] The historian Matthew Gambino found this sensibility at work on the wards of St. Elizabeth's Hospital in Washington, DC, the largest US mental institution.[96] Yes, these psychiatrists agreed that the same set of universally human psychic forces operated within the bodies of blacks and whites. But as white citizens within the society that generated Jim Crow and immigration restriction, they considered it "racially plausible"[97] that a uniquely black psyche would result when those universal forces interacted with inferior African American bodies. Within psychiatric institutions in 1936, this racial exceptionalism was a standard expectation, influencing how mental health workers perceived black patients.[98]

Most of psychiatry's dominant intellectual frameworks easily accommodated this racial determinism. The psychiatrist Adolph Meyer's psychobiology eschewed the mind-body dualism pervading US psychiatry prior to the 1920s. Meyerians understood any mental disease as a patient's failure to psychologically and biologically adjust to the demands of his or her living space.[99] This psychobiology easily accommodated racial determinism. Racialists imagined that a physical substrate unique to black physiology was responsible for any emotional differences between blacks and whites.

Racialist assumptions had also been encoded within the very underpinnings of psychoanalysis. Freud's theory of emotional development and disease causation was hewn from a nineteenth-century evolutionary framework associated with the child-study pioneer G. Stanley Hall and British anthropologists, including E. B. Tylor and James George Frazer of *Golden Bough* fame. Within this framework, individual maturation was equated with human evolution. Inferior races were the least evolved, which marked them as primitive.[100] Stuck at a stage of arrested development, primitives represented the ancient "history of the race," the childhood of humanity.[101] Freudian psychoanalytic theory was constructed from within this racial-evolutionary frame. Mental health was conceptualized as full emotional maturation and the expected destiny for most whites. Mental or emotional disturbances were considered reversions to earlier, less-developed states of mind.[102] Psychoanalysts even employed the racially loaded term "primitive" as a synonym for the immaturity that allegedly characterized the thinking of both children and the mentally ill.[103]

American racialists embraced these Freudian links between childhood, mental pathology, and arrested development. They extended the evolutionary metaphor even further, describing the black adult psyche as "a more primitive type of mind."[104] As members of a race that had not advanced out of the early stages of human evolution, African Americans were incapable of reaching the full psychological maturity expected of normal white adults. According to one racialist in the 1930s, the "primitive mind tends to mature fast but decelerates or ceases to develop at an early age."[105] Typical for the era, the psychiatrists John Lind, Mary O'Malley, and Arrah Evarts of Washington's DC's US Government Hospital claimed that the black race's inferior developmental potential left African American adults stunted at the emotional level of our early human ancestors, white adolescents, and the severely mentally ill.[106]

To assess whether someone has returned to normalcy, medicine requires some standard against which therapeutic progress can be measured. In the psychiatric literature, writers intimated that the well-adjusted adult was content, serious, rational, sober, and responsible. Quite possibly, this individual would be prone to anxiety. With expert help, such a person could be expected to manage those feelings. But this early twentieth-century definition of emotional health only reflected what clinicians expected of someone middle class, heterosexual—and white.[107] These emotional norms were never meant to describe blacks. In the psychiatric literature, some authors were aware that some of the characteristics they claimed were typical or normal for otherwise well-adjusted African Americans—whimsy, mania, mood swings, lethargy, visions, and trance states—would earn a white adult a diagnosis of severe mental illness.[108] So how did racialist clinicians determine if black patients had successfully recovered from mental illness when the standard of emotional health did not fully apply to them?[109]

Psychiatrists resolved this dilemma by judging psychological normality in whites and blacks by different standards—standards that framed African Americans as naturally childish and incompletely gendered. As Martin Summers and Elizabeth Lunbeck both discovered, clinicians tended to believe that "white abnormality approximated blacks' normal state of being."[110] The literature described the emotional makeup of children and black adults in the same terms. They were all excitable, fanciful, superstitious, secretive, rhythmic, musical, hypersexual, unrestrained, and in possession of a less-developed nervous system.[111] For white adults such a profile would be considered abnormal. Psychoanalysts expected that normal white adults had tamed their natural drives and instincts.[112] According to the historian Clare Corbould, these same experts imagined that those "primordial forces within all people were simply closer to the surface in black people."[113] Thought incapable of maturing to the same psychological level expected of normal white adults, blacks were biologically destined to remain in thrall to the human species' most animalistic passions. Even normal black adults were not expected to be anything more than perpetual children, a happy-go-lucky race of Peter Pans.[114]

Analogously, clinicians perceived an abnormal lack of gender difference between the emotional capacities of black men and women. Psychiatrists believed that biological sex differences caused white men and women to think, feel, and emote in gender-specific ways. These gender profiles reflected conventional American cultural assumptions about men and women's essential natures. Considering gender gaps to be a natural hallmark of evolution, clinicians expected the emotional gap between men and women to be quite pronounced within the white race. By contrast, they presumed that men and women from primitive races would demonstrate far more similarities in affect. Accordingly, racialists imagined that black women were as oversexed and aggressive as white men, and black men as emotionally overwrought as white women. Such an overlap between men and women's inner natures would have signified either immaturity or mental disorder among whites. But with primitive blacks, clinicians considered the lack of clearly gendered emotional states to be perfectly normal for their race.[115]

Bender, Bellevue, and Racial Agnosticism

Although racialism still pervaded US psychiatry entering 1936, not all psychiatrists accepted biological determinism uncritically, even on the wards of Bellevue Psychopathic. Black physicians and some other intellectuals concerned with the health of the African American psyche had already rejected racialism.[116] By the mid-1930s, younger white psychiatrists also began offering social and cultural explanations for apparent psychological differences between races. Yet just because these clinicians entertained alternatives to racial determinism, this did not mean they outright rejected either racialism or racism. Typically, these authors picked apart the holes in old racialist claims while still holding out the possibility that African Americans could be racial primitives. According to the historian Ellen Dwyer, the "psychiatrists [who] increasingly attributed psychiatric disorders to social and economic factors" also "remained unwilling to abandon altogether the notion of biologically based racial difference."[117] Throughout the sciences, what the historian Michelle Brattain called "racial agnosticism" continued to be fairly common even after World War II. On Bellevue's wards in 1936, the leading exponent of this noncommittal position on race was Lauretta Bender.[118]

Lauretta Bender was a relatively young but talented Bellevue clinician who had just begun actively engaging with the "Negro patient" question. Dr. Bender was a white native of Montana and the wife of the senior Bellevue psychiatrist and former Freud analyst and Paul F. Schilder. In 1934 she became the director of the Children's Psychiatric Division. During her twenty-two-year directorship, Bender gained notoriety as one of the first proponents of the controversial diagnosis of childhood schizophrenia. She had also been a paid consultant for DC Comics, publicly defending Superman and Wonder Woman against the crusading psychiatrist Fredric Wertham and other critics of the comic-book industry.[119]

Bender's first foray into her profession's longstanding conversation about the black psyche thrust her into a very public debate over one of the Great

Depression's most iconic African American figures: the Harlem cult leader Father Divine. Born George Baker, the four-foot-six-inch preacher proclaimed himself the Judeo-Christian deity's earthly incarnation. His followers lived communally in one of Divine's several nationwide compounds; his Harlem site had been designated the Peace Mission cult's headquarters in 1932. Between 1933 and 1938, Father Divine became a minor American celebrity. In the midst of the Great Depression, this cartoonishly short black man managed to amass a personal fortune and keep the denizens of his Harlem compound apparently happy and well fed. This diminutive New Yorker even exercised influence over the mayoral election in 1935.[120] Journalists, academicians, businessmen, and psychologists churned out books and articles about Divine, purporting to explain how he persuaded poor African Americans to make him so rich and powerful.[121]

Dr. Bender entered this public debate over Father Divine and his followers in 1935. Some commentators claimed that Father Divine easily manipulated blacks because they were naturally excitable and childlike. Bender contested these facile racialist explanations. Bender first became interested in this issue after a few followers of Divine had been hospitalized at Bellevue for mental and emotional illnesses in the early 1930s.[122] At the American Psychiatric Association's annual meeting in 1935, Bender first shared what she had observed of the black Peace Mission followers, publishing her findings between 1938 and 1940.[123] Given the interest in Divine, New York journalists quickly reported on her 1935 paper.[124] Bender's work on Divine attracted much attention. In line with her profession's disproportionate branding of African Americans as psychotics, Bender diagnosed most of the adult followers with mania.[125] Nevertheless, the way she wrote about these black patients was not how racialists typically presented African American cases in print.[126]

Bender asserted that race did not matter in the cases of Father Divine's black followers.[127] She explicitly challenged the racialist assumption that the primitive black psyche was "likely to recover quickly" from manic episodes, whereas whites and "less emotional races" needed more time to recover from full-blown manic psychosis.[128] She also contested the racialist nostrum that African Americans were immune to neuroses. Neurotic feelings and anxiety developed as repressed urges returned from the depths of the subconscious. Since racialists did not believe that the primitive emotional profile included repression, they expected that black folks could not become neurotic. In contrast, Bender's observations of black children led her to conclude that African Americans could experience guilt feelings over "sexual urges and other neurotic mechanisms." They could repress urges and develop psychosexual conflicts and neuroses.[129] In her 1940 article, she noted her patients' racial identities but—atypically for the period—proceeded to discuss the cases as though race was not a clinically significant factor.

Based on Bender's published and unpublished accounts of her encounters with African American patients, it becomes clear that this young psychiatrist was not swayed by racialist thinking about the African American psyche. Her talks and articles reveal someone surprised to find that the black patients she encountered did not possess the happy-go-lucky, anxiety-free psyche described by racialists. Bender's clinical experience suggested to her that the black race's emotional capacities and potential might be far greater than what her own profession had led her to expect. Bender and other Northern clinicians were seeing their black patients demonstrate neurotic symptoms that, at least according to the literature, they should not have been able to exhibit.[130] If her observations were correct, if blacks could emotionally suffer in the same way as whites, it meant that an African American's inner world was vastly different from the one psychiatrists had long imagined. Moreover, it would mean that blacks were deserving of access to a wider array of mental health care than was presently available to them.

How was Bender able to recognize and assert that African Americans had more emotional depth than the psychiatric literature indicated?[131] In marked contrast to the racial liberals featured throughout the bulk of this book, it was not because she had simply dismissed racialism out of hand. Yes, just like New York's racial liberals, Bender was unwilling to accept racial determinism as a given. But unlike them, she never rejected it as a scientific possibility. In questioning racialism's intellectual hold over psychiatry, Bender had not been motivated by the racial liberals' political commitment to social justice and racial equality. Whether racialism was correct or incorrect was not a political matter for her. It was a scientific one. In her view, racialism was a potentially valid scientific hypothesis that could only be confirmed or denied through careful investigation—not political conviction.

In a 1939 article, Bender was plainly struggling to explain why her experiences with African American children at Bellevue had deviated from the medical literature's portrayal of the black psyche.[132] Bender examined many of the antiracialist explanations found in both the psychiatric journals and the social science literature.[133] She explicitly stated that recent epidemiological studies had convinced her that racialism did not offer the best framework for understanding and treating African American patients. She wrote that "careful studies have tended to disprove . . . in most cases" that "differences between the white and negro races in mental and disease exist due to actual racial differences or to the primitivity of the negro race."[134] Bender specifically credited Malzberg's 1936 study with compelling her to accept that "social and economical [sic] conditions" could explain "most differences between the white and negro in mental and nervous disease."[135]

Some of the deracialized elements in Bender's approach to the black psyche came from cultural anthropology. Columbia University's Franz Boas had revolutionized the field at the turn of the century, proposing that biological race did not determine culture. Boasians assumed that human beings, regardless of their race, were born with the same innate human potential to create and invent.[136] This revolution in cultural anthropology changed the practice of psychoanalysis in the United States, inspiring the development of ethnopsychiatry. Ethnopsychiatrists asserted that each of the world's cultures had the power to shape the psychological potential that all humans shared into distinct psychological types.[137] Although Bender was not an ethnopsychiatrist, she cited the Boasian anthropologists Margaret Mead and Ruth Benedict's work on culture and personality as an influence on her deracialized depictions of Divine's followers.[138]

Although she found racialist understandings of the black psyche unsatisfying, Bender was still open to the argument that some aspects of the black psyche might be racially determined. In 1936, at the American Psychiatric Association's annual meeting in St. Louis, she declared: "Racial differences have to be considered" in diagnosing and treating a black patient.[139] Even in the 1939 article in which she claimed that racialism had been "proven" wrong, she carefully added that this only applied to "most cases." In that same article, she considered the possibility that blacks might be hardwired to express their inner "turmoil in racially distinctive ways," an idea that colonial psychiatrists in Africa also considered.[140] Between 1936 and 1939, she proposed that minor physiological differences between black and white bodies could lead the two races to channel their shared human emotional potential in divergent ways.[141] In 1936, she claimed that dance therapy was more effective with black children. According to Bender, black childrens' allegedly innate talent for dancing enabled "their bodies to express submerged feelings and anxieties with greater ease and clarity than could the bodies of most white children."[142] She was not ideologically wedded to this position, eventually returning in the 1940s to the antiracialist arguments she made about Father Divine's followers in 1935.[143]

In 1936, the institutional culture of US psychiatric institutions encouraged Bender's provisional approach to race. At Bellevue, Bender was surrounded by a senior group of male racialists. She actively collaborated with some of them, including her husband Paul F. Schilder and Frank Curran—both of whom considered the black psyche a site of primordial savagery and arrested development.[144] Her provisional approach to race did not constitute a threat to racialists since it did not outright repudiate their perspective. In her work, Bender did not treat antiracist alternatives to racial determinism as if they were ethically superior. Consequently, both cultural relativism and racialism coexisted on Bellevue's wards. Younger and older colleagues consulted one another on cases of black patients without antagonism. In such a climate, the black psyche retained its place as "the thing against which normality, whiteness, and functionality had been defined."[145]

Conclusion

In the 1930s, Bender's racial agnosticism may have been an advance in racial thinking, but it did not dislodge racialism and institutional racism from either psychiatry or urban social policy. Although there were fewer racialists than ever before on the nation's wards, they had been replaced with diffident young clinicians unsure as to how fully human their patients were. Clinicians who still considered racialism a potentially valid hypothesis never developed the firm conviction that blacks and whites were psychological equals. Although they did challenge racialism, these new clinicians did not outright reject it. This very slight shift in race thinking did not dislodge US psychiatry's long-standing racialism and racism. Racial determinism remained intact, unthreatened by the younger generation's uncertainty regarding the necessity of separate psychiatric norms for white and blacks. The over-institutionalization of African Americans in state hospitals, psychiatric wards, and reforms schools endured while segregated black communities still lacked their own local mental health care resources.

Psychiatry's handling of black patients would not change until practitioners deemed that racial determinism was unjust and then simply abandoned it. The next chapter explores how political changes within Mayor La Guardia's New York offered racial liberals the chance to inject an antiracialist and antiracist sensibility into mental health care. Suitable openings within the juvenile justice system enabled some younger psychiatrists to break free from psychiatric racialism while avoiding racial agnosticism's conciliatory stance. Buoyed by an uncompromising faith in the psychological equality of the races, these clinicians and their political allies in New York's Domestic Relations Court took advantage of any opportunity to craft racially inclusive policies and patterns of resource distribution. Working across disciplinary and departmental lines on behalf of black children in New York's system of courts and corrections, they laid the foundations of a powerful but "unevenly shared" new psychiatric approach to race.[146] For the origin of this new approach, we now turn to the courtroom of Justine Wise Polier.

Chapter Two

Everyone's Children

Psychiatry and Racial Liberalism in Justine Wise Polier's Courtroom, 1936–41

In her 1941 book *Everyone's Children, Nobody's Child,* the New York Children's Court judge Justine Wise Polier recounted the story of two children brought up on juvenile delinquency charges. After reviewing each child's psychiatric evaluation, Polier determined that Selma Martin and Daniel Johns were the victims of emotional neglect. Foster families had mistreated Selma. Abandoned by his mother, Daniel had been passed from place to place. Polier concluded that the "misbehavior of the children was directly traceable to their sense of insecurity." Both "had never known security in their natural homes" and each needed a stable home and "psychiatric care to help solve the child's problem."[1] Polier presented each case as being fairly representative of the emotional torment that neglected children in her court had experienced.[2] The decision to depict these youngsters and their psychological reactions as typical was an extraordinary move. Although Polier cited each case as an example of the average neglected child, these two children differed from most American children in one appreciable way: Daniel and Selma were black.

That a judge could produce a race-neutral psychological profile indicates that psychiatric authority and racial liberalism had already converged in New York's courts for juveniles. Two very significant historical shifts occurred. The first shift, the psychologization of crime, took hold first. By the 1920s, more and more children's court judges and staff considered juvenile delinquency a psychological problem requiring psychiatric care. Owing to this shift in perception, judges were no longer in the business of simply punishing misbehavior. When Polier arrived on the bench in 1936, children's court justices were increasingly expected to facilitate the diagnosis and treatment of the underlying emotional illness or conflict that caused children to commit crimes.[3]

The second historical shift, racial liberalism, developed as a response to New Deal liberalism's reliance on race-neutral solutions to problems of racial inequality. During President Franklin Delano Roosevelt's first two terms (1933–40), most citizens who answered to the label "liberal" believed that government had a duty to open up individual opportunities for employment and upward mobility through social engineering and universal entitlements.[4] Liberals tended to believe that economic relief programs, safety nets, and social services could reduce racial inequality if they were available to all. By the mid-1930s, some of them recognized that some social policies were not so color-blind in practice. These racial liberals found that state and municipal authorities routinely undermined the egalitarian potential of their ostensibly inclusive programs, administering them in racially discriminatory ways. Some of these politicians, policymakers, and civil servants—including Justice Polier—began to oppose institutional racism in the distribution of government resources. Hoping to transform the public sector into a truer instrument of equal opportunity, these individuals supported antidiscrimination legislation and insisted on racial fairness in the delivery of social services.[5]

Between 1936 and 1941, both of these trends—the psychologization of juvenile justice and the emergence of racial liberalism—intersected within Justice Polier's Manhattan courtroom. New York under Mayor Fiorello La Guardia, a political ally of President Roosevelt, was a likely candidate for such a convergence. The former New York Congressman transformed his city into a proving ground for interventionist New Deal social policy.[6] As La Guardia's administration actively encouraged the public sector's growth, Polier was able to expand psychiatry's role within the Children's Court and demand that this care be delivered in a racially unbiased way. For the new judge and her court personnel, the New York child welfare system's lack of equal space for African Americans with untreated psychiatric needs was not just an injustice. Polier considered it a health crisis requiring immediate redress. She assumed that black children and white children were all born with the same psychological potential and developmental needs. Withholding standard psychiatric care from black children constituted a real threat to their emotional health.[7] This outright rejection of racial discrimination automatically set Polier and her court psychiatrists—Drs. Marion E. Kenworthy, Helen Montague, and Max Winsor—apart from older clinicians. It also differentiated them from younger psychiatrists who still entertained the possibility that blacks were psychologically different enough to require a separate standard of care. In short, Polier's courtroom had become a space where blacks and whites were considered psychological equals and psychodynamic principles were applied universally without reference to race.[8]

What follows examines how Polier and her court staff developed policies and practices informed by psychiatric universalism. Psychiatric universalism—or the "psychiatric point of view," as Polier termed it—refers to the assumption that blacks and whites psychologically developed in the same way, with the same basic emotional needs and vulnerabilities.[9] With so few providers willing to accept black children, Polier struggled to find adequate psychiatric care for her black charges. The 1936–37 reports of the Domestic Relations Court's investigation of the New York State training schools offers the first evidence that Polier's staff expected caregivers to safeguard the mental health of African American children. As this expectation gained ground among her staff, Polier came up with a way for her court to offer some psychiatric treatment. With La Guardia's approval, she and the child guidance pioneer Dr. Marion E. Kenworthy created the Domestic Relations Court treatment clinic in 1937. A prime example of the "racially inclusive universalism of New Deal liberalism," the clinic was open to all children. Nevertheless, its creators expected it would primarily help those who had the least access to any mental health care—black Harlemites.[10]

In her own courtroom handling of African American children, Polier incorporated the so-called psychiatric point of view as much as possible. A close reading of a black incest victim's case reveals the judge making a sincere effort to evaluate the child's emotional needs in a race-neutral fashion. Despite Polier's best efforts, racism remained endemic within private childcare agencies, the state training schools, and the Board of Justices during her first six years on the bench. Race-based restrictions on the placement of black children often prevented her from freely adjudicating in a color-blind fashion. At the start of the 1940s, Polier found that she was not alone in her frustration over these policies. The chapter concludes as she and other like-minded La Guardia appointees on the Children's Court committed themselves to the fight against institutional racism.

Justine Wise Polier and the Emergence of Racial Liberalism, 1920s–1930s

Prior to her 1935 appointment, Polier had never given much thought to psychiatry. Within a short time, however, Polier came to expect that psychiatrists should help rehabilitate troubled children regardless of their race. The concept of "psychiatric universalism" was not what prompted or motivated Polier to see institutional racism as something worth battling. Well before her courtroom became a key site in the battle against psychiatric racism, Polier had been a committed antiracist.

Justine Wise Polier's own biography ably demonstrates the political influences that helped generate racial liberalism in the mid-1930s. According to her: "The conviction that democracy meant that all people have equal opportunity to live fully and not be subjected to the injuries and scars that stem from racial injustice was part of the air that I breathed in my parent's home." Her parents also instilled in her the obligation to do more than just be "sensitive . . . to the doctrine of racism."[11] Polier, born Justine Wise, was the child of two of the United States' leading Jewish advocates for victims of racial and religious discrimination. Since 1916, Justine's mother, Louise Waterman Wise, operated an adoption agency for Jewish orphans that municipal authorities had refused to place with gentiles. Her father, Rabbi Stephen Wise, was one of the initial leaders of the American Jewish Congress, a liberal Jewish American civil-rights organization formed in 1916. A committed antiracist, he was a cofounder of the National Association for the Advancement of Colored People.[12] Their examples taught her that racism was not to be tolerated. It was to be fought.

Once in college, the future Justine Wise Polier expanded her range of social-justice interests. She became concerned with labor issues and wealth inequality. Not content with studying the working poor in economics classes at Bryn Mawr, Radcliffe, and Barnard, she joined the labor force and the labor movement. After working in a Passaic, New Jersey, textile factory between 1924 and 1925, she organized a strike in 1926. Eventually she enrolled in Yale law school, where she became a labor-rights advocate, and married Lee Tulin, a criminology professor.[13] After passing the Connecticut bar in 1928, Justine Wise Tulin took a research position with the Rockefeller Fund, becoming an expert in worker's compensation law. From 1929 to 1935 she worked as an administrator and counsel within the workmen's compensation offices of New York City and the New York State Labor Department.[14] Lee Tulin died of leukemia in 1932. His widow retained his last name until she married the civil-rights lawyer Shad Polier in 1936.

Her long-standing interest in both racial justice and labor rights eventually led Polier to relief work related to the Great Depression. In April 1935, she began serving as the city Emergency Relief Bureau (ERB)'s legal aid. A self-described liberal since her undergraduate years at Bryn Mawr, she and other New Deal liberals believed in "government [that] engaged in planning and intervened in the economy to create jobs" and opportunity for individual advancement.[15] At the ERB, Polier championed "increased relief allowances" and "improvement of the relief system" for needy families.[16] She also learned of the racism rampant in public assistance. As someone with a strong sense of social justice, she was not willing to accept it. She expected that a universal entitlement ought to be doled out without regard to skin color. She was not alone in feeling this way. In fact, racial liberalism emerged as a political viewpoint when Polier and other like-minded citizens administering New Deal-era programs began insisting that governments had a responsibility to distribute their resources in a racially equitable manner.[17]

After the 1935 Harlem Riot, Mayor La Guardia was eager to repair relations with the African American community and appeal to those who shared Polier's viewpoint. He created opportunities for individuals eager to promote "equal treatment for blacks and whites" as a new policymaking criterion.[18] In July 1935, Polier received her chance to do that within the courts. That month, La Guardia appointed her the first female justice on the Domestic Relations Court (a combination of family and children's courts).[19]

Even before the 1935 Harlem Riot, La Guardia's administration had already been carving out spaces for racial liberals within the public sector. La Guardia was elected mayor as the Fusion candidate just two years earlier in 1933. The Fusion Party was an antimachine reform movement. Nominally Republican, its ranks also included citizens who voted Democrat in national but not local elections. In 1932, Roosevelt's successful run for the presidency attracted voters to the Democratic Party that New York City's Irish-controlled Democratic machine—known as Tammany Hall—had traditionally alienated on the municipal level. These excluded groups included liberal intellectuals, Jews,

African Americans, trade unionists—many along the left side of the political spectrum. Tammany Hall had long neglected the interests of these populations, denying them patronage and access to opportunities and resources. In 1933 La Guardia and the Fusion Party successfully courted those voters. Once in office, La Guardia rewarded some of his most ardent liberal supporters with political positions.[20]

At the time of her appointment, Polier and her father were political allies and close friends of La Guardia. Rabbi Stephen Wise had been an important part of the Fusion Party's success. In municipal politics Jewish New Yorkers had never firmly committed themselves to either the Democrats or the Republicans. Rabbi Wise's support helped steer more Jewish voters into La Guardia's camp in 1933. During his tenure as mayor, La Guardia made good on campaign promises he made to the Jewish community. He rooted out Tammany Hall cronyism, opening up employment opportunities to qualified candidates—including high-profile Jewish Americans.[21] Polier's appointment was one such opportunity.

Yet deciding where to place Polier was more due to her gender than her ethnicity or religion. Polier's assignment to the children's court was an enduring legacy of the politics of "maternal statecraft."[22] Since the Progressive Era, "maternalist" reformers created job openings for women in child welfare. Manipulating the widespread assumption that nature had destined women to care for children, women professionals carved a space for themselves within the US Children's Bureau, adoption agencies, juvenile courts, and other offices serving children.[23] Nevertheless, the sexist assumptions that justified the creation of a female niche within the child welfare system also limited women's expansion into other fields of employment. La Guardia knew his friend Justine's specialty was labor law. But no woman in New York had ever held a judicial post higher than magistrate. To limit potential objections to the appointment of a female judge, La Guardia chose a court for Polier that New Yorkers were likely to consider gender appropriate.[24]

Although family law had not been her field of study, Polier did not arrive on the bench entirely disinterested in child welfare issues. A widow since 1932, she was a single mother with a son, Stephen Wise Tulin. Given her experience as a labor activist and ERB legal aid, she knew the difficulties she encountered paled in comparison to the obstacles facing working poor women "lack[ing] the money, parental support, and education" she enjoyed.[25] The daughter of a maternalist adoption reformer, she understood that poor mothers lived with the threat that courts could take their children. Polier's mother had brought home Jewish orphans the city refused to place, fostering them until she found them adoptive parents.[26] This experience led Polier to believe that children belonged with families or small agencies, not large custodial facilities. It was obvious that Polier was going to have trouble consigning any child—black or white—to some warehouse.

Once on the bench, Polier was initially troubled by the racial segregation endemic to New York's child welfare system. Since the Progressive Era, children's court judges theoretically wielded the authority to place delinquent and neglected children wherever they saw fit. But the childcare industry's peculiar restrictions limited Polier's ability to place children at her own discretion. Manhattan possessed no public facilities of its own. Instead the courts relied on private caregivers. Most of them were sectarian. They refused to take children from other faiths.[27] Private agencies also retained the right to exclude children on the basis of race. Before 1938, all of New York City's Protestant institutions refused to take black delinquents.[28] Consequently, there was an artificial scarcity of local childcare options available for the black children in Polier's courtroom. On top of it all, what public facilities were available to African American children rarely offered adequate mental health services.[29]

Psychiatric Universalism and Juvenile Justice, 1936–37

There was never any guarantee that Polier would interpret racial disparities in psychiatric access as evidence of racial injustice. Undoubtedly, the rapid expansion of psychiatric authority within American juvenile justice did make that more likely to happen. Entering the 1930s, the psychologization of New York's Children's Court was well underway. Psychiatrists and social workers actively drove that process. The New York School of Social Work began teaching psychodynamic theory in the 1920s, graduating the first US psychiatric social workers. Some of them found work in the courts.[30] As a court justice, Polier had access to a diagnostic clinic staffed by the psychiatrist Dr. Montague and a team of psychiatric social workers.[31] Thanks to both Montague's tutelage and the availability of cutting-edge social-work courses, Polier's case workers and probation officers had all learned to think about juvenile delinquency in psychodynamic terms—as a symptom of an underlying psychological problem.[32]

Polier's own receptiveness to psychiatry made it more likely that she would take an interest in race-based mental health disparities. Polier actively participated in the therapeutic turn within juvenile justice. Since the Progressive Era, children's courts and correctional facilities became increasingly dedicated to reforming rule-breakers rather than meting out punishments.[33] Throughout the 1930s, the court staff increasingly regarded juvenile rehabilitation as a "therapeutic matter."[34] As Polier and her staff understood it, unresolved psychological problems made it hard for some delinquents to regulate their emotions and behavior. If a correctional facility could resolve those problems with a psychiatrist's help, the child might learn to exercise more self-control.[35]

Although juvenile justice had been psychologized, it did not necessarily follow that all court authorities automatically expected psychotherapy to work with black delinquents. To even make the claim that African Americans deserved equal access to psychiatry, one first had to imagine that blacks were capable of benefiting from such care. When Polier and other judges began deferring to the expertise of psychiatric authority, many mental health professionals still considered the black psyche to be racially exceptional. Racialist clinicians and case workers thought it unlikely that traumas or repressed urges were responsible for causing delinquency within the uninhibited black race. According to Regina Kunzel and other historians of social work, most case workers expected that only white cases of delinquency would have psychological causes. In their view, immorality, culture, or even biological race caused juvenile delinquency among blacks. Such cases would not require psychiatric attention. Psychotherapy's effects would be negligible.[36]

Nevertheless, Polier did not have those preconceptions. Without racialist preconceptions or psychiatric training, she felt free enough to imagine the human psyche as a space that biological race had no part in shaping. The Domestic Relations Court's 1936 and 1937 investigations of the state reform schools reveal that Polier and some of her staff already regarded the rehabilitation of black delinquents as psychological in nature. In May 1936 the court Board of Justices appointed a Committee on Institutions to evaluate the Hudson State Training School for Girls and the Warwick State Training School for Boys. By August, that new committee's task took on greater urgency when a State Department of Welfare hearing revealed that Hudson racially segregated its students.[37] Such revelations were particularly distressing to Polier. Most of those black students were Harlem residents her court had placed.[38] Warwick's student body was also disproportionately black. African American males—mostly from Harlem—comprised over 60 percent of Warwick's population. Polier was concerned that racism might be rampant there as well.

Polier and her diagnostic clinic psychiatrist, Dr. Montague, took the lead, placing their stamp on the committee's investigation of the reform schools. Between December 1936 and June 1937, the court sent two teams of investigators— including Polier and Montague. According to its mandate, the teams gathered data that would enable the court to "set certain standards . . . which will assure to the children the best treatment available at that time."[39] Not surprisingly, the liberal expectation that public resources should not be allocated on the basis of race became one of these certain standards. The Hudson report corroborated the state's findings regarding racial segregation in that school.[40] In contrast, the Warwick report depicted a school with a "definite policy of racial amity in mind."[41]

Polier and others within the Domestic Relations Court expected that standard care for delinquents would address their emotional needs.[42] On each campus, the court visitors inquired into the available mental health care. They also studied how well these institutions integrated child psychology into their educational and disciplinary routines. Writing about the Hudson school administrators, the investigators lamented their use of corporal punishment and their open contempt for child-guidance precepts, pronouncing: "There is no psychiatric care [there] as the term is generally understood."[43] In contrast, the visitors found that the Warwick faculty did not denigrate psychiatry or defend corporal punishment.[44] They seemed to demonstrate more "open mindedness."[45] The committee was impressed that Warwick even had a psychiatric clinic, regarding it as an "exceptionally efficient medical unit."[46]

Significantly, these reports clearly indicated that the Committee on Institutions expected reform schools to foster the emotional well-being of all juvenile delinquents—black or white. These reports suggest that the psychological turn in juvenile justice and the development of racial liberalism seem to have already mapped onto one another. Nowhere in the reports is there any suggestion that Montague, Polier, or any of their caseworkers thought of African Americans as racial exceptions to white psychological norms. In decrying Hudson's resistance to a psychodynamic understanding of delinquency, the investigators implied that the rehabilitation of even black children primarily took place on a psychological level.[47]

The court visitors expected that reform schools had a duty to attend to the psychological needs of even the black juvenile delinquents, but the committee concluded that neither school lived up to the challenge. According to the reports, Hudson's deficits were much greater. Still, even Warwick did not meet Polier and Montague's standards. Although the Warwick school psychiatrist Dr. Max Winsor wanted his office to operate as a child guidance clinic, few faculty referred students for such purposes. Polier suspected that Warwick was not as therapeutic or racially egalitarian as she had been led to believe. The campus was too orderly. The staff had been too well coached, a reflection of the fact that the court visits had been announced in advance.[48] Nevertheless, an interview with Winsor gave Polier hope that he might eventually serve as a good ambassador for psychiatry there, perhaps helping Warwick to meet the court's modern standards of childcare.[49]

The Domestic Relations Court Treatment Clinic, 1937–45

The state training school investigations taught Polier that the correctional system did not adequately meet the emotional needs of African Americans.[50] With little power to alter the state training schools, Polier devised a way to offer psychiatric therapy to the black children she was forced to send upstate. She proposed that the Children's Court provide treatment itself. Just short of two full years on the bench, Polier already thought of the rehabilitation of juvenile delinquents as largely a therapeutic process.[51] To provide black children with such care, Polier reached outside the court. In assembling the Domestic Relations Court treatment clinic in 1937, she relied on a small cadre of psychiatrists and philanthropists, all of whom seemed to think that black juvenile delinquents should have access to some psychiatric care.

As far as the treatment clinic's creation is concerned, one good thing came of Polier's disappointing state training school investigations. Without those official trips she might not have met the Warwick psychiatrist Max Winsor. He was a fellow Manhattanite with an interest in social justice and progressive education. Winsor had a medical degree from Columbia, experience in the labor movement,[52] and a talent for explaining the psychiatric point of view in layman's terms.[53] Polier was quite taken with Winsor's desire to convert Warwick's staff to his "mental hygiene point of view and to a form of discipline which will be in accordance with these principles."[54] His conviction that psychodynamic principles should suffuse both corrections and education struck a real chord with Polier. Once Polier made a serious effort to offer psychotherapy through the Children's Court, Winsor was one of the first people she contacted for assistance.

The psychiatrist Dr. Marion E. Kenworthy played an even more crucial role in the creation of Polier's treatment clinic. A child guidance pioneer, Dr. Kenworthy helped shaped Polier's understanding of psychiatry's usefulness in the courtroom. Polier's second husband, Shad, had introduced the two women. He was a member of the NAACP Legal Defense Fund and an aspiring leader within the American Jewish Congress. Having found a kindred political spirit in Kenworthy, Shad believed that his wife could only benefit from a friendship with this clinician. He was right. Kenworthy had been central to the histories of psychiatric social work, mental hygiene, and child guidance in New York. A leading proponent of a team-based child guidance approach, she helped integrate psychology into social work. In the 1920s she cofounded the New York School of Social Work's psychiatric social work program. Through the psychiatric social workers she had trained, Kenworthy exerted a major influence on Polier's courtroom well before the two women even met.[55]

Dr. Kenworthy quickly became Polier's mental hygiene mentor. Primarily interested in combating juvenile delinquency with psychiatry, Kenworthy helped the National Committee for Mental Hygiene and the Commonwealth Fund establish the US child guidance movement. She had even served as the initial director of New York City's first child guidance clinic in 1922. Polier had nothing but respect for Dr. Kenworthy, referring to her as the "mother of child guidance." Kenworthy recommended that the court offer on-site treatment to at least some children. Polier embraced the suggestion.[56]

To make such a clinic possible, Polier realized that she would have to expand the juvenile court's already wide powers. Polier argued that a children's court judge had a duty to act as a social engineer and change the existing child welfare system when it no longer served the "best interest of the child."[57] Ever since Chicago created the first children's court in 1899, juvenile justices possessed wide powers to redistribute community resources to the benefit of their young charges.[58] As psychodynamic thinking influenced the practice of adjudication, Polier broadened the bench's powers to include court-ordered psychiatric care.[59] For Polier and other young La Guardia-appointed justices, serving the best interests of the child now meant that a judge should base his or her placement decisions on each child's specific emotional needs.[60] Polier argued that the court's broad "authority" to act in loco parentis enabled her to "call attention to the gaps in community facilities" and to "secure new services or to induce established agencies to extend themselves to meet new needs."[61]

Since Polier found it necessary to secure psychiatric treatment for some children, she relied on like-minded psychiatrists to meet those new needs. Polier and Dr. Montague, the court's diagnostic clinic psychiatrist, enthusiastically accepted Dr. Kenworthy's suggestion that the court provide short-term, on-site therapy. In October 1937, Polier successfully convinced her Domestic Relations Court superiors to open a short-term treatment clinic as an annex of the court diagnostic clinic.[62] Opened in November, it operated on an experimental basis for eight years. To run the clinic itself, Polier secured Dr. Winsor's services, and Dr. Kenworthy staffed it with her students.[63]

The new clinic provided treatment under constrained circumstances. The inevitable graduation of Kenworthy's social-work students led to chronic understaffing and constant turnover. In such a milieu, patients could not establish much of a relationship with any one clinician or caseworker. Owing to both the clinic's outpatient character and the severe time constraints placed on cases, therapy often "focused on the child's immediate emotional problem" as opposed to its more deeply rooted causes.[64] Yet during those years, the clinic managed to provide 626 children, most of them African American children from central Harlem, with short-term therapy that they would not have gotten elsewhere.[65]

Polier staffed and financed this new clinic without much public funding.[66] Luckily, she secured the financial backing of fellow racial liberal Marshall Field III, one of America's wealthiest men. Field was heir to the Marshall Field's department store fortune in Chicago. In the Roaring Twenties, he had led a hedonistic life. According to his biographer, he eventually "suffered a psychological crisis, underwent psychotherapy, and emerged with a profound life-commitment to social justice."[67] Polier met this politicized version of Field through his attorney Louis Weiss, a New Yorker with connections in the spheres of political activism and psychoanalysis. As "something of an advisor to [Field] on social causes," Weiss encouraged Field to meet with Polier. Polier educated Field to the racial injustices in the child welfare system.[68] Galvanized, Field became a key asset to Polier. He not only helped bankroll the clinic, but his philanthropic Field Foundation (founded in 1940) also eventually helped finance other liberal programs the city refused to fund.[69]

Part of the reason the treatment clinic needed outside funding was that it had powerful enemies entrenched in the court. Some older justices, especially Herbert O'Brien, a staunch political ally of the Catholic lobby and the Tammany Hall machine, disapproved of the treatment clinic. Regarding psychiatry as an unwanted interloper within both the courts and childcare, O'Brien claimed that he "objected to having the supervision of Catholic children surrendered to any social school or group of irresponsible people who are not part of the Court, or that the work of the Court be placed in the hands of an outside agency."[70] Polier threatened to give mental health professionals the chance to design childcare standards that private agencies might be forced to follow. More important, her courtroom regularly challenged old justifications for the racial segregation of both childcare and jurisprudence. One of those challenges was psychiatric universalism.

Universalism in the Courtroom: Judge Polier and the Emotional Development of African Americans

Justine Wise Polier's own handling of African American cases best indicates that her court had embraced a race-neutral understanding of psychodynamic theory.

By the late 1930s, psychiatric universalism—or the psychiatric point of view, as she styled it—informed both Polier and her court clinic's handling of cases involving black Harlem youth. Although she was a layperson, Polier's appropriation of psychiatric concepts had a great impact on the lives of many Harlem children. In 1939, 58.4 percent of the 2,301 children in the Domestic Relations Court were categorized as "colored" or "Negro," and most of them hailed from central Harlem.[71] Polier and her court thus provided thousands of black Harlemites before World War II with their first experience of psychiatry. Given that, it is instructive for us to examine how race mattered within her courtroom.

With her African American cases, Polier tried to apply general psychodynamic principles in a race-neutral fashion. To assess how successful she was, we first need to gauge Polier's basic understanding of human psychology. In developing her own psychodynamic courtroom approach, Polier relied on Dr. Montague and Dr. Kenworthy. She also educated herself, regularly consulting the child guidance literature.[72] During the 1930s, Polier familiarized herself with "the work of education, medicine, psychiatry, and social science in order to meet needs that become patent through study of child after child."[73] The judge generally relied on the practical advice of lay mental health professionals, including psychiatric social workers in child-guidance clinics and juvenile courts.[74]

Borrowing ideas from these various mental hygiene experts, Polier constructed her own "special kind of court room approach" to juvenile delinquency.[75] In her 1941 study of New York's juvenile court system, *Everyone's Children, Nobody's Child*, Polier detailed what she called her "individualized approach,"[76] a style of adjudication reliant on mental hygiene precepts.[77] Polier accepted the psychodynamic proposition that juvenile delinquents were generally emotionally deprived children who misbehaved because their lives offered few outlets for expressing unmet needs for "emotional security."[78] Over the course of the late 1930s, Polier learned to read delinquent behavior as a warning flag alerting her that a child might have an emotional problem.[79] To help her properly "individualize" such a case, Polier relied on the court's probation officers, social workers, clinic, and even Bellevue Hospital.[80] By individualization, Polier meant that she expected her staff and other mental health professionals to help her to "study the background of the child, to evaluate his problems in the light of that background as well as in terms of the immediate offense that brings the child to court, and finally to determine what type of treatment is most likely to achieve his adjustment in society."[81] Polier argued that the failure to match a child with the right services could harm both the individual and society.[82]

In the search for the right services, Polier was receptive to the opinion of outside psychiatric experts—just as long as they were not racialists.[83] She did encounter well-respected Manhattan psychiatrists who treated African Americans as if they possessed a racially distinct psyche. In September 1942, Polier remanded a black teen to Bellevue's adolescent psychiatric ward (Ward PQ-5) for observation.[84] Dr. Frank Curran, head of the adolescent ward, found that the young man had an IQ of 65 and was "uncooperative" and preoccupied with sex. He was nervous, prone to hallucinations, heard voices, and harbored suicidal and homicidal thoughts. Curran also observed that the teen "talks in a very bizarre fashion," but did not elaborate on what that meant. Curran was fairly certain that the subject was "psychotic at this time." Yet officially, he chose to classify him instead as a "case of Undiagnosed Psychosis." Something caused Curran to hesitate in making a diagnosis. Curran's report to Polier made very clear as to what that something was.[85]

Curran admitted that his black patient's racial identity made it difficult to render a diagnosis. He explained that "with his limited intelligence and his negro ancestry, the symptoms which he has are not considered as pathological as if they had occurred in a white boy of higher intellectual endowment." He assumed that the teen's race played some essential part in shaping the basic organization of his personality. But he was not certain if the otherwise abnormal behaviors he witnessed were perhaps normal for blacks.[86]

In contrast, Polier and her court clinic rejected racialism and embraced psychiatric universalism.[87] Universalism was quite different from the general proposition that psychiatry could handle the black mind. Racialists also believed that they knew what was best for black patients. But when Polier advocated "psychiatric treatment for children of all races" within her court, she meant a psychiatry that treated the psyches of blacks and whites as equivalent terrain.[88] Given her assumption that blacks and whites were psychological equals, Polier expected that courts and child-welfare agencies had a duty to meet the emotional needs of black children "at least to the extent to which they are met for white children."[89]

For universalists such as Polier, racial determinism compromised a clinician's ability to individualize an African American patient's case. Expecting that the black psyche would defy psychological norms, Curran and other racialists treated a black patient as a racial type rather than a single unique case. Universalism permitted the normalization of the black psyche. Essentially, universalists such as Polier imagined that psychiatry could fully describe and explain black emotional life without any need to account for alleged racial peculiarities in the African American psychological makeup. Polier and her handpicked staffers assumed an individual from any race would possess an autonomous human self with a distinct, singular personality. Whereas racialists expected psychological differences between races, the universalists in Polier's courtroom anticipated that differences would only exist between individuals—regardless of race.

Although new, the universalist approach to psychiatry was not unique to New York or the United States. Within roughly the same time period, a few British colonial psychiatrists in Nigeria started to abandon racialist beliefs in an inferior black psyche.[90] A decade earlier, mental health professionals and criminologists working in Boston court clinics also adhered to universalism. Drs. William Healy and Augusta Bronner found that the general child-guidance approach—a combination of mental hygiene, psychobiology, and psychoanalysis—worked well with patients of all "races and nationalities." In their work, no racial group had its own basic personality or psychological type. The normal child, they assumed, could be African American.[91]

As psychiatric theory, universalism never achieved the status of explicit doctrine, partly because its adherents naturalized the concept so quickly.[92] Polier and her fellow racial-liberal clinicians Kenworthy, Montague, and Winsor did not explicitly theorize and publish their positions on race and human psychology. None of them proclaimed the race-neutrality of the normal human psyche as though it were a new discovery. For racial liberals serving African Americans in interracial institutions, universalism was a shared leap of imagination that became an unspoken article of common sense for them.[93] They never sought or demanded proof for their new a priori truth.[94] They just took it for granted that blacks and whites were equally endowed with the potential to develop a normal human psyche.

The institutionalization of psychiatric universalism within Polier's court began in a simple way. Dr. Montague's clinic staff took psychodynamic principles, most of which had been developed with whites, and merely applied them without alteration or adjustment to African American children. In the late 1930s, the diagnostic clinic examined the cases of two delinquent teenagers, one a "fourteen year old colored girl" from the working-class and the other a white male whose mother was a wealthy celebrity. Even though the details of the children's lives were dissimilar, the clinic concluded that they had been damaged in the same way. Examining each child through a race-neutral lens, the clinicians agreed that their emotional conflicts required the same solution: a "normal and stable family life."[95]

In recommending that even black children required a normal family life, Montague's staff did not mean normal for just African Americans. When the case workers used the term "normal family life" they meant the middle-class nuclear household stereotypically associated with whites. Racial liberals assumed that this middle-class family structure was optimally suited to foster "mature emotional, physical and intellectual growth" in any human being, regardless of his or her race.[96] Montague's staff considered the middle-class nuclear family a superior lifestyle, reflecting the class bias endemic to racial liberalism. Notwithstanding, it is significant that the staff was just as confident that African American children had the potential to grow to full maturity within that family setting. Consequently, the clinic recommended foster-home placement for both teens, assuming they could equally benefit from a "normal" middle-class environment.

Polier and her court staff were confident that black children could become emotionally mature adults. They possessed such a conviction because they did not share the racialists' perception of black adulthood. Well into the postwar years, many within New York City's legal system and psychiatry itself still conceived of the black race as a less developed one whose adulthood was closer to the white race's adolescence.[97] In psychodynamic terms, (white) human adulthood was characterized by emotional depth, introspection, stability, and self-control, a complex process that developed in timed stages. According to Lauretta Bender, racial determinists believed that an African American was "a biologically primitive organism" whose "primitive mind tends to mature fast but decelerates or ceases to develop at an early age."[98] For these racialists, even a mentally fit black adult was destined to evince less maturity than a white adult. This belief in the black race's stunted development helped reinforce stereotypes of black adults as childish and incapable of controlling their puerile feelings and desires. Well into the postwar era, the image of African Americans as perpetual children continued to justify disinvestment in black childhood development.[99]

In contrast, Polier and her staff assumed that African Americans were capable of becoming fully mature adults.[100] In promoting black emotional growth as a goal worthy of public investment, they expected that black adults would be as psychologically complex and mature as white adults. Reimagining the black adult psyche as a completely human space enabled antiracist psychiatrists to see neglected and delinquent black children as salvageable human beings. According to mental hygienists, adult criminality arose because critical emotional needs were left unmet during childhood. Theoretically, if more children experienced happier childhoods there would be less adult misery and crime. Nevertheless, meeting a black child's unmet emotional needs could only prevent adult crime if the black race was capable of producing self-possessed adults. Since that is precisely what Polier believed, she became convinced that the city could reduce crime in Harlem by investing in the emotional potential of its most vulnerable black children.

Recognizing Trauma and Vulnerability in African Americans: The Case of Joetta

In fact, the liberal faith in the black psyche's salvageability rested on a strong belief in the black race's emotional vulnerability. African Americans were long considered happy-go-lucky and naturally immune to stress and strain. This alleged lack of psychological depth and emotional range traded on expectations that African Americans were less complex beings, less evolved, incompletely human. In one sense, the racial liberals' act of reimagining African American inner life as a site of emotional pain also worked to locate the black race's humanity in its susceptibility to mental suffering. Blacks and whites were both fully human because their emotional development was so fragile. Justice Polier's court record demonstrates that she believed mistreatment could impede the maturation of any child. The following case of sexual assault and its psychological effects clearly demonstrates that a race-neutral understanding of psychodynamic theory informed Polier's jurisprudence. It also highlights just how much the liberal fight against institutional racism hinged on the concept of "black emotional damage."[101]

By the 1930s, psychodynamic psychiatrists had introduced a new interpretation of childhood sex experience. Since the Victorian era, most Americans conceived of such experiences in a moralistic framework, regarding children as nonsexual beings and sex as a morally corrupting force. Incest and statutory rape robbed children of their innocence, dooming them to lives of unrestrained sexual activity or "sex delinquency."[102] Freudians, however, rejected the idea that sex ruined a child's chances of becoming a successful adult. For them, children were not sexual innocents. They were inherently sexual beings whose development was psychodynamic rather than moral in nature. Claiming that even normal children desired sexual contact, they argued that intercourse with adults would not necessarily harm a child—at least not psychosexually.[103]

In the late 1930s, New York was at the forefront of this psychiatric reappraisal of intergenerational sex. In 1937 Lauretta Bender conducted the first psychiatric study of American children that had engaged in sex acts with adults. Well into the 1970s, psychiatrists generally contended that sexual intimacy with adults would not irreparably sabotage a child's psychosexual and emotional development. As Elizabeth Pleck and other historians have noted, these clinicians failed to take into account the often violent, coercive, and unequal nature of these "relationships" and the deep betrayal of trust involved. A few psychiatrists in the 1930s, including Bender, did acknowledge that certain aspects of intergenerational sex experience—especially a sense of guilt—could psychologically harm some children. These clinicians did think it possible that sexual contact with adults could thwart the emotional development of some vulnerable children, especially if a psychiatrist did not help them cope with their conflicted feelings.[104]

Polier incorporated some of these new psychiatric insights into her courtroom approach to incest. But there was a limit to her reliance on psychodynamic theory. The judge was never comfortable with the psychoanalytic argument that children desired sexual contact with adults so much that even incest would not damage them emotionally. Writing about the issue in 1941, Polier indicated that she—like most Americans—thought of children as sexual innocents. Given that presumption, she readily accepted the clinical observation that sex crimes, especially incest, could be deeply upsetting for a child.[105] Polier gleaned from the psychiatric reports she read that incest victims tended to feel guilty about what happened to them. According to Polier, incest was most devastating because of a "sense of confusion and conflict that arises from the child's emotional relationship with the offender."[106] Afraid of family disapproval, children kept their feelings secret. Repressing such an event might "lead to sexual precocity and promiscuity or to a complete revulsion against every aspect of sex expression." As Polier understood it, the unresolved emotional results of incest could compromise a child's chance to develop into a healthy adult.[107]

Yet by the 1940s, most child development experts doubted that forced sexual intercourse with adults could ever emotionally scar a black child. According to the historian Lynn Sacco, early twentieth-century judges and psychiatrists tended to think of incest as common among blacks but rare for whites. Consequently, a black child's claims of statutory rape or incest were more likely to be taken seriously. Yet while authorities were more inclined to accept that a black man might have had sex with his daughter, they were also less inclined to think that such acts would traumatize that black child. The historian Stephen Robertson found that the psychiatrists who contended that sex with adults could harm children were only "concerned about the ways in which a white child's progress toward sexual maturity might go awry."[108]

Even in New York City, many clinicians outside of Polier's courtroom did not fear that black children could be damaged by unwanted sex with adults. Because primitive races were expected to reach sexual "maturity rapidly and at a less complex level,"[109] racialists expected African Americans to reach sexual maturity in late childhood rather than in adolescence or even adulthood. For racialists, sexual contact between black children and adults was no cause for alarm. They expected that intergenerational sexual contact would not stunt a black child's psychological growth or prompt lasting feelings of guilt or shame.[110]

Contrary to conventional wisdom, Polier believed that sexual violence could emotionally damage black children. In 1939, Polier applied universalism in reevaluating a sexual-assault case involving an eleven-year-old black girl from Harlem. Polier referred to the young girl twice in print, each time using a different pseudonym, either Anita or Joetta.[111] Joetta's stepfather sexually assaulted her the day after Christmas in 1938. After Joetta contracted gonorrhea from the rape, the first judge (not Polier) who heard her case removed the girl from her home. In June 1939, the court remanded her to the Catholic House of the Good Shepherd, a detention facility for so-called wayward women. These included rape victims, women with sexually transmitted diseases, accused prostitutes, and single mothers between the ages of sixteen and twenty-one years.[112] Because of her age, Polier argued, Joetta should have been fostered, returned home, or placed with other neglected children.[113] Instead, because of the stigma attached to both her sex experience and the sexually contracted disease, the eleven-year-old was placed with adults. This was general practice in sexual-assault cases. Children's courts had few other placement options since private agencies refused to expose the "innocent" to those with "sex experiences, even when they were the victims of criminal attacks."[114] Finding this practice psychologically unsound, Polier argued that "removal from home meant punishment to this child at a time when she needed comforting" for her emotional shock. Polier asserted that she was in "dire need of personal, affectionate care."[115]

In September, the court sent Joetta to Bellevue Hospital, where Dr. Lauretta Bender provided what Polier called the first "understanding picture of the child."[116] In the 1930s, Bender had been one of the only psychiatrists to publicly assert that the sexual development of black children and white children followed the same patterns.[117] She struck the same race-neutral tone when evaluating Joetta. This pioneering child psychiatrist determined that incest had caused her emotional harm. Bender found Joetta rightfully bitter, confused, and terrified about her sexual experiences, her gonorrhea, and the "painful, punitive, and derogatory" treatment she suffered at the hands of authorities. She described Joetta as having "been exposed to rather distressing psychic traumas" that "resulted in giving [her] a decidedly inhibited and bitter reaction against all sexual experience."[118] As the historian Lynn Sacco has shown, psychiatrists and legal authorities in the 1930s were more likely to believe African Americans girls' allegations of incest owing "to professional and popular insistence that father-daughter incest occurred only among the poor, working class, and people of color."[119] Perhaps this racial bias had led Bender to believe Joetta's story. But even if it had, at least Bender's description of the traumatic effect of rape deviated from the racialist expectation that sexual intimacy with adults would not harm black children.

Polier's published analysis of Joetta's case relied heavily on Bender's sympathetic, race-neutral account. When writing about this young person, Polier depicted Joetta as angry and confused about being punished for "an unfortunate incident for which she was not to blame." The judge noted her difficulty opening up to adults and her repulsion at the mere mention of anything sexual.[120] Polier's description of Joetta's emotional state perfectly matches her 1941 profile of a typical rape victim. Having given Joetta's case file the type of reading racialists reserved for cases involving white rape victims, Polier determined that this young black Harlemite was neither immoral nor the product of an immature race. Instead, she was an emotionally scarred victim in need of sympathy and care, preferably within a loving home. According to Polier, Joetta's reactions and treatment needs fell within the normal range expected of any child traumatized by incest—white or black.[121]

That Polier deemed Joetta's case typical rather than exceptional again demonstrates her race neutrality. As well, Polier's sense that black psychological development was a fragile process prone to derailment became a foundational part of racial liberalism. That human maturation could be so easily thwarted injected a sense of urgency into the liberal campaign against racial inequality in mental health care. Rather than divert attention away from issues of institutional racism, this early liberal focus on black vulnerability and pathology initially helped bring attention to the modern state's long-standing neglect of the black community. The universalists' readiness to find only pathos and suffering within individual black lives did eventually distract policymakers and activists from the structural and political causes of race disparities. Nevertheless, the liberal desire to shield black children from any further emotional damage generated a powerful new argument: government-supported racism might constitute a mental health risk.

Universalism and Racial Justice in Child Placement, 1938–41

Intellectually spurred by universalism and buoyed by her courtroom experiences, Polier began arguing in the 1940s that racial discrimination could do psychological harm to vulnerable black children. As noted earlier, Polier arrived on the court with a strong sense of justice and an expectation that public services should be delivered with efficiency and fairness. Not surprisingly, Polier initially perceived the lack of court-appointed child services for Harlem blacks as first and foremost an unjust distribution of resources. But over the course of her six years on the bench, Polier eventually argued that race-based denials of psychiatric services could emotionally damage a black child's personality, preventing such children from becoming stable adults.[122]

What prompted Polier to craft this more nuanced argument was a 1938 change in policy. Before that year, it had been much easier for Domestic Relations Court judges to classify and place children as neglected rather than delinquent. Nevertheless, a mounting conservative backlash succeeded in pushing New York City's system of justice and corrections to enforce a stricter distinction between neglected and delinquent children, with the latter understood as simply malefactors rather than victims.[123] By 1938, agencies that cared for neglected children began to rigidly define a "delinquent" as a misbehaved child. Reserving the right to refuse court-appointed children, these voluntary agencies rejected any child adjudged delinquent.[124] This institutional bifurcation forced the hand of judges, pressuring them to act as angels of retribution, punishing all lawbreaking children.[125]

This hardening of the line between children classified as delinquent or neglected adversely affected Polier's charges. Neglected and delinquent children were placed in different institutions. In the 1930s, the courts generally placed neglected children in foster homes and shelters. There, some sort of child guidance was available. In contrast, the private Children's Village was the only agency that accepted delinquent boys under the age of twelve. Given the lack of placement options, preteen delinquents were often sent to reform schools intended for adolescents.[126] Reform schools did not always provide adequate child guidance services. So by 1938, a finding of delinquency greatly diminished a child's chances of receiving therapeutic services.

The stricter division of the neglected and delinquent created a severe shortage of placement options for African American children. In July 1938, a committee of justices found that spots for blacks were dwindling fast. Space was still available for black delinquents at the state training schools, but neglected black children were out of options. Whites-only agencies were off-limits. The Colored Orphan Asylum and Valhalla's Brace Farm (the only private facilities taking neglected blacks) were full. Agencies that placed black children in foster homes all refused to take any more.[127] The committee lamented that there were "literally no places to which the Court can send Negro children who are in need of immediate removal from their homes." Since a disproportionate ratio of black children appeared before the court, the situation, the committee noted, was "critical."[128]

This placement crisis became so critical that Polier found it increasingly difficult to be race neutral in cases of neglect. The shortage of space for neglected nonwhites encouraged the court to pronounce them delinquent. In the 1938 case of one thirteen-year-old Puerto Rican male who lived with his aunt on 114th Street in Harlem, Polier made what she considered the right assessment of this "colored" child's needs. His aunt had brought him to court on a delinquency petition, accusing him of stealing ten dollars. Polier felt that if the aunt's dubious accusation was true, it was only a symptom of a larger problem. In scanning his file, she noted that he had been abandoned and repeatedly ran away. His mother had returned to Puerto Rico, his father was incarcerated on Riker's Island, and the aunt did not want the teen either.[129] She connected these details, creating her own picture of the adolescent's emotional state. Profiling his personality as that of a typical runaway, Polier concluded that family neglect left the teen emotionally insecure.[130] She wanted to classify him as "neglected" since his "delinquency has stemmed from neglect here, if this is delinquency. This boy has no real home" and he needed stability.[131]

The trouble was that when Polier "correctly" classified the Puerto Rican teen as emotionally neglected, none of the whites-only agencies would agree to take him. Early in the twentieth century, childcare agencies identified children of Caribbean descent within America's racial binary of "colored" and "white." Officials considered this thirteen-year-old Puerto Rican teen to be darker skinned, so they racially categorized him as "colored." White institutions rejected him as a rule. As per the policy of racial matching, private agencies did not place neglected black children in white foster homes.[132] And few "colored" foster homes existed.[133] Polier was exasperated with these institutional handcuffs. Informed by the psychiatric point of view, Polier was convinced that the teen was not a delinquent. He was a victim of neglect. She concluded that "with this Puerto Rican or colored child we have no place for him to treat him as a neglected child which is, in my opinion, the only way we should treat him."[134]

Despite Polier's insistence that this was a case of neglect, the probation officer recommended placing the Puerto Rican teen as a delinquent. He argued that more bed space was available for "colored" delinquents. Throughout the late 1930s and early 1940s, it became common for judges to make a ruling of delinquency in cases involving nonwhite victims of neglect.[135] Since few agencies accepted neglected "colored" children, judges often had little choice but to return them to their allegedly neglectful homes. To avoid doing that, many judges made a "finding of 'delinquent' on the basis of some slight evidence of misbehavior, so as to allow a black child to be sent to a public institution for delinquent children."[136] Either way, whether assigned to a state reform school or sent home, such children were unlikely to get the child-guidance services Polier believed they needed.

Writing for a popular audience in 1941, Polier charged that this sort of institutional racism could psychologically scar African American children. She argued that the neglect of a black child's emotional needs actually fostered juvenile delinquency in Harlem.[137] That she had become confident enough to publicly criticize her own institution was partly a reflection of racial liberalism's growing presence on the bench. In 1939 La Guardia appointed Jane Bolin—a prominent NAACP leader—to the Children's Court, making her the first female African American judge in history.[138] Dudley F. Sicher rounded out the trio of La Guardia appointees. He joined the Domestic Relations Court full time in 1939 after a temporary stint in 1937. In addition to being a close friend of La Guardia, he was an antiracist Jewish American active in the American Jewish Congress.[139]

With those two crucial 1939 appointments the black-Jewish alliance emerging in New York City took root within the Domestic Relations Court. Nationwide, this alliance of leftists, liberals, and labor was crucial to the civil-rights movement's wartime phase. At this radical moment in the black freedom struggle, issues of economic justice and equal access to state resources took center stage.[140] Not surprisingly, Sicher and Bolin joined Polier's battle against institutional racism in mental health care. Very early on, Sicher expressed his dissatisfaction with the lack of psychiatric care for black children.[141] In 1940, Sicher wrote Polier: "The placement of Negro children has become such a cruelly baffling problem as to call for some affirmative action by our Board [of Justices]."[142]

Conclusion

At the time, the Hon. Justine Wise Polier and her fellow liberals on the Domestic Relations Court were not yet powerful enough to implement substantial affirmative action on behalf of their young African American charges. Certainly La Guardia's political support created the opportunity for Polier to advocate racial fairness in the delivery of mental health care within New York's systems of juvenile justice and child welfare. And she made the most of it. Between 1936 and 1941, Polier's courtroom became a space in which judiciary personnel tended to assume that whites and blacks were psychological equals. Even the judge's own case record demonstrates that she imagined and acted as though both races were endowed with the same capacity to emotionally suffer and then recover with the aid of psychotherapy. Consequently, Polier and her staff expected that the children in her court—regardless of skin color—might have psychological problems and developmental needs that required immediate psychiatric attention.

Polier's court was but only one node in the child-welfare system. Her power to implement change within that whole system was limited. Throughout her first six years on the bench, institutional racism restricted her ability to adjudicate in a color-blind fashion. In the face of racist private agencies refusing to take Harlem's black children, Polier tried using the public sector to provide delinquent and neglected African American youth with access to psychiatry. With the aid of her court clinicians between 1936 and 1937, Polier investigated the level of care the New York State training schools provided students and successfully pushed her court's diagnostic clinic to offer short-term psychotherapy. Still, conservative opposition on the Domestic Relations Court, the lack of direct oversight over the state reform schools, and the hardening of the line between delinquent and neglected cases further hampered Polier's ability to provide black youth with psychiatric care.

As a Children's Court judge, Polier was only legally bound to serve the best interests of the children in her court. With so many restrictions, she often found herself unable to do that for her black charges. Some of them needed psychiatric care, but there were few opportunities for them to receive that care. Although the child-welfare system had failed these children, Polier began to consider whether it could do something to prevent other children from ever coming to the law's attention. Might it be possible to identify the black children who were most at risk for juvenile delinquency in Harlem? Unfortunately, the court could not take any affirmative action in this regard. Prevention was outside its jurisdiction. Nevertheless, there was another institution that could gain access to all of Harlem's children, keep track of their behavior, and even offer early psychiatric diagnosis and treatment: the public school.

Chapter Three

Psychiatry Goes to School

Child Guidance and the Prevention of Juvenile Delinquency, 1940–42

In his 1965 memoir *Manchild in the Promised Land*, the former Harlem gang member Claude Brown recounted the day he appeared in Domestic Relations Court. In 1948 Brown had been caught robbing a store on 147th Street. The presiding justice that January day was Polier's colleague Jane Bolin. Not quite eleven years old, young Claude had heard of her. Regularly featured in the black press, Judge Bolin was a well-known African American role model. A force for antiracism in the 1940s, she was a member of the NAACP's Board of Directors and a tireless advocate for women, children, and Harlem.[1]

Claude Brown remembered Jane Bolin differently. He recalled that as a child he did not see this extraordinary woman as his advocate, but as his adversary. "From the minute I laid on eyes on the mean queen, I knew she wasn't going to send me home, and she didn't." Bolin sent Brown to a private reform school in the Catskill Mountains, the Wiltwyck School for Boys. Bolin did not conceive of her decision as punitive. Brown experienced it as a form of punishment. She had deprived him of his freedom, taking him away from his family, his gang, and his neighborhood. Seeking a reason why the court would punish him in this way, ten-year-old Claude attributed his fate to Bolin's disposition. She was not a "soft-hearted judge," but a "mean old colored lady." Claude the author recalls regarding Bolin as a bully who "wanted to show the people there how bad she was" by restricting the freedom of others—including his.[2]

Brown's account reveals that the liberal struggle for racial equality was often a story of increased government interference in the lives of African Americans. To assert that social-justice movements could result in less freedom from government authority might seem counterintuitive. Such a claim would not seem as controversial to historians of other ostensibly humanitarian efforts. Since the 1990s, scholars have generally come to accept that "a story of humanitarian intervention is also a story of domination."[3] To promote the just distribution of a service or resource, state authorities have often developed more intensive power relations with neglected populations. As Claude experienced, greater racial equity in juvenile justice meant fewer black youth released back onto Harlem's streets and more of them institutionalized under a psychiatrist's legally mandated supervision.

Bolin and the Domestic Relations Court's racial liberals expected that increased psychiatric authority over black lives would promote mental health and prevent crime within Harlem. For these judges, meeting those goals was a matter of racial fairness and safety. Since the Progressive Era, crime prevention resources had been "unevenly distributed among people of different racial categories."[4] Central Harlem's arrest rate was high, but its access to mental hygiene and child guidance—key crime prevention resources—was still meager heading into the 1940s. Psychiatrists deterred crime by helping individuals to manage their desires and conduct. But as noted in chapter 1, racialists framed criminality as a black racial trait. Some law-enforcement officials claimed that African Americans' natural impulsivity and lack of introspection made them prone to crime.[5] Black crime was natural, unpreventable. Why bother devoting public resources to help blacks control their emotions and behavior when nature had rendered them incapable of doing that in the first place?

Polier and the supporters of the Domestic Relations Court treatment clinic did believe that African Americans could become emotionally stable, law-abiding citizens. Given this assumption, they saw the lack of public investment in the mental health of potential black offenders as both an unjustified racial disparity and a major oversight in crime prevention. In the summer of 1940, Justice Polier convinced La Guardia's administration that increased public investment in the psychological development of black youth would make New York safer. She argued that the city could best avert crime by using public resources to promote mental health within the black community. Polier then called for an unprecedented expansion of psychiatric authority within Harlem, offering child-guidance experts the opportunity to surveil and intervene in African Americans' personal lives as never before.[6] This expansion did not come through the courts. Instead it developed through the public schools.

Between 1940 and 1942, race-neutral psychiatry spread outside of the Domestic Relations Court and into four of central Harlem's junior high schools—P.S. 136, 139, 184, and 194. Administered by the Bureau of Child Guidance (BCG) psychiatrist Dr. Max Winsor, the Special Child Guidance Unit in Harlem placed psychiatric resources in the uptown public schools with the highest statistical rates of juvenile delinquency. An ambitious Board of Education experiment, the Harlem Unit featured P.S. 194's Joint Kindergarten Project. Run by Justice Polier's close friend Dr. Viola W. Bernard, the Harlem Unit's organizers expected the Joint Kindergarten Project to collect psychological data on P.S. 194's students and make it available to the Domestic Relations Court. As designed, the Harlem Unit was supposed to identify, treat, and track young African American children at risk for juvenile delinquency. Nevertheless, resistance from both teachers and parents reduced the Harlem Unit's effectiveness. Additionally, the various civil servants and philanthropists behind Dr. Winsor's program determined that Harlem's public schools could not accommodate male students with severe behavioral problems.

In search of psychiatric care for those young black men, Polier and other individuals involved with the Harlem Unit took administrative control of the Wiltwyck School for Boys in 1942. The private reform school in the Catskills happened to be one of the only independent institutions that accepted black New Yorkers. Liberal support for this private facility should not be read as a rejection of statist solutions to racial inequality. Yes, Polier and her fellow antiracist activists were certainly willing to look outside of the public sector for other sources of psychiatric care. But this does not mean that these racial liberals no longer believed that public resources should be equally available to all. Rather, their commitment to Wiltwyck simply reveals impatience with the child-welfare system's slow pace of change.

Max Winsor and Social Psychiatry in Harlem's Public Schools, 1938–40

Entering the 1940s, color-blind psychiatry maintained a niche within New York's juvenile justice system. But the Domestic Relations Court judges Polier, Bolin, and Sicher had very limited authority to further promote psychiatry's expansion within Harlem's black community. As children's court judges, the three could only order interventions in a family's life once something had gone seriously wrong—if a child had committed a crime or had been abandoned. For many troubled African American children, Dr. Helen Montague's court clinic downtown on 22nd Street often afforded them their first and only encounter with psychiatry. As a devotee of mental hygiene, Polier felt those children should have seen a psychiatrist much sooner. As far as she was concerned, early exposure to child guidance could have prevented these young people from ending up in court. Nevertheless, there was little the three justices could do to mandate such preventive care. They had no substantial legal authority to identify, monitor, and facilitate the psychiatric treatment of children who had not been brought before the court.

A key hire within Harlem's public schools offered Polier and her fellow judges a chance to increase psychiatry's presence within central Harlem. In 1938, the BCG hired Dr. Max Winsor, formerly the Warwick Training School's psychiatrist, as the new director of its two-year-old Special Child Guidance Unit in Harlem. The Harlem Unit was one of three new child guidance facilities the BCG had opened in neighborhoods with high rates of juvenile delinquency.[7] In the Harlem Unit, Winsor served as a roving child psychiatrist for central and west Harlem's public schools. He had access to the very children the Domestic Relations Court could not reach: young African Americans who had never seen the inside of a courtroom.

Winsor, a native New Yorker, arrived in Harlem's schools with a long-standing preference for progressive education's child-centered approach. This is not surprising, given Winsor's liberal tendencies and the city's reputation as the American epicenter for pedagogical theory and research. While an undergraduate at Columbia University in the 1920s, Winsor became a disciple of the progressive educators John Dewey and William H. Kilpatrick. Both advocated that education move away from rote learning to a focus on each individual child's learning process.[8]

Perhaps even less surprising, Winsor's brand of progressive education held that schools should also help facilitate and monitor each student's emotional development. In the 1920s, a movement to study child development merged with progressive education, producing a new field, education research.[9] Education research was an interdisciplinary profession producing progressive pedagogy informed by the latest scientific findings about how children thought and behaved. By the 1930s, education researchers were heavily influenced by mental hygiene and child guidance. From these fields, they gleaned that children were ever-changing emotional cauldrons undergoing a natural process of maturation. Based on this insight, education researchers urged teachers to recognize how a child's learning capacity would be limited by his or her level of emotional maturity. Women in Winsor's own family, his wife, Charlotte, and her sister Barbara Biber, modeled this educational research for him in their pioneering work with Manhattan's Bank Street College, founded in 1916.[10] As a mental hygienist Winsor already believed that psychiatric principles could help reform everyday life. He readily accepted that a school should help protect and foster a child's emotional development as part of its educational mission.

Given his pedagogical expectations, Winsor "was angry, deeply angry at the things that are wrong with the schools" in Harlem.[11] Even after all the attention that La Guardia's administration had paid to Harlem's public schools after the 1935 Harlem Riot, most of them remained overcrowded, underfunded, and ill-equipped.[12] Some progressive attempts had been made to update a few schools, most notably P.S. 24 on East 128th Street. In 1935 that school implemented the Board of Education's experimental "activity program."[13] Under the direction of the city's first African American principal, the feminist writer and social-justice activist Gertrude Elise McDougald Ayers, P.S. 24 developed a more child-centered pedagogy. It fought racial discrimination in student tracking, invited greater community involvement, created an intercultural program, and discouraged corporal punishment.[14]

P.S. 24 was an exception. What struck Winsor most about the other Harlem schools was the severe institutional neglect. The facilities were out-of-date and insufficient. The textbooks, pedagogy, and even the pedagogues were just as inadequate. Winsor decried the typical Harlem teacher's ignorance of the latest child-development findings and continued reliance on corporal punishment.[15] What is more, he was particularly dismayed that the city continued to assign white teachers with unabashed racial prejudice to classrooms filled with African American students.[16]

Speaking as a practitioner of social psychiatry, Winsor claimed that the typical Harlem school had generated a harmful "emotional climate"[17] not conducive to learning or living.[18] Since the 1930s, the term "social psychiatry" referred to clinicians determined to improve the mental health of communities, not just individuals.[19] Social psychiatrists employed child guidance, mental hygiene, epidemiology, and social engineering in an effort to identify and prevent the social factors responsible for predisposing a population to emotional maladjustment. With the characteristic optimism of a New Deal-era social engineer, Winsor was convinced that psychiatrists and the state should work together to make their communities healthier.[20] As his wife said of him: "He was much more than a technician in psychiatry. . . . He did not try to adjust people to the world."[21] Instead, Winsor believed that institutions should adjust themselves to meet the emotional needs intrinsic to all humans. He felt that Harlem's school setup did not take into account what made children of any race feel comfortable and engaged. According to Winsor, the net effect of this psychological neglect was a hostile emotional climate that sabotaged the students' cognitive and emotional maturation.

In his first two years as Harlem's roving psychiatrist, Winsor tried to ameliorate the emotional climate of Harlem's schools. Despite his limited staff and solitary office, he did provide some children with therapy, usually those whose misbehavior earned them a clinic referral. Just as he had done at the Warwick State Training School, Winsor taught his staff the psychiatric point of view—a race-neutral approach to modern psychology. In his jargon-free style, he taught a few courses for teachers on the fundamental precepts of mental hygiene. According to fellow psychiatrist Dr. Viola Bernard, "many originally skeptical educators . . . came to accept the mental hygiene approach as he presented it."[22]

Although he may have scored a few personal victories with teachers and students,[23] Winsor knew that it would take more than one psychiatrist and one clinic to change Harlem's schools. All combined, the Harlem district's forty public schools contained close to one hundred thousand students cramped into small, aging classrooms. The Harlem Unit's resources were much too meager to permit any kind of comprehensive mental hygiene program. Winsor had only one office and one school psychologist, one clerical worker, and one social worker to help him handle this large region. Winsor chose to spread his services throughout the forty schools. He never could spend much time in any one of the forty schools, so individual treatment could never be intensive. Consequently, the Harlem Unit was unable to devote enough attention to the Harlem schools in which the risks to mental health were highest.[24]

Max Winsor's Proposal, 1940

But by mid-1940, Winsor managed to link his efforts in the schools to the battle against juvenile delinquency. Having worked in corrections for three years, Winsor was well aware of the racially disproportionate rate of black children brought to court on delinquency charges between 1935 and 1938.[25] A racial liberal dissatisfied with pat old racialist explanations, Winsor finally had a chance to investigate this statistical trend. Granted access to the case files and statistics of Warwick State Training School, the Domestic Relations Court, and the BCG,

Winsor made a startling epidemiological correlation in 1940. He found that over half of the young men sent to Warwick for delinquency came from just three Harlem schools: P.S. 139, 171, and 184.[26]

Winsor recommended that the BCG concentrate its Harlem services in those three subneighborhoods where delinquency was apparently epidemic. Winsor believed that central Harlem's high levels of socioeconomic distress produced children more emotionally prone to delinquency.[27] Having worked in Harlem, he also recognized that the region across 110th Street was not a monolithic den of pathology. Instead, Winsor knew that Harlem was composed of neighborhoods with widely varying socioeconomic profiles and different levels of institutional disinvestment in schools. He theorized that this clustering of male delinquents in three specific Harlem neighborhoods was an epidemiological signpost. It alerted him to the unhealthiest neighborhoods and the most insufficiently progressive schools. Interpreting the data in this way, Winsor felt that distributing scant child guidance services throughout all forty Harlem schools made little sense. Instead it seemed more logical to concentrate the BCG's psychiatric services in the schools with the most deleterious emotional climates.[28]

In making this policy recommendation, Winsor recognized that schools might be able to facilitate color-blind psychiatry's expansion into Harlem in a way the Domestic Relations Court could not. Governmental support for child-guidance services was premised on psychiatry's potential as a crime prevention tool.[29] Winsor believed that psychiatry could help schools identify which black children were at greatest risk for becoming adult criminals. He also was convinced that it could help them avoid that path in life.

Three factors account for Winsor's certainty that psychiatry could prevent delinquency in Harlem's schools. First, Winsor assumed that the environmental risks that had generated juvenile arrests rates in 1938 would remain constant, producing the same results within the next generation of black children. This faith in epidemiology's predictive power enabled child-guidance professionals such as Winsor to believe it was possible to "control the future by engineering the earliest years of life."[30] Second, since children spent so many years in schools, these places were uniquely positioned to collect longitudinal data about changes in the personality, affect, family history, and behavior of every child—not just the ones who had already seen the inside of a judge's chambers.[31] Third, Winsor had the utmost confidence in the universality of his profession's linear models of normal personality development.[32] Although child-guidance experts individualized each case, they still expected that certain internal needs common to all would have to be met if a child was ever to become a healthy adult. Psychotherapy was supposed to help the emotionally ill meet those needs. Since Winsor considered normal human maturation to be a race-neutral process, he was confident that psychiatry could put black youth on a path of healthy maturation.

Eventually, all of these felt certainties pushed him inexorably into public policy.[33] Winsor proposed a special child guidance unit providing intensive clinical and classroom services in Harlem's problem schools. In early 1940, he introduced this idea to Dr. Frank O'Brien, the BCG's director. O'Brien strongly supported Winsor's contention that more psychiatry in these three Harlem public schools could both treat and even prevent delinquency among African Americans. Since its creation, the BCG operated on the premise that the public school had a responsibility to help combat juvenile delinquency—with child-guidance experts taking the lead of course.[34] Guided by this stated mission, the BCG had been working since the 1935 Harlem Riot to expand its coverage of schools with black students—the very reason Winsor's Harlem Unit existed in the first place.

Under O'Brien, the BCG seemed to support Polier's conviction that child guidance and mental hygiene would work with all children regardless of race. Politically, it made sense for the BCG to embrace racial liberalism. This department was still new. It lacked political capital among New Yorkers wary of psychology. Asserting that psychotherapy would work with all children—including blacks, the race most associated with crime since the Progressive Era—was one way to make the BCG seem necessary.[35] Seeing Winsor's proposal as such an opportunity to gain more public support for the BCG, O'Brien told the BCG's original director, Marion E. Kenworthy, that he was hopeful that it would "demonstrate quite objectively the inroads that child guidance services can make in reducing delinquency, at least evaluated in terms of institutional commitments."[36]

Unfortunately, the BCG was underfunded in the early 1940s. Its tiny budget could not accommodate Winsor's project.[37] With the wartime American public already leaning toward more retributive approaches to criminal justice and child-rearing, it became increasingly difficult for the BCG to maintain public support for its modern methods of childcare.[38] To fill the gap in financial and political backing, Winsor desperately looked for help. With the Domestic Relations Court treatment clinic in mind as his model for a quasi-public treatment facility, Winsor turned to the woman who created that model: Justine Wise Polier.[39]

The Liberal Politics of Change:
Polier, La Guardia, and Winsor's Proposal

Winsor's proposal enabled the Domestic Relations Court to finally expand psychiatric authority more equitably into Harlem. Judge Polier provided four related reasons for why she championed Winsor's plan. First, she imagined that his project would make psychiatric services more available to the Harlemites the private childcare agencies had rejected on grounds of race or religion.[40] Second, Polier hoped that these clinics could serve as a base of operations for the sort of efficient, coordinated, and racially just child-welfare system the court had been unable to develop itself.[41] Third, public schools might eventually even serve as a kind of central registry cataloguing personal information about New York students' psychology. She hoped that access to such a detailed history of a child's emotional development could help children's court judges make better decisions.[42] Fourth, and perhaps most important, she shared Winsor and O'Brien's hope that early diagnosis and psychiatric intervention in Harlem schools could help the city to identify, track, and prevent younger "children who are now living in the New York area that has the highest delinquency rate" from ever appearing in her courtroom.[43]

That Polier was looking for ways to provide African American children—not just those in her courtroom—with greater access to psychiatric care illustrates that racial liberals were actively seeking to reduce the racial slippage in psychiatry's expansion within American life. Winsor essentially offered Polier's court and its allies a chance to serve as social engineers, intervening in the lives of black children that not been ensnared by the juvenile justice system. By the time Winsor had approached her about his Harlem proposal, Polier felt that it no longer made sense to only concern herself with the psychological well-being of her courtroom's young black Harlemites. To her, their racially disproportionate presence on the court docket represented the future for thousands of other emotionally vulnerable Harlem children, a future made possible by psychiatry's weak presence in Harlem. New York's relative inattention to the emotional needs of Harlem's black children was remediable, and Winsor offered them the most promising potential fix.

Nevertheless, Polier's willingness to throw the weight of her court behind Winsor's proposal was not just a product of her racial politics. The increasing acceptance of courts as policymaking bodies and agents of social change also informed her decision. In 1941 she argued that just as the children's court judge should "develop special treatment to meet the needs of children who appear before the Court, he should at the same time stimulate the development of more adequate care for all children through schools, hospitals, private and public agencies."[44] Polier and other New Deal-era liberals began claiming that judges could use these powers to protect the welfare of all children, dramatically enhancing the court's potential as an instrument of social engineering.

This approach to juvenile justice rested on an argument developed in the Progressive Era: government intervention was legitimate as long as it served the public interest.[45] Whenever the community lacked the resources needed to serve the public interest, Polier claimed that judges were obligated to act as policymakers, creating those missing services themselves. By the 1940s, the New York public had a vested interest in reducing juvenile delinquency. It just lacked the requisite resources, especially in Harlem. In Polier's estimation, she had little choice but to make Winsor's proposal a reality.[46]

With the aid of individuals who helped create the Domestic Relations Court treatment clinic in 1937, Polier quickly secured staff and three years' worth of private funding.[47] Kenworthy and the New York School of Social Work provided the requisite psychiatric social workers. In March 1940, Marshall Field III agreed to provide Polier with most of the estimated funds. Through the help of her husband Shad, Polier then secured a financial commitment from the prominent Jewish philanthropist Marion Ascoli, a daughter of the Sears Roebuck tycoon Julius Rosenwald.[48] A well-connected new clinician in the

Domestic Relations Court, Dr. David Levy, provided a substantial monetary contribution. Levy was married to Marion Ascoli's sister Adele, a philanthropist herself. Together Ascoli and the Levy family pledged $15,000, enough to hire a full child guidance team.[49]

Private funding made the proposal attractive to authorities in the New York public school system. Substantial charitable support convinced the BCG director Frank O'Brien that Winsor's proposal was feasible. He agreed to make "this proposed new unit in Harlem possible."[50] Emboldened, Winsor sought to get the public school system's approval as quickly as possible. To do that, Winsor realized that Polier might have to do more than raise funds. True to her expansionist view of judges as policymakers, Polier agreed to lobby the school authorities herself and promote the proposal as its primary sponsor. Given that a judge from a prominent family was making the proposal, the public schools' Board of Superintendents and Board of Education were more likely to take the project seriously. Polier did even more than simply make a formal proposal to the two school boards. Upon Winsor's request, Polier asked for Mayor La Guardia's political assistance in the fight against juvenile delinquency.[51]

In response to this overture from Justice Polier, his family friend and valued political ally in the Jewish community,[52] Mayor La Guardia quickly agreed to sponsor the policy. La Guardia's support made the difference. New York City's school authorities approved the program in October.[53] Even though La Guardia had begun trimming the annual school budget in 1939, generating harsh criticism from within the ranks of his liberal base, the Board of Education and Superintendent Harold G. Campbell were all La Guardia appointees.[54] Campbell knew how proud La Guardia was of the acclaim the public school system's experimental programs had achieved among education experts. Campbell and his cohort played this to their advantage. Advisers within La Guardia's administration believed that progressive education projects enhanced the city's reputation. Shrewdly, the Board of Education encouraged the development of such experiments, ensuring Campbell a bigger share of the city budget in the early 1940s.[55]

Notwithstanding, the proposal's adoption is not evidence that racial liberalism had suddenly been institutionalized within the New York public school system. In formally pitching Winsor's proposal to school authorities, Polier did not try convincing them that the black psyche was a fully human space requiring a race-neutral style of psychiatry. Instead, she was very careful to sell the proposal as a cost-effective way to reduce juvenile delinquency and the "rate of court appearances and institutional commitment" in one of the city's most troubled regions.[56] Given the way she sold the project, the school authorities who approved the plan were not being asked to endorse liberal ideas about racial equality. They were presented with an opportunity to help a La Guardia-appointed judge potentially lighten her future caseload and reduce the expense of incarceration.[57] Winsor now had his project. This did not mean that all the officials who approved the proposal necessarily shared Winsor's belief in the psychological equality of blacks and whites. But in permitting this program, school authorities did permit egalitarian racial ideas and practices to take hold.

The Harlem Unit, 1940–42

What the Board of Education had approved was a privately financed "three year child guidance service program in the Harlem district . . . established and administered in accordance with the plan proposed by Justice Polier."[58] Superintendent Campbell appointed an advisory committee to supervise the Special Child Guidance Unit in Harlem. It included not only the BCG's Drs. Winsor and O'Brien and members of the Board of Superintendents, but also three of Polier's close associates—Dr. Kenworthy, Marshall Field, and the child psychiatrist David Levy, famous for coining the phrase "overprotective mother" in 1929.[59]

For the most part, funding for the program came from private sources. As with the Domestic Relations Court treatment clinic, the city did provide facilities, office equipment, and a few staff members in joint positions. The Board allowed Winsor to devote time to both his BCG and Harlem Unit duties.[60] In the main, private backers provided the money used to staff Winsor's Harlem Unit. Incorporated as the private Foundation to Further Child Guidance in the Field of Public Education, the philanthropists Field, Ascoli, and Adele Levy paid the salaries of all ten members of the unit's child-guidance team.[61]

Although the child-guidance team's roster was not finalized until February 1941, the Harlem Unit began operation in fall 1940. The Advisory Committee assigned the Harlem Unit to three junior high schools: P.S. 136 for girls, P.S. 184, and P.S. 139. All three generated high rates of delinquency. The latter two had been among the ones Winsor identified as having produced a majority of the city's male delinquents.[62] The regular Harlem Unit still provided the other thirty-seven Harlem schools with child guidance, but these three received the most intensive diagnostic and therapeutic services.

Because Winsor's project was designed to demonstrate whether the extension of psychiatric authority into central Harlem could reduce delinquency within its young male population, P.S. 139 and P.S. 184 received the bulk of attention. Each school was given unique access to its own part-time psychiatrist, a full-time psychiatric social worker, a psychologist, a pediatrician, and a team of social-work students.[63] In 1941, P.S. 139's Harlem Unit saw 74 cases, providing services ranging from brief consultations to more intensive clinical services. From February 1941 to May 1942, the Harlem Unit handled 108 cases at P.S. 184. Fifty-two of these cases involved psychiatric consultations, psychological testing, and pediatric exams. Despite time constraints and logistical problems, 11 cases received individual psychiatric therapy. Owing to both personnel constraints and the lack of priority given to girls in the project, the Harlem Unit handled only 30 cases at P.S. 136 between February 1941 and May 1942. Between September 1940 and June 1942, the School of Social Work students had a hand in 136 of the cases at these schools, helping to provide 87 students with intensive treatment.[64]

Looking to inject its clinical mission into the school's day-to-day operation, the Harlem Unit's staff tried forging a relationship with the faculty. The Harlem Unit's staff assumed a pedagogical role, introducing teachers and principals to both the psychiatric point of view and its usefulness in the classroom. In conferences with Harlem principals, Winsor presented lectures on topics such as "The Use and Misuse of School Records." The psychiatric social workers, Rose Goldman at P.S. 139 and John Rockmore at P.S. 184, even established significant working relationships with their respective school's liaison teacher (a prototype of what later became known as the guidance counselor).[65]

As Winsor's advocates, these liaison teachers helped make it possible for the Harlem Unit and the psychiatric point of view to infiltrate the classroom and influence school policy. The liaison teachers often consulted with the Harlem Unit, relying heavily on Winsor's child-guidance team as they identified problem children and assessed their needs. When helping to make decisions regarding grade promotion and class placement, P.S. 139's liaison teacher referred to both the school psychologist's test results and the social worker Rose Goldman's advice. The liaison teachers actively promoted the psychiatric point of view among the teachers. At P.S. 184 Murray Sachs organized a Teacher's Mental Hygiene Discussion Group. Liaison teachers even managed to bring some school procedures into better accordance with mental hygiene principles.[66] For example, P.S. 139's liaison teacher successfully abolished the detention policy on the grounds that it was "doubtful whether the results [of detention] to personality adjustment . . . were anything but destructive."[67]

Psychiatric Universalism in the School System

Plainly, racial liberals had taken new steps to make psychiatric services and ideas more available within Harlem. Yet it is not enough to simply note the number and kind of services and mental hygiene principles that the Harlem Unit introduced into these two Harlem schools. Demonstrating that so many students received a certain quantity of care does not tell us whether the people involved in the project subscribed to psychiatric universalism in administering such care. We have already noted that Polier employed race neutrality in her courtroom cases. This section examines how Winsor and his staff made race matter within their clinical encounters in Harlem's schools.

Max Winsor's writings between 1942 and 1943 indicate that he treated black children using basic principles culled from the study of white children. An article he wrote for the July 1943 issue of the *Atlantic Monthly* perfectly demonstrates this point. In this article, he wanted to prove to readers that child guidance was the most medically sound way to rehabilitate delinquent children. To convince his audience that unmet emotional needs produced bad behavior, he presented the real-life case of Rhoda, an adolescent referred to Winsor's clinic for stealing.[68] The article recounted how his clinic determined that her theft was symptomatic of an undiagnosed emotional problem. He made it very clear that his clinic used the same investigative techniques and displayed the same "respect for her personality" it would give any case. Yet Winsor never informs the reader that Rhoda was a Harlem resident or that his cases were primarily African American. Although he did not divulge Rhoda's race, the likelihood is strong that she was a black student. That Winsor felt he could make a general point about all children's personalities using a black Harlemite's case demonstrates his commitment to psychiatric universalism.[69]

Nevertheless, being committed to clinical universalism did not mean that Winsor practiced a literally color-blind psychiatry. Universalists did not completely ignore a child's race. They did not even try to do that. Rather, Winsor and other racial liberals were merely blind to the possibility that biological race could determine a patient's psychological development. As a social psychiatrist, Winsor was not blind to the social fact of race. Social psychiatrists assumed that folks with similar circumstances might share many of the same formative experiences. They considered blackness a fairly reliable social index of racial inequality and injustice. So as a social fact, a patient's blackness could alert a clinician to the possibility that her psyche may have been exposed to social conditions and pressures unknown to a white child.

For example, Winsor suggested that racism had emotionally harmed some of Harlem's black children. Writing in the *American Journal of Orthopsychiatry* in 1943, he explicitly identified a boy named Richard as a "Negro" from a poor neighborhood.[70] He did not make note of this child's race and economic status because he felt the black child's basic psychological apparatus differed from a white child's.[71] Rather, Winsor identified Richard's race only because his neurosis had been compounded by the "special doubts that we have imposed on Negroes." The child's race itself was not the source of the special doubts. Rather, the source was a purely social factor: racial discrimination.[72]

For Winsor, black looks clinically served as an external sign that racial discrimination—society's "special doubts"—might have negatively impacted some "Harlem children." Winsor clearly indicated that this impact, usually a feeling of "unconscious or conscious rejection," was not racially specific to blacks.[73] Instead, Winsor assumed that a black child responded emotionally to discrimination in the same that any child would react to some other noxious emotional stimulus. Although he did not offer any additional theoretical explanation on this matter, it is clear that he imagined that racism could emotionally harm some of his patients.[74]

Like many racial liberals, Winsor was sure that most Americans would learn to see things his way if only they spent some time in Harlem. In his June 1942 report on the Special Child Guidance Unit in Harlem, Winsor intimated that the New York School of Social Work students had a unique on-the-job opportunity to gain "an understanding of, and sympathy with, the problems of an area like Harlem." He hoped that they would learn to see that what happened to Harlem's children could happen wherever the same social conditions prevailed. Ultimately, he hoped that the experience in Harlem would help these future social workers become "oriented in the needs of the underprivileged, not restricted to Harlem."[75] Evidence indicates that some psychiatrists and psychiatric social workers did in fact practice psychiatric universalism while on this project. For one of Winsor's two white part-time psychiatrists, Dr. Viola W. Bernard, the experience working with black students fundamentally shaped her psychiatric approach well after she left the clinic.

Dr. Viola W. Bernard and the Harlem Unit, 1940–42

Viola W. Bernard's two-year stint as one of the Harlem Unit's two part-time psychiatrists fulfilled her third-year of psychiatric residency. As a Jewish American woman graduating from Cornell Medical College in 1936, she experienced difficulty securing quality internships and residencies in child psychiatry. As was common for the era, entrenched white male prejudice—in the form of both quotas and informal checks on Jewish and female applicants—prevented Bernard from securing the sort of prestigious opportunities someone with her class ranking and Ivy League diploma should have received. Child psychiatry was not a highly regarded field in the 1930s. Some of its gatekeepers claimed that the presence of Jews and women in their ranks explained their specialty's low status. Seeking to raise child psychiatry's standing, they recruited white males for residencies, internships, and fellowships, and discouraged applicants from undesirable social groups.[76]

Owing to entrenched resistance to someone of her ethnicity and gender, the first spots she managed to get were lackluster to say the least. She first interned between 1937 and 1938 in the underfinanced Jersey City Medical Center with a chief surgeon who, Bernard quickly found out, "really hated women."[77] Yet after spending her first psychiatric residency with a little-known clinician in Westchester County, New York, her training opportunities dramatically improved. In 1939, she landed a second-year residency at the New York State Psychiatric Institute and was accepted for analytic training at the New York Psychoanalytic Institute.[78] The next year, she began studying psychosomatics with Columbia-Presbyterian's Dr. George Daniels.[79] Thanks to Max Winsor and the approval of the American Board of Neurology and Psychiatry, Bernard completed her third residency under a unique arrangement, doing two "half years" as a part-time psychiatrist in the BCG's Harlem Unit.[80]

Although the actual process is not clear, evidence does suggest that Dr. Kenworthy and Polier had brought Winsor's project to Bernard's attention. Bernard had befriended Kenworthy as a teen, well before she became interested in medicine. As Bernard recounts, the "mother of child guidance" encouraged her to go to medical school, stimulating her interest in psychiatry. Once in medical school, she stayed in close contact with her mentor. Since Cornell Medical College did not offer enough instruction on psychodynamic psychiatry, she audited one of Kenworthy's courses at the New York School of Social Work. Bernard's friendship with Kenworthy also offered her something that generally only white men with her ambition tended to possess: a well-respected professional contact. Kenworthy networked on Bernard's behalf, securing her acceptance for psychoanalytic training and perhaps putting a good word in for her with Winsor.[81]

Bernard was also a close friend of Justine Wise Polier. Their parents had introduced them in 1934 when Bernard was a student at New York University and Polier was working in the New York Workman's Compensation Bureau. Both were young, highly educated, socially conscious Reform Jews from prominent New York families. Each had been raised in cosmopolitan social circles that prized philanthropy, compassion for the downtrodden, and open-mindedness. Their families encouraged them to defy social convention and pursue advanced degrees. Both women had also been exposed to progressive models of education, including the New York-based Ethical Culture movement, a heavily Jewish but nonsectarian humanist organization promoting antiracism, free thought, and social responsibility.[82] According to Bernard, she and Polier "became aware of each other's shared values and when we developed professionally, we did so in an intertwined way." Most likely, Polier introduced Winsor and Bernard, facilitating the latter's employment in Harlem.[83]

Bernard was attracted to the Harlem Unit partially because she already had some prior experience working with patients from diverse backgrounds. As a medical student she had done clinical work in obstetrics at the Bronx's Berwind Clinic. Bernard worked with working-class Italian women and their families, sometimes in their own homes. In the Jersey City Ambulance Corps in 1937 she "got a great exposure to many kinds of settings and lifestyles of poor people and of ethnic ranges of people." According to Bernard, her work in the Bronx and Jersey City "gave me experience I had lacked in my own middle class upbringing." Seeing and interacting with people from a variety of "life arrangements" helped her to better understand why her mentor, Dr. Kenworthy, ascribed so much importance to environment in the formation of personality. Bernard felt that these experiences encouraged her to develop a lifelong interest in how social, psychic, and somatic factors worked together to forge personality and behavior patterns. Years later, she argued that these experiences were akin to "field work in social psychiatry."[84]

Bernard immediately embraced Winsor's own brand of social psychiatry. What impressed her most was the highly sociological character of his theory and practice. Since she was also undergoing training in psychosomatic medicine and psychoanalysis, Bernard was particularly open to Winsor's "whole child" approach. Even before going into psychiatry, she had studied Eastern philosophy and was very interested in links between mind, body, and culture. Because medical schools offered no courses on sociology or mental hygiene, she was keen to learn more about the social dimension of psychosocial development.[85] Winsor offered Bernard a way to analyze the environment's role in shaping the psyche.[86] His example inspired her to develop her own social-psychiatry approach. Bernard theorized that individual personalities developed as the result of a complex interplay between "instinctual needs," family relationships, and "social and cultural influences."[87]

What is more, Bernard quickly realized that Winsor's political commitment to Harlem informed his sense of how the "social" mattered. In a 1970 letter to Winsor's widow, Dr. Bernard praised Max Winsor for having "taught me so much about the spirit and practice of child psychiatry in Harlem."[88] The spirit was one of social justice and racial liberalism. She had recognized that Winsor was not a detached clinician. He was an advocate "who cared very much about the Harlem children served by that Unit."[89] The young psychiatrist was not turned off by Winsor's passionate contempt for racial prejudice and class inequality. Rather, Bernard "wanted his value system and abilities."[90] In an obituary she wrote for Winsor, she praised him as "courageous" and "warm-hearted."[91] Even prior to joining the Harlem Unit she had already committed herself politically to making psychiatry more racially inclusive. In 1939, as a resident at Westchester's Grasslands, she had formed a committee protesting the dearth of African American psychiatrists.[92]

Under Winsor's tutelage, psychiatric universalism became an essential part of Bernard's published work in the early 1940s. Bernard's first publication regarding her work in Harlem appeared in the July 1942 issue of *Mental Hygiene*. In the article, Bernard offered a series of guidelines that teachers could use to help them detect the early signs of emotional instability. Although she worked largely with black Harlemites, she did not identify the students' races or schools. Although she did not unpack her racial assumptions for the readers, Bernard's article suggested that both white children and black children psychologically responded to environmental stimuli and regulated their emotions in ways intrinsic to all humans. She intended for her guidelines to help teachers anywhere identify all problem children, not just potential black delinquents.[93]

P.S. 194: The Joint Kindergarten Project

Dr. Bernard did have a number of opportunities to work with teachers and students during her two years in the Harlem Unit. In 1941, she spearheaded a subproject within Winsor's larger program. With the principal and the BCG's approval, Bernard initiated the Joint Kindergarten Project in P.S. 194, a Harlem elementary school with a majority African American student body. The project's staff included Bernard, the school psychologist Jeanette Vosk, a social worker, and the kindergarten and first-grade teachers of P.S. 194. Through the Joint Kindergarten Project, P.S. 194 received the most intensive and collaborative services the Harlem Unit offered any school.

The Joint Kindergarten Project turned out to be the Harlem Unit's most concerted effort to extend psychiatric authority into New York's African American communities.[94] It was primarily designed to detect potential emotional problems among the youngest students in Harlem's public schools. Polier eagerly supported the program in P.S. 194. She was convinced that her courtroom would contain fewer emotionally disturbed black teens if the city found a way to identify and treat them in early childhood. Kindergarten was the first public institution all children were obligated to enter. Bernard recognized that these kindergarten classes thus offered the first real opportunity to systematically monitor and gather information on potential delinquents. With a system of psychological monitoring and data collection in place, school and court authorities could potentially identify, track, and manage the emotional development of troubled young Harlemites. Pooling the data-collecting resources of her joint staff, Bernard aimed to assemble a "whole-child" profile, itemizing each kindergarten student's "total needs, assets, and liabilities as early as possible in his or her school experience."[95]

In pursuit of this whole-child profile, the clinical staff gained remarkably invasive access to every P.S. 194 kindergartner in 1942. Jeanette Vosk performed psychological tests and observed children within the classroom, and a social worker took case histories and interviewed families.[96] Bernard met with some children, sometimes in their own homes, providing Bernard with her first glimpse of black private life.[97]

Bernard imagined that this surveillance might eventually be of use to Polier and other public authorities interested in promoting emotional health within black Harlem. Bernard hoped that the knowledge produced in these psychological profiles could be securely maintained in a master file, if not a central registry. The data would be available to the police, the courts, and other agencies interested in a specific child. The amassing of psychological data on individual children was not an Orwellian bit of speculative fiction. In 1944, Washington, DC, developed such a central register, and other cities—including New York—followed suit by decade's end.[98] Armed with this knowledge, Bernard expected her child-guidance team to tailor specific educational and clinical services for potential delinquents. Such personal attention could help each student internally regulate his or her own affect and behavior, potentially reducing police arrests, court caseloads, and incarceration in the future.[99]

In an effort to produce as much data as possible about the inner life of Harlem children, Bernard encouraged teachers to share their classroom observations with BCG staff.[100] In after-school conferences, her staff tried to explain how teachers could become Bernard's eyes and ears in the classroom, offering lessons on how to spot patterns of interest to the psychiatrist. Apparently during the first two conferences, Bernard's staff presented general theoretical principles of mental hygiene and Bernard demonstrated these principles with a discussion of an individual case.[101]

Teacher and Parent Resistance to the Harlem Special Child Guidance Service Unit

Although teachers were willing to change their classroom conduct and priorities, some of them found the clinic's lessons difficult to put into practice, which sabotaged Bernard and Winsor's efforts.[102] Bernard observed that "teachers want clinic staff to be less theoretical and give more practical suggestions for handling specific difficulties." They expected the clinic to give them a list of distinct "types of problem behavior" and a clear protocol for dealing with the children that fit each type. As a firm believer in the mental hygienist's "need for individualizing the child," Bernard could not fully accommodate the teachers' need to place children into discrete types. According to Bernard, the basic philosophy behind the project was that similar "symptoms do not stand for the same thing in each child, so methods of handling cannot be generalized." In the absence of either clear behavioral categories or explicit procedures, some of the teachers remained uncertain about what the clinic wanted them to pay attention to in their classrooms. Because of this conceptual confusion, the teachers were generally unable to provide Bernard's clinic with the "specific details of observed behavior" needed to assemble a picture of the "whole child."[103]

Part of the confusion may have stemmed from Bernard's race neutrality. In presenting the cases of three kindergarten students, W.G., J.H., and H.T., the clinic staff argued that each child's misbehavior was the result of a "multiplicity of causative factors." In each of the three case presentations, the staff examined what it considered the relevant causal factors. Race was never included.[104] Similar to her mentor Winsor, Bernard felt that racial identity could clinically matter, but only as a source of social stress for blacks. Given that the majority of students at P.S. 194 were black, the chances were good that at least two of the three students were black. Nonetheless, in the process of individualizing each case, Bernard and her staff assumed that biological race did not fundamentally shape a child's development. Not surprisingly, Winsor and Bernard criticized teachers who saw their black students' misbehavior as evidence of racial inferiority. Most of Harlem's teachers were white. Some of them were racially prejudiced. Bernard warned that a bigot could weaken "the emotional fortitude of those ostracized," undercutting his or her ability to reach black students.[105]

Obviously such stern criticism would have alienated prejudiced teachers. Racists were probably not alone in their resentment of the Harlem Unit and its presence in the classroom. Winsor and Bernard's harsh criticism, their mandatory afterschool meetings, and their lack of practical advice may have also have turned off instructors who saw themselves as artisans or craftsmen struggling to maintain authority over their workshops. In addition to the unwanted pressures from parents and principals, Harlem teachers now had psychiatrists and their support staff meddling in their domains, unwanted interlopers undermining the chief product of their labors: an orderly classroom.

Yet teachers may not have been the only source of resistance. Some African American parents could have been as well. The evidence for this assertion is not as clear. No record remains of the clinical interactions between parents and the Harlem Unit, not to mention Bernard's home visits. Other historians have shown that some black families, many of them recently from the rural American South, had their own culturally satisfying explanations for juvenile delinquency.[106] Among African American urbanites with strong roots in the harsh, devoutly Christian, and sometimes violent worlds of the rural Caribbean and the US South, corporal punishment was still considered the most effective remedy for such habitual willfulness.[107] When spankings or "whuppings" did not "straighten out" a stubborn child, Harlemites could fall back on a number of popular explanations. The trope of the "bad nigger," defined by Al-Tony Gilmore as one "who adamantly refuses to accept the place given to blacks in American society," was still available.[108] As well, some preferred supernatural or magical explanations for intransigent behavior and difficult dispositions. These ranged from the devil's own influence to folk conjurers and curses.[109] In Claude Brown's autobiography, his mother and aunt speculated as to why he was "so damn bad," debating whether a West Indian root doctor or "some old person" had placed a spell or the "bad mouth" on him.[110]

Although evidence is scant for this as well, parents may have been resistant to what psychiatrists had to say about their children because white psychodynamic clinicians could not effectively communicate with them. Claude Brown recalled that his mother, a recent Southern transplant, was not sure if a Bellevue psychiatrist was trying to "say Sonny Boy was crazy." Astutely, she recognized that the confusion was not her fault, but the result of miscommunication. She explained, "You know, mosta those white doctors don' know how to talk to colored people anyway."[111]

The archival evidence suggests that Bernard was aware that working-class black folks might be unfamiliar with psychodynamic psychiatry. In 1944, two years after the Harlem Unit closed, Bernard served as a consultant for the Harlem office of the Community Service Society, a Manhattan antipoverty charity founded in 1939. Regarding the case of a black male teen with depression, Bernard worried that if she and the social workers were not careful about how "analysis itself and the arrangements for it are interpreted to the boy and his family . . . I'd feel analysis might seem too alien to them" and they would refuse treatment for him. Bernard offered that the parents would be more likely to agree to the sessions if the caseworker emphasized that the son was going to receive the "proposed psychotherapy . . . in recognition of his assets and potentialities rather than abnormality or pathology."[112]

Significantly, Bernard made such comments before she met the parents. She expected resistance. But she was sure she could gain their confidence if she told them their son was receiving psychiatric care "because of his promise as a valuable person" not because he was "crazy."[113] It is possible that Bernard's two years in the Harlem Unit had taught her that the black experience with psychiatry had largely been a punitive one. Given that experience, black parents were likely to mistrust the intentions of Bernard and the Harlem Unit. Perhaps some perceived these otherwise well-intentioned civil servants as simply the latest agents of the criminal justice system they hoped their children could avoid.

The Wiltwyck School for Boys' Psychiatric Promise, 1942

In addition to the problems posed by resistance, Bernard and some of the Harlem Unit's supporters recognized that public schools could not accommodate the needs of some deeply disturbed children. Writing to a fellow psychiatrist about one such black male student at P.S. 139 in Harlem, Bernard imagined that "to leave him where he is and to reenter his neighborhood school" would be "intolerable" for the boy, his classmates, and the staff. She predicted that a return to court on a charge of juvenile delinquency would be "almost inevitable" if he continued to remain at home in Harlem.[114] As late as 1941, however, only private childcare agencies cared for delinquent and neglected children with severe emotional problems. Almost every one of those institutions still exercised the legal right to bar children of color. The Warwick State Training School for Boys was the only public institution that could have taken them. Warwick was primarily for delinquent teenagers. It was a dangerous place for young children. In desperation, Polier and her fellow racial liberals looked outside the public sector to place troubled preteen African American boys.

In 1942 Polier and several other like-minded civil servants, acting as independent citizens, forged a relationship with a relatively new not-for-profit facility. In 1937 the New York Protestant Episcopal City Mission Society established the Wiltwyck School for Boys as a sectarian reform school. Located to the north of the city in rustic Esopus, a small village in the Catskill Mountains, the Wiltwyck School was the only place the Domestic Relations Court could send delinquent black males too young and emotionally vulnerable to handle Warwick. Although Wiltwyck was small and largely custodial in function, Polier and Bolin routinely assigned their black Harlem charges there.[115]

Motivated by a shared desire to keep this institution open, many of the same people behind the Domestic Relations Court treatment clinic and the Harlem Unit took administrative control of the Wiltwyck School. Some of these activists—including Polier, Kenworthy, and Field—had advised and funded the school during its formative years. In 1939, upon learning that the City Mission Society could not afford to keep the school open, Bolin and other individuals affiliated with the Domestic Relations Court stepped in to save the only agency that would accept the Claude Browns of Harlem. On June 11, 1942, a board composed of court personnel and their allies assumed directorship. The new board included Field, Ascoli, Kenworthy, Bernard, and the Levys, as well as justices Polier and Bolin.[116]

As Wiltwyck's new administrators, these philanthropists, psychiatrists, and judges hoped to transform this largely custodial facility into a therapeutic one. Drs. Bernard, Winsor, and Kenworthy lent their psychiatric expertise to the staff on matters of intake, individual casework, and administrative procedure. From the start of this new era, Polier, Bolin, and the Board of Directors insisted that the proper care of delinquents, black or white, included attention to their emotional needs. To this end, the new board immediately hired trained caseworkers, the consulting psychiatrist Dr. Virginia Moore, and the African American social worker Robert L. Cooper as the school's executive director.[117]

Even in their first year of running Wiltwyck, Bernard and her colleagues were confident that the school could eventually rehabilitate Harlem's delinquents. Very early on, the consulting psychiatrist Moore conceived of "Wiltwyck as a preventorium—to prevent the development of serious delinquencies."[118] While still toiling in the Harlem Unit, Bernard informed Moore that one of her male patients might benefit from the Wiltwyck "experience in living, if the latter is directed by psychiatric considerations."[119] Bernard's optimism about Wiltwyck's therapeutic promise reflected the amount of control she and her fellow board members could potentially exert over this reform school's setup. As a psychiatrist with the Harlem Unit, she and her team of psychological experts did not have that same freedom. They had marginal influence on the administration of any public school in which they worked. A clinician had more authority to influence the operation of a private institution like Wiltwyck. To be sure, Bernard and her fellow racial liberals were still committed to transforming the public sector into an instrument of equal opportunity. Nonetheless, the amount of institutional control the voluntary private sector offered was certainly quite appealing.

Conclusion

Between 1940 and 1942, color-blind psychiatry and the promise it offered extended its reach beyond Polier's courtroom. Polier and a cadre of antiracist psychiatrists, philanthropists, and children's court officials earnestly believed that central Harlem's relative lack of access to mental health care constituted an egregious racial injustice. For these juvenile delinquency experts, the expansion of psychiatric authority into Harlem held out the possibility of reducing the disproportionate number of black children on the children's court dockets. Toward that end, Dr. Max Winsor's Harlem Special Child Guidance Service Unit and the Wiltwyck School for Boys provided more institutionally based opportunities to promote mental health among central Harlem's black youth.

Nevertheless, these well-meaning civil servants within the Domestic Relations Court and the Bureau of Child Guidance did not fundamentally alter New York's systems of juvenile justice, child placement, and education. By 1942, some African American children certainly had received greater access to child-guidance services. Polier, Winsor, Bernard, and their colleagues intended to facilitate a clinical experience that would be humane, race neutral, and relevant to their patient's lives in Harlem. Despite their good intentions, there was much that New York's color-blind psychiatrists could not control. Clinical encounters with African Americans took place within the legally mandated confines of a school, a court clinic, or a correctional facility. These were institutions where children and parents had no right to refuse encounters with psychiatric authority. Like Claude Brown, some experienced these moments as coercive intrusions into their lives. Additionally, psychiatrists in such institutions were expected to work with other public employees and officials, some of whom actively resisted race-neutral psychiatry. Psychiatric authority had extended its reach within Harlem, but it was not always received with a hearty welcome.

Entering 1942, there were still plenty of spaces where color-blind psychiatry was entirely unwelcome. Private facilities retained the right to racially discriminate against Harlem's black youth. After the Pearl Harbor attack of December 1941, Polier, Winsor, and Bernard began losing what little political backing LaGuardia had lent the expansion of psychiatric authority within the courts and schools. As his administration's support waned, these public servants turned to civil society. Significantly, they made appeals to the community they were most intent on helping: Harlem.

Chapter Four

Psychiatry for Harlem

Wartime Activism and the Black Community's Mental Health Needs, 1942–45

After two years with the Special Child Guidance Unit, Max Winsor felt that he had not done enough to fight mental health disparities in Harlem. In November 1941, Winsor wrote to Viola Bernard, admitting that he had "tended to narrow interests, contacts, and hopes to the Unit's work since coming to the Bureau."[1] He worried that this kind of insularity might impede the larger fight against institutional racism.

In late 1941, Winsor, Bernard, Justine Wise Polier, and others within both the Domestic Relations Court and the Bureau of Child Guidance realized that their ability to reform their institutions from the inside was limited. When public funds were not sufficient to finance the Harlem Unit or the Domestic Relations Court clinic, Polier and her fellow civil servants relied on philanthropy. But private contributions were not enough to sustain social programs in one of America's largest cities. As La Guardia sought to appeal more to his conservative Italian base during his third mayoral term, Polier could not always count on him to continue supporting her progressive policy experiments. Given these limits, racial liberals realized that they might have to call on civil society to place political pressure on the mayor.

Between 1942 and 1947, proponents of social justice in juvenile justice and public education forged an alliance with leaders from Harlem's black freedom struggle. They found support for their institutional reform efforts within a pivotal new civil-rights organization, the City-Wide Citizen's Committee for Harlem (CWCCH). Assembled in 1941, the CWCCH was composed of private citizens and African American community leaders. This group initially sought to understand and prevent crime in central Harlem. The CWCCH welcomed input from school and court officials with experience tackling youth crime in Harlem. CWCCH leaders such as the Harlem YMCA's Channing Tobias were eager to work with local authorities willing to promote racial justice. Polier, Winsor, and Bernard fit that bill, offering them the opportunity to promote the emotional health of black children as a matter of civil-rights import.

Thanks to the advocacy of Polier and other racial liberals, the CWCCH incorporated color-blind psychiatry with juvenile delinquents into the wartime civil-rights movement. Once appointed to the CWCCH Subcommittee on Crime and Juvenile Delinquency, Polier, Winsor, and Bernard secured the organization's support for three of their antiracist policy efforts in the courts and schools. Two of these proposals were enacted. One was the 1943–45 Harlem Project, an expansion of the Harlem Special Child Guidance Service Unit. The second was a 1942 municipal law forbidding childcare agencies from discriminating on the basis of race. Only Polier's 1945 bid to renew the Domestic Relations Court treatment clinic's funding failed. The CWCCH's political backing signified that the child-welfare system's small pocket of resistance to psychiatric racism had become part of New York's organized struggle against racial injustice.

The CWCCH's engagement with the issue of race and psychiatry amounted to more than just the local civil-rights movement's adoption of the white racial liberals' agenda. In endorsing the African American psyche as an acceptable site for making civil-rights claims, Harlem's black activists helped reshape what that meant. Up until World War II, Polier and her allies' racial-justice efforts focused narrowly on meeting the mental health needs of Harlem's black youth. The scope of Polier, Winsor, and Bernard's racial-justice efforts had been limited to children's issues since they all worked within New York's child-welfare system. As these public servants engaged with Harlem's black freedom struggle, a movement oriented primarily toward the needs of adults, they expanded their antiracist agenda. Collaborating with Harlem's civil society, Polier, Winsor, and Bernard developed programs and goals they could not conceive from within the confines of the child-welfare system. In particular, the CWCCH helped Dr. Bernard learn that black adults also faced mental health inequalities. These racial disparities included Harlem Hospital's lack of a psychiatric ward and New York's severe dearth of black psychiatrists—a problem Bernard tried to resolve by actively recruiting African Americans into the psychiatric profession between 1942 and 1947.

The remainder of the chapter examines how the CWCCH's political support emboldened Justice Polier's wartime fight against institutional racism in New York's childcare system. In 1944 the CWCCH lent its public support to Polier's indictment of the Children's Shelter, an overcrowded facility where many emotionally neglected black youth had been housed. After a public exposé, the shelter closed. The next year, Hubert T. Delany, a left-leaning CWCCH leader and new La Guardia appointee to the Children's Court, helped Polier launch a second investigation of the Warwick State Training School. This time, the judges found evidence that the reform school neglected its black charges' mental health. In each case, municipal authorities recognized and penalized these instances of institutional racism. Despite these minor victories, it was not certain whether any institutions besides Harlem school clinics and the Domestic Relations Court had adopted a race-neutral understanding of the black psyche. Nevertheless, the wartime collaboration between racial liberals and Harlem's civil-rights leaders enabled Polier to put pressure on some of the childcare providers that had prevented her from serving the best interests of emotionally troubled black children.

The City-Wide Citizens Committee for Harlem

Thanks to the Harlem Unit, racial liberals in the child-welfare system found proponents of psychiatry within Harlem's community organizations. In 1941 Winsor initiated such connections by incorporating the Board of Education's liaison teacher program into the Harlem Unit.[2] Winsor encouraged these liaison teachers to locate organizations willing to allow the BCG psychiatrists to work with African American clients off school grounds. Subsequently, the liaison teachers connected Winsor's unit to private Harlem agencies including the Community Service Society, the YMCA, the YWCA, and the Urban League.

These new African American community contacts offered Polier and other reformers in the courts and schools a chance to directly engage with central Harlem's civil society at a critical moment in the black freedom struggle.[3] According to the historian Martha Biondi and others, New York City was one of the wartime civil-rights movement's most important staging areas. Nationwide, a "black popular front" of liberal and leftist black leaders pursued fair employment and economic justice for African Americans.[4] In New York, the movement "sought to redistribute economic and political power within the increasingly divided metropolis."[5] In their effort to erase the racial inequities within the expanding modern state and the increasingly segregated urban landscape, wartime black activists forged political alliances in "Northern cities involving Jewish and Protestant liberals, Communists, Socialists, segments of the New York intelligentsia, and segments of the Northern philanthropic establishment."[6]

Serious coalition building between this black popular front and New York's systems of education and juvenile justice did not take place until the winter of 1941–42. This alliance first developed in response to the press's irresponsible reporting of a Harlem "crime wave" in November 1941. During the war, city newspapers transformed small surges in petty crime in Harlem into "crime waves," playing on the fears of white readers. The Police Department imposed a massive dragnet on petty thieves and loiterers in Harlem. The number of African Americans in custody sharply spiked. The press corps erroneously concluded that this jump in arrests meant that Harlem was more crime-ridden than ever.[7]

Harlem's African American leaders did not let these charges go unchallenged. Since the 1920s, Northern civil-rights activists had been publicly railing against the politicization of racial differences in crime rates. Summoning arrest rates as evidence of the black race's innate criminality, racialists divested black neighborhoods of critical crime prevention tools on the grounds that black crime was biologically driven and unpreventable.[8] Black luminaries skeptical of this political abuse of race-based crime statistics included the Brotherhood of Sleeping Car Porters' A. Philip Randolph, the NAACP's Walter White, and the Urban League's Lester B. Granger.[9] Long active in the interwar black freedom struggle, they recognized that persistent small-time crime in Harlem was merely a symptom of a larger, intensifying problem: the enduring inequalities facing disproportionately black communities across the African Diaspora.[10]

Set on opening a dialogue on crime, prominent Harlem leaders met with close to 250 of the "leading citizens of the white and Negro community."[11] The November meeting produced the interracial CWCCH, an advocacy group composed of academics, civil servants, ministers, activists, and community leaders, all of whom felt that the "Negro problem in New York" was in urgent need of resolution.[12] For them, the CWCCH was chiefly an act of local citizenship. Yet owing to New York's central place within the wartime black freedom struggle, the CWCCH's efforts were also of interest to activists elsewhere confronting their own "Negro problem."[13]

In line with how civil-rights activists in Detroit or Oakland analyzed their "Negro problem," both the CWCCH and New York's racial liberals traced central Harlem's social problems to racial inequality in the distribution of socioeconomic resources.[14] According to CWCCH leaders such as Walter White, crime and other social ills could not be cured until racial disparities declined.[15] Charging that government should help ensure African Americans equal access to economic and educational opportunities, the CWCCH urged the La Guardia administration to become a truer mechanism of redistributive racial justice.[16] Unsurprisingly, Polier, Winsor, and Bernard agreed that equity in public policy could reduce crime.[17] The interests of the CWCCH, Justice Polier, and the Harlem Unit's psychiatrists dovetailed. Collaboration was likely.

Winsor and Polier not only joined the CWCCH but they were also appointed to its Board of Directors.[18] It makes sense that the CWCCH offered them leadership roles. During World War II, New York's civil-rights leaders were willing to work with political and institutional insiders, especially those who were not opposed to redistributing their public agencies' resources.[19] Polier and Winsor were civil servants with substantial power over the lives of central Harlem's black youth. Even more important, for almost four years they had been using their positions to establish racial fairness as a policy guideline within the La Guardia administration. Since juvenile delinquency was such a pivotal issue for the CWCCH, the inclusion of Polier and other sympathetic insiders gave civil-rights leaders the chance to potentially influence New York's systems of education, corrections, and juvenile justice.[20]

Juvenile Delinquency as a CWCCH Issue

In early 1942, the CWCCH began identifying Harlem's neglected needs, proposing strategies "designed to increase support for racial justice measures in city government."[21] The CWCCH divided its membership into topical subcommittees. Winsor and Polier joined the Subcommittee on Crime and Delinquency. Two other veterans of the Harlem Unit also attained positions of prominence in the Subcommittee on Crime and Delinquency. On Judge Polier's recommendation, the CWCCH included Viola Bernard on this subcommittee of "leading judges, social workers, and others" in January 1942.[22] The psychologist Dr. Caroline Zachary, the new BCG director and a Harlem Unit adviser, also joined the subcommittee in early 1942. Many of the African American Harlemites who served as CWCCH leaders held all four in high regard. Dr. Tobias considered Winsor "among the few friends who live outside Harlem who has taken the time to fully identify themselves with the interests of our people."[23]

Once entrenched within the Subcommittee on Crime and Delinquency, Polier, Winsor, Bernard, and Zachary helped shape the CWCCH's conception of Harlem's battle against crime. Initially, crime was the cornerstone issue of the CWCCH.[24] Even the other subcommittees on health, housing, education, and recreation sought ways to prevent adult crime in Harlem. Owing to their positions as juvenile-justice and public-education insiders, however, these four New Yorkers did not exclusively focus on Harlem's adult crime as they served on the subcommittee. They concentrated much more on fighting juvenile delinquency.

The CWCCH Subcommittee on Crime and Delinquency issued reports predicting that crime would decline in central Harlem if more was done to prevent juvenile delinquency. The early reports reflect Winsor and Polier's contention that juvenile delinquency had increased in 1941 and early 1942, especially in Harlem. Like many social experts nationwide, Polier and Winsor had fully expected child crime to increase in wartime.[25] Supported by statistics gathered from the Children's Court, Polier and Winsor found that juvenile court arraignments rose in 1941. They also determined that Harlem's black population produced more delinquency arrests than any other racial group in the city. In general, the subcommittee attributed this to Harlem's status as a disinvested area, arguing that institutional racism, employment discrimination, and a racially segmented housing market bred delinquency and eventually adult crime. The subcommittee reduced its thesis to a handy equation: "Poverty plus discrimination plus crowding equal[s] crime!"[26] Polier and the other subcommittee members even agreed with the CWCCH proposition that only a "large-scale social reconstruction" of New York City could alter the conditions that had generated crime in central Harlem.[27]

Nevertheless, these racial liberals working with the CWCCH presumed that such a radical restructuring was not forthcoming any time soon. Instead, Max Winsor and his fellow veterans of the Harlem Special Child Guidance Service Unit used their subcommittee posts to advance their ongoing battle against racism in the delivery of children's mental health services. Within their first two months on the CWCCH Subcommittee on Crime and Delinquency, Winsor, Bernard, and Zachary initiated and led a special subdivision called the Committee on Psychiatry. In its March 1942 report, the committee's recommendations clearly reflected the priorities and interests of the child-centered social institutions it represented.[28] Max Winsor's Committee on Psychiatry argued that an increase in child-guidance services in Harlem would help prevent outbreaks of juvenile delinquency. According to the committee, central Harlem's dearth of mental health services for troubled children unjustly denied all of its black residents a less crime-ridden future. Winsor pressed the CWCCH to throw its support behind the Domestic Relations Court and BCG's efforts to supply Harlem with those resources.[29]

There was a tone of real urgency in the Committee on Psychiatry's 1942 plea. Both Polier and the BCG's Dr. Zachary worried that they could no longer count on Mayor La Guardia to support psychiatry's expansion into Harlem. During World War II, the public funding for child guidance and other local mental health services declined as Americans became disenchanted with psychiatry as a crime prevention tool. With rates of juvenile delinquency rising in Great Britain following the 1941 blitz, the stateside press prepared the public to expect the same spike in misbehavior once the United States entered the war.[30] In 1942, adult crime rates declined nationwide, but rates of juvenile delinquency did appear to rise.[31] Nationwide, a moral panic over this apparent wartime outbreak of youth crime ensued. La Guardia turned the local iteration of this panic to his political advantage.

Some conservative New Yorkers blamed this apparent wave of juvenile delinquency on a wartime decline of the male-headed family. According to this perspective, children misbehaved whenever their authoritarian fathers went off to war, leaving only mothers and childcare workers armed with child psychology to coddle and spoil them. La Guardia astutely picked up on white working-class skepticism toward psychiatry's effectiveness as a crime prevention tool. This skepticism was especially widespread among Roman Catholics, including Italian Americans and Irish Americans. In the 1941 mayoral campaign, he had lost support among that segment of the public, winning reelection by only a slim margin. Eager to regain that support, he echoed their demands for a harsher crime-fighting approach in the midst of war. Formerly he had supported progressive education and the development of mental hygiene programs. But from 1942 through 1945, he publicly singled out the Children's Court as soft on criminals and encouraged traditional "punishment as the only effective method of treating delinquent youth."[32] He openly criticized the court's use of psychiatry, complaining that psychiatrists were unable to "tell the character of a child."[33]

Once the United States entered the war in December 1941, the La Guardia administration began slashing mental health services from the city budget.[34] Psychiatric services in the judicial system were particularly hurt. In addition to the decrease in municipal funding, Works Progress Administration (WPA) assistance had disappeared. Thanks to La Guardia's active partnership with President Roosevelt and his New Deal coalition, the Domestic Relations Court had depended on the WPA since 1935 to help fulfill its staffing needs. Yet between 1939 and 1942, fiscal conservatives in Congress scaled back this expensive federal program. In 1943 the WPA dissolved.[35] By war's end, the Children's Court diagnostic clinic lost its full-time staff, leaving it with only three part-time psychiatrists, each working less than thirty hours a week. Not only had the quantity of services declined but the quality also suffered. According to Polier, the part-time clinicians tended to produce shoddy "conveyer belt reports" littered with careless misdiagnoses.[36]

Despite the cutbacks, the number of children requiring mental hygiene services rose dramatically. For example, between 1941 and 1945, Children's Court cases increased by 57 percent in New York City.[37] Just as the volume of emotionally unstable children increased, available resources declined. Overcrowding as much as fiscal cutbacks helped decrease the relative proportion of psychiatric services. In 1943 both Bellevue's children's ward and the Warwick State Training School for Boys stopped admitting delinquent children referred by the Children's Court.[38]

Harlem's black community was hit hardest by these austere measures. Bellevue and Warwick were two of the few institutions that offered troubled black youth the possibility of psychiatric care. When those two institutions stopped taking new clients, the courts had to place black male delinquents in temporary shelters (such as the Society for the Prevention of Cruelty to Children's shelter on East 104th Street) with no psychiatric facilities. Some, including ninety male teens between January and April 1944, waited in adult prison cells.[39]

The Mental Health Needs of African American Children and Adults

The Domestic Relations Court's racial liberals and their allies in the BCG were deeply dismayed by the 1942 municipal budget cuts. Nevertheless, most of these judges and psychiatrists were not in a strong enough position to publicly criticize the socially conservative turn within wartime politics. They were employees of public institutions that had fallen out of favor with both the voting public and the mayor's office. Hoping to regain La Guardia's support, they could not oppose his budget cuts on their own. But as an independent voice in civil society, the CWCCH was free to politicize their grievances for them. But before these mental hygiene advocates could expect Harlem civil-rights activists to make the public allocation of mental health funds their priority, they had to explain how this issue mattered to the black community. In other words, Polier had to persuade the CWCCH that her fight against La Guardia's budget cuts was in Harlem's best interest.

To this end, Bernard tried convincing key CWCCH leaders that increased mental health care spending would help central Harlem. She argued that New York City's mental health services were an essential part of the effort to prevent delinquency and crime in Harlem. On April 14, 1942, Dr. Bernard wrote Walter White, the CWCCH cochair and executive director of the NAACP, arguing that La Guardia's proposed budget cuts would increase "Negro juvenile social maladjustment, of which delinquency is such a conspicuous part." Bernard stressed that the spending cuts in mental health care "particularly involves the Negro children, because their needs for this kind of service are greater, and the resources to meet them, less." Because of poverty and the racism of private agencies for children, Harlem depended on public institutions as a "coordinated whole" to meet its mental health needs. She asked White to consider that a budget cut affecting "any cog in this coordinated whole threatens the effectiveness of the whole machinery." Without a childcare system shorn of institutional racism and equipped to restore Manhattan's troubled black youth to mental health, Harlem's rates of delinquency and crime were sure to rise.[40]

Though her letter to White highlighted just how much the budget cuts would affect Harlem's African American children, Bernard and her Committee on Psychiatry colleagues recognized that they would have to include the mental health needs of adults within their liberal agenda. This was a crucial adjustment on their part. In seeking CWCCH support for the expansion of color-blind psychiatry, Polier and her allies realized that they would have to convince civil-rights activists of its relevance for all of Harlem—not just troubled children. In the Committee on Psychiatry's March 26, 1942, report, Winsor, Bernard, and Zachary warned the CWCCH against marginalizing the psychiatric point of view, arguing that solving Harlem's problems depended on the "essential integration of mental hygiene with the work" of all committees.[41] Since these other committees focused on the immediate needs of Harlem's adults, Winsor, Bernard, and Zachary sought to persuade the CWCCH leadership that increased psychiatric services would also address adults' emotional needs.

Prior to 1942, most of the Committee on Psychiatry's members had only been concerned with the mental health needs of young African Americans. Nevertheless, Winsor and his cohort did not have to make much of an imaginative leap to consider the black adult psyche in antiracialist terms.[42] As racial liberals, they already expected that mature black adults could exist. These veterans of the Harlem Special Child Guidance Service Unit and Polier's courtroom would not have tried to promote the emotional development of black children had they considered them incapable of becoming normal adults.[43]

Nevertheless, beyond this rather indirect concern with the emotional capacities of black adults, racial liberals in New York's public schools and Children's Court had never addressed the mental health needs of *actual* black adults. Polier, Winsor, and Bernard worked within a child-welfare system obsessed with juvenile delinquency. Once troubled children grew up, they fell outside the jurisdiction of the schools or juvenile court. With little to no professional contact with emotionally ill black adults, these racial liberals' efforts to reduce health disparities narrowly focused on the needs of black children.

Working with the CWCCH, racial liberals began to actively consider the mental health needs of the black Harlemites that most concerned wartime civil-rights activists: adults. Throughout the 1940s, the CWCCH became best known for its efforts to promote fair employment and fair housing—struggles that aimed to improve Harlem by equalizing economic opportunities for black adults, especially black male breadwinners.[44] The CWCCH cochair Algernon Black, president of Manhattan's Ethical Culture Society, actively committed the CWCCH to the fight against housing discrimination and labor fairness.[45] Given the CWCCH's interest in solutions that could benefit the black family as a whole, Polier and her allies on the Subcommittee on Crime and Delinquency became more than advocates for Harlem's children.[46] They became advocates for Harlem.

Intent on making color-blind psychiatry more relevant to the black freedom struggle, the Subcommittee on Crime and Delinquency identified five mental health goals for central Harlem, two of which focused on adults. Each proposal constituted a cog in the very sort of racially equitable childcare machinery that Dr. Bernard had urged Walter White to envision. Bernard, Zachary, and Winsor initially included each of the five goals in the Committee on Psychiatry's 1942 report. The first three goals were extensions of Polier and Winsor's ongoing efforts to end racial inequality in New York's childcare system. They included a successor to the Harlem Unit, increased funds for the Children's Court treatment clinic, and a law banning racism in childcare agencies.

The final two goals were new. They reflected these civil servants' newly heightened awareness of black adults' needs. These two recommendations called for an outpatient psychiatric ward at Harlem Hospital and the active recruitment of black psychiatrists.[47] According to Winsor and his team, Harlem's lack of both hospital space and employment opportunities for adults interested in mental health careers constituted racial injustices the CWCCH ought to address.[48] With Polier's active support, these suggestions found their way into the Subcommittee on Crime and Delinquency's 1942 report and two CWCCH reports dated 1943 and 1944, respectively.[49]

The CWCCH embraced the Subcommittee on Crime and Delinquency's comprehensive mental health agenda. CWCCH leaders were persuaded by Dr. Bernard's argument about the harm the recent city budget cuts posed to Harlem. At a meeting of social agencies held at the offices of the Russell Sage Foundation—an organization that promoted the development of social programs since 1907—the attorney Frank E. Karelson spoke on behalf of the CWCCH. Karelson decried the La Guardia administration budget cuts in the very terms set by Dr. Bernard. Karelson argued that "as the budget stands now it means juvenile delinquency in Harlem will go up," suggesting that racial liberals in education and juvenile justice had successfully injected their psychiatric point of view into the black freedom struggle's assessment of Harlem's needs.[50]

Preserving the Domestic Relations Court Treatment Clinic—for Harlem

Throughout the war, the CWCCH backed racial liberals' efforts to make psychiatric care more available to black children in court. Reeling from the 1942 budget cuts to the judicial system's mental health allocation, Polier urged the CWCCH to help her save her court's psychiatric treatment clinic.[51] As representatives of the Subcommittee on Crime and Delinquency, Winsor and Bernard argued that the court clinic aided Harlem's fight against juvenile delinquency and that it was the only resource of its kind for black children. "More Negroes reach the Children's Court, in part because fewer community resources are available to them than to the white group. Accordingly, the Negro children are particularly dependent on the clinical facilities attached to the court, which are insufficiently staffed."[52] Defending the court clinic as one of the only spaces where black Harlemites could receive psychotherapy, Winsor and Bernard urged the Subcommittee on Crime and Delinquency to help it secure funding and permanent status. Not only did this subcommittee accept the recommendations,[53] but the CWCCH was so convinced that the clinic's survival was in Harlem's best interests that it even created the Advisory Committee on Treatment of the Psychiatric Clinic of the Children's Court.[54]

After the Harlem Riot of August 1, 1943, the La Guardia administration did increase its support for social programs intended to serve Harlem's best interests. Unlike the Harlem Riot of 1935, this insurrection was ignited by a confirmed incident of excessive police force. The white police officer James Collins shot and wounded Robert Bandy, a uniformed soldier who had interfered in the arrest of another individual. He was shot in the back. A twelve-hour uprising—immortalized in Ralph Ellison's *An Invisible Man*—ensued, resulting in extensive property damage in central Harlem. Some Harlem leaders interpreted this event as a reaction against racial inequality. In response, La Guardia instituted rent control, passed fair-employment legislation, and promised more public housing.[55]

The Domestic Relations Court's mental health programs did not receive any of this postriot largesse. Whereas La Guardia tried to appear sympathetic to black Harlem leaders, East Harlem's Italian community tended to see the Harlem Riot as a crime wave rather than a form of political expression. Not surprisingly, those constituents expected that La Guardia could best prevent a future riot with draconian law enforcement and less coddling of criminals. Still eager to appeal to his ethnic white base, La Guardia continued to ignore the Domestic Relations Court's requests to renew its experiments with psychiatric services.[56]

Entering 1945, La Guardia's final year in office, the CWCCH urged the mayor to keep the clinic open. The previous three years, CWCCH activists encouraged philanthropists, prominent medical organizations, politicians, and even court officials to support Polier's clinic. Those efforts bore little fruit.[57] Support waned even within the clinic's political base, Children's Court liberals. La Guardia's budget cuts and wartime demonization of psychology in the courts had demoralized Polier's colleagues.[58] Eventually the CWCCH finally refused to continue alone in this fight "without some clarification as to the question of City support."[59] After one last attempt to sway La Guardia in April, the Children's Court treatment clinic discontinued operations in September 1945.[60]

The Harlem Project, 1943–45

Nevertheless, the CWCCH did help racial liberals create some new psychiatric services for children in central Harlem. Max Winsor and Viola Bernard felt that the Harlem Unit had not adequately met Harlem's psychiatric needs. In 1942 Winsor reported that "the needs for service in all these schools is much greater than anticipated. When we first began no one was in a position to help us with an estimate of how much and what kind of clinical service any such school is in need of."[61] He was sure that additional clinical resources would help meet those needs.

In March 1942, Bernard, Winsor, and Zachary advised their fellow CWCCH members to support a larger successor to the Harlem Unit.[62] Winsor and his colleagues wanted to see what would happen if mental hygiene experts could influence the administration of a public school.[63] This proposal was a clear expression of the managerial ethos that had dominated the American approach to business, social policy, and problem solving since the Great Depression began.[64] Simply put, racial liberals wanted to reshape public schools into instruments capable of improving what Winsor dubbed the "emotional climate" of central Harlem's toughest streets.

The public school system approved this new child guidance program in 1943. Its approval is a bit surprising, given that progressive ideas in corrections and juvenile justice had become suspect within New York politics. Of course the promise of substantial private funds from the nonprofit Hofheimer Foundation and the New York Foundation made it easier for school authorities to endorse the plan.[65] But taxpayers also helped foot the bill. Evidently the public schools had managed to protect this experiment from the financial cutbacks that the Domestic Relations Court faced. There were two reasons why this happened. First, since 1934, the Superintendent of Schools' office had consistently and successfully ascribed any success in the city's public schools to its nationally recognized programs in progressive education and mental hygiene.[66] Second, during La Guardia's term in office, the Board of Education had successfully "insisted . . . that the schools were a quasi-independent body."[67] As such a body, the Board of Education was unwilling to bend to La Guardia's current assault on mental hygiene and risk sabotaging the school system's reputation for modern pedagogy. By September 29, 1943, both the Superintendent of Schools' office and the Board of Education successfully approved the two-year program known as the Harlem Project.[68]

The City-Wide Citizens Committee helped facilitate the Harlem Project's integration into the local community. The Harlem Project leadership contained a large number of CWCCH members, including Winsor, Polier, and Bernard—all of whom pushed Harlem's civil-rights community to discuss the program's progress at meetings.[69] The Harlem Project staff not only enlisted the help of local private agencies, but it also included some Harlem organizations as vital partners in the "new program." In searching for such partners, Polier and Winsor drew from a talented pool of CWCCH compatriots. Dr. Tobias was one of Dr. Winsor's strongest supporters. Tobias was not only a leader in Harlem's YMCA and NAACP branches, but he was also a political ally of Marshall Field III, the philanthropist who helped fund the Harlem Special Child Guidance Service Unit and the Domestic Relations Court treatment clinic. The well-connected Tobias became a valued member of the Harlem Project's Joint Advisory Committee, helping to broker aid from both local agencies and the Field Foundation.[70]

Even though colleagues of Max Winsor and Justice Polier monopolized the leadership of both the Harlem Unit and the Harlem Project, the latter was a separate venture.[71] First, the Harlem Project operated in three other schools, Junior High School 120 in Mount Morris Park, Junior High School 161 on 111th Street and Lexington Avenue, and P.S. 10 on St. Nicholas Avenue and 116th Street.[72] Second, the Harlem Project attempted to change how schools served students, altering the curriculum and adding new specialized faculty. The Project aimed to help schools identify and "contribute fully to [the] emotional and social adjustment" of potential delinquents.[73] As the third and most key difference, the Harlem Project worked on the premise that aberrant family dynamics generated most of Harlem's juvenile delinquents.

Ironic as it might seem, the race neutrality of the Harlem Project's researchers is what enabled them to latch onto this condescending perspective. The Harlem Project's Research Committee, which Polier chaired, claimed that its therapeutic efforts were undone every afternoon as the children left the school clinic and returned to their families. Most mental hygiene experts also tended to blame parents for the behavioral problems of white children. The Harlem Project's racial liberals believed that black misbehavior had similar causes. They fully expected that the homes of Harlem's juvenile delinquents were not conducive to emotional health.[74] It was not because of bad biology. Instead, Harlem suffered from a glut of "inadequate parents."[75]

As social justice advocates, the Project staff claimed to sympathize with the parents they criticized. Like other CWCCH affiliates, they agreed that any family disorder in black Harlem was generally a result of racial inequality rather than either race or choice. Project researchers stated that such "pervasive economic and social evils as result from segregation and prejudice" made it difficult for poor black parents to forge emotionally stable families.[76] Yet despite their purported sympathy for working-poor Harlem parents, Polier and her Harlem Project colleagues sought to shield their own children from them. Having identified the black working-class Harlem parent as the immediate cause of a delinquent's emotional instability, the Project attempted to take over child-rearing duties. The Project's leaders expected that for some of these "slum children," clinical adjustments could be sustained if the children spent most of their time in emotionally healthier communities.[77] These racial liberals hoped to create such a community within each target neighborhood.[78] The Research Committee intended for school to serve as the "community center" of the ideal community central Harlem ought to have. Students would spend as much time as possible there to counteract the influence of their pathological families.[79]

The Harlem Project did expand the function of its three target schools, opening each of them as an ersatz community center. Through the all-day school program, the Harlem Project arranged to keep the school open after regular school hours and in the summer. In all three schools, the New York Foundation and the Board of Education jointly hired counselors, teachers, and social workers to design and run the all-day programs. The day personnel ran after-school recreational programs. These programs were conducted in the school building and on the playgrounds. For three hours each weekday, the substitute parents led students in games, sports, crafts, music, clubs, and enrichment programs. In the summer, the schools became all-day community centers for neighborhood children. Staff provided meals, daycare for infants, activities, and field trips to Bear Mountain and other resorts. At P.S. 10—where the aspiring novelist Ann Petry worked in an afterschool program, gathering material for *The Street*, her bleak novel about wartime central Harlem—64 children in 1944 and 139 in 1945 even received the chance to attend summer camps in the countryside. In the evenings during the school year and the summer, the three schools remained open for adult education classes and teen recreation.[80]

As the war wore on, labor issues beset the Harlem Project. Addressing the CWCCH in 1944, some of the Project's workers and leaders complained that too many of the teachers were both racially prejudiced and opposed to modern psychology.[81] Owing to wartime teacher shortages, the Board of Education was never able to fully staff the Project's classrooms. All three schools even relied on Project personnel to "cover classes" for missing teachers.[82] Making matters worse, there was never enough money in the budget to keep the schools open all day.[83] Even if there had been, the custodians' union, justifiably worried about the exploitation of its members, refused to keep the schools open all day or all summer. Consequently, the Harlem Project never became what Winsor had intended: an effort to socially engineer a more healthful emotional climate in Harlem.[84]

In Search of Black Psychiatrists for Harlem

Working with the CWCCH, Polier and her cadre of antiracist mental health professionals proposed policies intended to reduce racial inequity in the distribution of mental health care resources. Most of their plans included African Americans only as recipients of care. In contending that Harlem needed more black mental health care providers, the Committee on Psychiatry deviated from this pattern. With that recommendation, these New York racial liberals managed to align their agenda with one of the wartime civil-rights movement's primary goals: the full and equal employment of African American adults.

US psychiatry was a profession with few black faces. Entering 1942, the number of African American psychiatrists and medical students undergoing psychiatric training was quite small. That year there was only one board-certified black psychiatrist in Manhattan. According to Bernard, less than twenty of the three thousand psychiatrists in the United States were listed as "Negro."[85] Most medical schools, teaching hospitals, and the American Medical Association (AMA) actively discriminated against blacks interested in allopathic careers. Even during World War II, most black physicians, residents, and interns worked and trained at historically black hospitals. In response to mainstream medicine's denial of equal care to black Americans, many black communities had created and run their own private hospitals. Owing to the Great Depression, the slow integration of municipal and private hospitals, and civil-rights activists' growing disapproval of separatist solutions to racism, almost half of all black hospitals closed between 1923 and 1944. As the number of black hospitals declined during World War II, opportunities for black physicians decreased when the AMA approved fewer internships and residencies at the remaining facilities.[86] Given this dire situation, some racial liberals felt that something had to be done before America's small supply of black psychiatrists dwindled even further.

The CWCCH Committee on Psychiatry offered an integrationist solution to the dearth of black psychiatrists. In its February and March 1942 reports, the committee stated that Bellevue and other public hospitals ought to accept black psychiatric residents. As integrationists, the BCG and Domestic Relations Court's racial liberals were very much interested in rooting out racism from psychiatry and opening up opportunities for black medical students to train and work in formerly all-white psychiatric departments.[87]

The psychiatrist Dr. Viola Bernard, a Jewish American woman, felt most strongly about the issue. Of all the racial liberals in the fight against psychiatric racism, she actually incorporated the need for black clinicians into her personal and professional agenda. Since 1941, she had already been working to raise awareness about the dearth of African American psychiatrists. She, Grassland Hospital's Dr. Thomas Brennan, Harlem Hospital Mental Hygiene Clinic's Dr. Harold Ellis (New York City's only board-certified black psychiatrist), and Dr. Ellis's wife (a nurse) had joined a short-lived committee on this matter. The Committee on Mental Hygiene for Negroes initially formed in 1939, the brain-child of a black former psychiatric patient from White Plains, New York, Rose Kittrell. Kittrell intended the group to improve and expand psychiatric care for African Americans. From 1941 to 1943, the Committee on Mental Hygiene for Negroes explored recruitment strategies, discussing what black psychiatrists could possibly do for Harlem.[88]

Bernard believed that an increase in black psychiatrists would benefit the nation's segregated black communities in two ways. First, the addition of "some well-trained Negro psychiatrists" would "help . . . meet the deplorable inadequacies in psychiatric care for the Negro community."[89] Owing to the "extreme delicacy of the doctor-patient relationship" in a psychiatric case, Bernard felt that "having only white psychiatrists available creates a wall at the outset." Anger over racial discrimination might deter an African American patient from opening up to a white psychiatrist. Such a patient might be far more comfortable with someone of her own race. A clinic with a racially diverse staff would be able to address that particular need, one Bernard claimed might be common in black Harlem.[90]

Second, Bernard argued that black psychiatrists might help white psychiatrists understand their nonwhite patients better. She and other racial liberals took it on faith that psychodynamic models of the normalized (white) human self could equally describe a black citizen's inner life. Nevertheless, Bernard recognized that this presumption was flawed. She argued that almost all of the psychiatric theories about how the human mind operated "are doubtless traceable to the fact that conclusions are too often based on data from a middle-class white group, interpreted by investigators of the same social group." Bernard questioned the universal applicability of a model based on such a racially and socially "incomplete sampling" of the human population. Should a white middle-class model of "inner, subjective life" be a template for all others? How would one really know what was culturally learned and what was natural, what was normal and abnormal about an African American's behavior?[91]

Bernard claimed psychiatry needed to construct a new model of the human psyche by drawing on "work between investigators of different ethnic and social derivation." Only then could psychiatrists discover truly universal principles of the mind. Consequently, "the psychiatric body of knowledge needs the contributions of colleagues who represent the whole community, including its Negro members." Enhanced by the perspective that black psychiatrists might be able to offer, Bernard anticipated that psychiatry might improve its ability to assess the needs of black patients in central Harlem.[92]

Starting with her work on the Committee on Mental Hygiene, Bernard began recruiting potential black psychiatrists. Bernard understood that African American medical students did not have equal access to information about the opportunities available for advanced medical training and financial aid.[93] In the 1940s, white male physicians generally shared such information with those in their social circles: other white men. As a Jewish woman, Bernard knew this white male advantage firsthand.[94] Bernard also knew that it was possible for someone else on the inside to share this information with individuals in an otherwise disadvantaged position of informational access. Bernard had professionally benefited to some degree from her prior friendship with Dr. Kenworthy.

Bernard was determined to become a similar point of access for black psychiatric hopefuls. She gave talks to audiences of African American medical students. She kept in touch with medical professionals who knew of prospective psychiatric candidates. Throughout the 1940s, she was confident that she knew every black psychiatrist-in-training nationwide. She kept detailed lists of them on file. For some of these aspiring psychiatrists, Bernard had served as a recruiter, source of career information, and recommender.[95] She established her first documented connection at Howard University Medical School in July 1943 with a black medical student named Charles B. Wilkinson.[96] Three years later, Bernard sought residencies for him in "neurology, psychiatry, and psychosomatic medicine."[97]

She learned about many of her recruits through a nationwide grapevine of racial liberals. For example, Clarence Pickett, a Pennsylvania community-service organizer and friend of Dr. Brennan, first introduced Bernard to one of her top recruits, Dr. Margaret Lawrence. In 1946, Pickett told Bernard about the Meharry Medical College graduate's intention to train in child psychiatry with New York Hospital's prominent pediatrician Dr. Benjamin Spock. Pickett sold Bernard on Lawrence's racial and gender significance, writing that "she is particularly interested in eventually becoming a child psychiatrist and, if she does, will be one of the first Negro women in this field . . . you ought to know each other."[98]

In some cases one of her recruits led her to other potential recruits. One recruit, Lt. Garnet Ice, a black Marine Corps army physician, wrote to Bernard while he was receiving special training at Bellevue.[99] Although he himself did not eventually pursue a career in psychiatry, he kept in touch with Bernard. He even introduced her to the Detroit intern James L. Curtis.[100] Upon Ice's recommendation, she added Curtis to a typed list of African Americans interested in psychiatry, helping him secure psychoanalytic training in New York.[101]

Bernard networked with officials willing to sponsor the training of black psychiatrists. For example, Bernard made contact with Dr. Franklin McLean, a Chicago physiologist who set up the National Medical Fellowships fund in 1946. The fund supported postgraduate training in medical specialties for minority physicians.[102] That year, she also learned of an administrator in the Veterans Administration that had been breaking down racial barriers for black psychiatric residents. Dr. Florence Powdermaker was the director of the VA's postwar residency training program for psychiatrists, awarding stipends and placement opportunities. To her surprise, Bernard discovered that Powdermaker was "most interested and effective in regard to the training of Negro psychiatrists." At the 1946 APA meeting, Powdermaker told Bernard that "she welcomes the submission of any Negro psychiatrists who are interested in training to be sent directly to her." She doled out stipends regardless of race and even helped place awardees with the only three VA training centers that accepted African Americans.[103]

Using these connections, Bernard created "suitable openings" for African Americans seeking psychiatric residency.[104] Bernard later recalled that her "office became a sort of unofficial vocational counseling center for would-be black psychiatrists" between 1942 and 1944.[105] In 1944, she helped Dr. Charles Brown net a National Medical Fellowship and become Bellevue's first African American psychiatric resident.[106] By 1945 Bernard took on the dual responsibility of screening all of New York's black candidates for the National Medical Fellowship and securing them psychiatric residencies through the VA.[107] In this way, she tried to locate fellowships and residencies for three black medical students, all of whom became notable Harlem Hospital psychiatrists: Dr. Elizabeth B. Davis, Dr. June Jackson Christmas, and Lt. Ice's friend, Dr. James L. Curtis.[108]

Unafraid to make use of her professional position, Bernard broke down racial barriers for her recruits. By 1946, she had already become a well-established psychiatrist with a long list of highly respectable affiliations. Besides having a private practice and consulting job with numerous agencies, she had become a professor at the Columbia University College of Physicians and Surgeons. Bernard even helped found the university's Psychoanalytic Clinic for Training and Research. Using these various positions, she created professional entry points within New York for some of her top recruits. Rutherford B. Stevens and Margaret Lawrence were two of the people she helped to obtain positions in psychiatry.

Bernard helped secure employment positions and professional development opportunities for Dr. Rutherford B. Stevens. Dr. Stevens had completed a VA residency at Karl Menninger's famous clinic and published an article in the *American Journal of Psychiatry* on his VA work with black soldiers.[109] After he arrived in New York, Bernard "sponsored him in obtaining" positions with the CSS and the Northside Center for Child Development, Harlem agencies that she worked for in some capacity.[110] She also introduced him to the liberal wing of psychiatry, creating a position for him within the racial-justice-oriented Group for the Advancement of Psychiatry's Committee on Social Issues in 1946.[111]

The case of Dr. Lawrence best illustrates what Bernard herself described as her "expressed interest in furthering the efforts of qualified Negro physicians to seek and secure psychoanalytic training."[112] Bernard opened several doors for Margaret Lawrence, Manhattan's first black female psychiatrist. Under circumstances that are not entirely clear, Bernard successfully persuaded her former head resident Nolan D. C. Lewis to break the Psychiatric Institute's long-standing pattern of racial exclusion and accept Lawrence as its first African American in 1947.[113] Once she had secured this residency for Lawrence, Bernard, as a Columbia University professor, successfully recommended Dr. Lawrence for analytic training there.[114] Since psychoanalytic training required that the trainee undergo analysis herself, Bernard pushed the process along by handpicking another racial liberal to serve as her analyst.[115]

In her final year of participation within the CWCCH, Bernard urged its leaders to support her professional recruitment efforts. She argued that her work in this area would necessarily help achieve another of her goals for Harlem: an expanded mental hygiene clinic at Harlem Hospital with both inpatient and outpatient services. In 1945 she told the CWCCH member Wolf Schwabacher that if Harlem was to have its own mental hygiene clinic, it needed more black psychiatrists. She argued that even though a "need for a mental hygiene clinic in Harlem is unquestioned . . . the chief difficulty lies in the shortage of suitable Negro psychiatrists to head it up." Although Bernard's efforts in breaking down racial barriers within psychiatry did not depend on the CWCCH in any direct way, she still insisted that the CWCCH recognize central Harlem's need for black psychiatrists.[116]

Combating Racial Discrimination in the NYC Child Welfare System

The CWCCH did actively help Polier and other racial liberals on the Domestic Relations Court achieve one of their long-standing goals: the systematic desegregation of New York City's private childcare agencies. Even though these charities received public funds to take neglected children placed by the Domestic Relations Court, they still retained the right to reject children on the basis of skin color. La Guardia's three appointees to the bench—judges Polier, Sicher, and Bolin—had long complained of this discriminatory arrangement. The bench's entrenched religious conservatives ensured that it remained inviolate, however. Entering the 1940s, it was clear that the court was not going to reform itself anytime soon.

In 1942 the CWCCH helped end this impasse. The organized black freedom struggle provided racial liberals with the political muscle needed to legislate racial fairness into New York's child-welfare system. In 1941, A. Philip Randolph's threat of an all-black March on Washington convinced Franklin D. Roosevelt to create the Fair Employment Practices Commission, and Harlem legislators successfully proposed equal-employment bills in the New York State Assembly.[117] The CWCCH also advocated legislation as a means to achieve racial justice. Convinced that racism within the juvenile-justice system constituted a breach of civil rights, the CWCCH helped Polier alter the terms of the city's arrangement with the private agencies. With the aid of both Poliers, the Subcommittee on Crime and Delinquency drafted a "Race Discrimination Amendment" to the charitable institutions' appropriation of the New York City budget. On April 27, 1942, the Board of Estimates unanimously voted to accept the change. The rule mandated that any private agency that rejected a child on account of race would lose its city funding.[118]

At Justice Polier's insistence, the CWCCH even monitored how the Race Discrimination Amendment worked. In October 1942, the first month the amendment took effect, all but five Protestant agencies agreed to accept at least some black children. On October 13, the CWCCH Subcommittee on Crime and Delinquency lodged a formal complaint against those offenders with William Hodson, the city's Commissioner of the Department of Welfare.[119] Not surprisingly, Polier's professional interest in the enforcement of the law kept this issue on the CWCCH agenda. Polier suspected that most agencies ignored the new law, so the CWCCH subcommittee kept track of the numbers of services that complied with the Race Discrimination Amendment. On October 23, 1943, the subcommittee found that "125 Negro children are now in institutions where they would not have been before the race discrimination amendment was passed."[120] Later, Polier discovered that private institutions, such as Children's Village, did circumvent the law. They refused black children on specious yet technically nonracial grounds, a pattern that many New York agencies continued to follow well into the 1960s.[121]

Nonetheless, CWCCH support emboldened Children's Court judges to criticize private childcare agencies. Polier took part in an investigation of the Children's Shelter.[122] Operated by the private Society for the Prevention of Cruelty to Children (SPCC), the Children's Shelter had been only a temporary shelter. Yet during the 1943 overcrowding crisis, the Shelter became the Children's Court's top long-term placement option for young black Harlemites.[123] In October, allegations of staff neglect and rampant misbehavior among the predominantly black residents caught the court's attention. The court formed an investigatory committee that included Polier and other CWCCH members.[124]

In January 1944, Polier coauthored the Committee on Institutions' scathing indictment of the Children's Shelter. The committee alleged that the facility did not adequately care for its interracial population.[125] Unsurprisingly, the psychiatric point of view informed her committee's expectations.[126] The investigators condemned the institution for containing "no social workers, no recreational leaders, no psychiatric facilities."[127] They concluded that the SPCC management was "uninformed . . . as to the essential standards of child care" and had "wrought incalculable harm to thousands of children entrusted to its care."[128]

After the release of the report to the press in 1944, the city shut down the Children's Shelter, removing the overwhelmingly black clientele to a new municipal shelter. Nevertheless, this did not mean that Polier's championing of black children's emotional needs won over the La Guardia administration. Even though the committee's report did factor into the mayor's decision, this is not evidence of a wholesale institutional shift in childcare standards. The committee also reported that the SPCC neglected the children's basic physical needs. Perhaps those allegations had struck the proper chord with authorities.[129]

Nevertheless, by war's end, the assumptions behind color-blind psychiatry gained a more solid footing within the Domestic Relations Court. La Guardia's 1942 appointment of Hubert T. Delany, a rising leader in Harlem's black freedom struggle, further increased the presence of liberals and leftists on the bench. A Harlem resident since 1919, he was the first black graduate of Yale Law School. As a civil-rights activist, Delany understood the black freedom struggle in broad terms. He opposed and battled a wide range of injustices—from job discrimination to police brutality and European imperialism.[130] Even before he joined the bench, Polier counted him an ally on the NAACP, the leftist National Lawyers Guild formed in 1937, and the CWCCH, where he proved an able proponent of her pro-psychiatry agenda.[131]

With Delany's assistance, Polier decided to solve the Warwick State Training School mystery: namely, did it actually practice racially progressive childcare? Superintendent Herbert D. Williams had skillfully dodged allegations of misconduct, rough discipline, corporal punishment, and racism since 1937. Yet on April 28, 1945, Polier and Delany finally caught his staff in the act. When the CWCCH veterans Polier and Delany arrived unannounced that day in Warwick, it became clear that a "surprised" assistant superintendent Simon Fletcher had not been coached for the visit. Unsure as to what he was supposed to conceal, he inadvertently confirmed some of the judges' worst fears. He admitted that, as head disciplinarian, he regularly ignored the emotional needs of his largely black population. He never consulted the clinic on problem cases, relying on fear and humiliation to punish his charges. He even went so far as to ridicule students in front of the judges.[132] They then put all of this damning information in a report. Within months, former and current Warwick employees came forward, affirming the allegations.[133] Whistle-blowers even leveled new charges, accusing Fletcher of regularly administering corporal punishment and disciplining black and white youths differently.[134]

The Board of Justice's reaction to the report signaled a change in thinking within the juvenile-justice system. Acting Presiding Justice W. Bruce Cobb defended the veracity of Delany and Polier's accusations. In the face of both the Warwick administration and the State Department of Social Welfare's claims that the judges had distorted the facts, the Board of Justices stood by their colleagues.[135] Simon Fletcher acceded to mounting pressure and resigned his post. According to Polier, Fletcher's successor "asked the [school's] psychiatrist and a social worker to end the reign of terror enforced by his precedessor [sic]."[136] Polier's expectation that modern childcare ought to be delivered without reference to race had apparently gained some institutional acceptance within New York's system of child welfare.

Conclusion

During World War II, Justine Wise Polier, Viola Bernard, and Max Winsor convinced Harlem leaders that racial inequality within the child-welfare system merited the civil-rights movement's attention. The City-Wide Citizens Committee for Harlem's timely support enabled them to continue battling institutional racism in mental health care despite severe budget cuts threatening the Bureau of Child Guidance and the Domestic Relations Court between 1942 and 1945. Even though the CWCCH could not save Polier's Domestic Relations Court treatment clinic, the organization placed its stamp of approval on several successful policies. With the Harlem Project, African American children received psychiatric care in their neighborhoods. With the passage of the Race Discrimination Amendment to the city budget in 1942, it was now more difficult for private agencies to reject black children placed by the court. Emboldened, Polier even launched new investigations of discriminatory childcare providers. In promoting these public-policy initiatives, the CWCCH integrated the ongoing battle against race-based health disparities within the local black freedom struggle.

Racial liberals within the BCG and the Children's Court did not simply impose their own vision of Harlem's mental health needs on the CWCCH. Instead, their wartime experience with local black activists expanded the scope of their agenda. Moving beyond a singular focus on the African American children their institutions served, these civil servants finally considered the mental health disparities facing African American adults. Bernard even made the recruitment of black psychiatrists her personal mission.

When the war concluded, more and more psychiatrists assumed that blacks and whites shared the same psychological capacities. Although this assumption was a growing national trend, it was definitely more pronounced in New York, where it had already informed public policy, psychiatric practice, the psychiatric literature, and even mental hygiene films. In one sense, published work treating the black psyche in race-neutral terms amounted to psychiatry's recognition of the black community's "common humanity." Yet this "universalist recognition" was not an unmediated process.[137] Including African Americans within the human race as equals involved a definite shift in the way psychiatrists imagined the black race fit within the most fundamental of all human social frameworks: gender.

Chapter Five

The Quiet One

Racial Representation in Popular Media and Psychiatric Literature, 1942–53

The Quiet One debuted in New York City in 1948. This Academy Award–nominated film tells the fictional story of Donald Peters, a young African American sent from Harlem to live at the Wiltwyck School for Boys in the Catskill Mountains. Hailed by most critics as an authentic and medically accurate portrayal of juvenile delinquency,[1] the film was produced on location with the full cooperation of Wiltwyck, a private reform institution run by Justine Wise Polier, Viola W. Bernard, and other New Yorkers committed to preventing juvenile delinquency in central Harlem's black community.

Despite otherwise rave reviews, at least one New York psychiatrist expressed dissatisfaction with the film. Hilde Mosse was among the city's growing number of race-blind clinicians. She had experience treating Harlemites. Mosse branded *The Quiet One* a "misleading" deception, claiming it grossly distorted the reality of central Harlem's slums. Because "the audience is led to believe that they are seeing a film about juvenile delinquency in general," rather than one about the special emotional challenges facing African Americans growing up in a racist society, Mosse wrote off the film as a dangerous misrepresentation of both black life and delinquency in Harlem.[2]

In the Northern civil-rights movement, many antiracists expressed concern with media representations of race. By the late 1940s, social scientists challenged racial prejudice and the depiction of African Americans in popular culture. Some historians have understood these efforts as separate from and even at odds with efforts to change the lives of actual blacks. They argue that racial liberals combating racial stereotypes tended to see racism as a personal problem, focusing on eliminating simple racial prejudice rather than confronting institutional racism. In this view, the civil-rights movement was split between those who sought to change the hearts and minds of whites and those who sought to alter life outcomes for African Americans.[3]

Nevertheless, this model of a bifurcated civil-rights movement may not be the best way to understand why Bernard and Mosse were both so interested in the media representation of race. In fact, their efforts to combat racist imagery were inseparable from the battle against psychiatric racism. The issue of racial representation only arose when the circulation of racist ideas "denied some individuals and groups the possibility of participating on a par with others" in New York's system of mental health care.[4] As long as ideas of black inferiority justified the neglect of the emotional needs of Harlem's residents, the predominance of those ideas constituted an unjust barrier to the equal allocation of medical resources.

Antiracist clinicians used the mass media to generate support for new private institutions, largely because efforts to meet blacks' emotional needs through the public sector had stalled. Confronted with entrenched racism and a Cold War climate inhospitable to the interracial expansion of social services, activists hedged their bets and sought out mental health alternatives.[5] Private facilities such as the Wiltwyck School and Hilde Mosse's Lafargue Mental Hygiene Clinic were supposed to compensate for governmental neglect of Harlem's needs. To solicit funds for these new institutions, their promoters relied on advertising, print media, and even film. These antiracists attempted to convince potential donors to invest in private psychiatric care for black Harlem.

What follows examines both the content of antiracist representations of blackness and the controversies they engendered. It illuminates how Wiltwyck's administration used advertising and film to convince potential donors that its black reform-school students deserved access to psychiatric care because their race was psychologically capable of benefiting from it. To defuse crude stereotypes about blacks and Harlem, African American children were depicted in ways that downplayed both race and place. Through *The Quiet One* and other projects, Wiltwyck's boosters hoped that white audiences would recognize the common humanity of blacks and whites in their shared possession of emotional depth, psychological potential, and internal suffering. Also highlighted in this chapter is the role that the reification of gender conventions played in the process of reimagining the black race as the white race's psychological equal.

Some antiracist psychiatrists disagreed with the Wiltwyck boosters' decision to ignore differences of race and place. In postwar New York, not everyone who accepted psychiatric universalism was a racial liberal. Racial liberals—such as Bernard and the Wiltwyck directors—expected that racial inequalities in wealth, health, and social outcomes would end once government authorities made opportunities for individual advancement more available to African Americans. Not all color-blind psychiatrists in New York were so convinced. The Lafargue Clinic leaned further to the left than did Wiltwyck's Board of Directors. Lafargue's staff believed that America's economic, political, and social systems required a more thorough restructuring before racism's effects could be undone. Dr. Mosse argued that *The Quiet One's* refusal to acknowledge and explain the existence of racial inequality actually squandered a teaching opportunity. The Lafargue clinical team wished that audiences had been shown that Harlem's juvenile delinquency rate was not the effect of some weakness in African American families, but rather the symptom of far more serious structural flaws within American society.

New York's antiracist clinicians did not agree on the best way to portray black delinquents on-screen. They did agree that the psychiatric literature should not include ideas they deemed racist. The last section of this chapter treats their vitriolic response to *The Mark of Oppression*, a landmark civil-rights-era text. Dr. Abram Kardiner and Lionel Ovesey's controversial book argued that racism irrevocably damaged black psyches. Despite their political disagreements, Wiltwyck supporters and Lafargue Clinic staff all refuted this popular work, charging it with racism. Both camps felt that the book's focus on black psychological difference jeopardized efforts to increase African Americans' access to psychotherapy. Claims of intractable racial difference had long justified the denial of equal opportunities. These New Yorkers countered such claims, encouraging a medical discourse of psychological sameness between the races. By changing the way race was represented, antiracists aimed to change the way resources were distributed.

Selling Wiltwyck as a "Therapeutic Environment"

When Polier and other professionals from New York's courts and schools became the Wiltwyck School's Board of Directors in 1942, they wanted to give preteen black offenders a therapeutic alternative to the abysmal state training schools.[6] The board envisioned an institution that could adequately handle the psychological needs of central Harlem's delinquents. Despite the directors' optimism, questions soon emerged as to whether Wiltwyck actually was a "therapeutic environment."[7] Conflicts between caseworkers and administration over protocol and procedure continued over the course of the next five years, leading to the departure of the entire casework department at the end of 1947.[8]

In 1948, two outside surveys declared Wiltwyck therapeutically ineffective. Deputy Commissioner Lee Dowling of New York State's Department of Social Welfare criticized the school for failing to integrate mental hygiene principles into its everyday operation.[9] Ironically, he claimed that Wiltwyck had committed some of the same psychologically insensitive violations that certain Wiltwyck board members had accused the state training schools of perpetrating. Dowling deplored the prevalence of corporal punishment and the lack of both "psychiatrically trained caseworkers" and lay counselors with any mental hygiene training.[10] A similar survey by Dr. Fritz Mayer of Ohio's Bellefair reform school put it more bluntly: "Wiltwyck is not a treatment institution at this time . . . but is mainly a custodial institution."[11]

Amid these allegations, administrators continued to tout the school's devotion to the psychological rehabilitation of troubled African American youth. Wiltwyck's Board of Directors, composed largely of individuals who supported the Harlem Project and the Domestic Relations Court treatment clinic, had been careful about how it presented the institution to potential allies and donors. Throughout the 1940s, board members consistently portrayed the school's mission as a therapeutic one, even as its staff deviated from that in practice.[12]

In a 1945 letter to another clinician, Bernard described Wiltwyck as a school for "Negro boys under twelve, where we are trying to do a progressive mental hygiene job, including psychiatric and case work service."[13]

Owing to its dependence on philanthropy, Wiltwyck administrators shaped how the school was portrayed in the media. In 1945, the novelist and Harlem resident Richard Wright agreed to write a fund-raising brochure championing Wiltwyck's therapeutic effect on young, damaged black psyches.[14] The board created a fund-raising and public relations department to help sell the public on the institution's therapeutic promise, and administrators continued to generate positive press accounts. In 1944, the Brooklyn YMCA administrator Hans Maeder wrote the Wiltwyck director Robert Cooper, thanking him for allowing a visit to the campus. Maeder was impressed to find "mentally and socially maladjusted boys at ease and in happiness," and he detailed the school's impact on the boys he met there.[15] Cooper thought that Maeder's glowing account would "make excellent publicity material."[16]

Maeder's story became the basis for an article published in the board member Marshall Field III's left-liberal New York newspaper, *PM*. The story made an impact. It generated letters of support from readers and donations for the school, yet failed to produce a deluge of new benefactors.[17] *PM* catered to a small niche of liberals and radicals already inclined to see Wiltwyck's value.[18] But what about more conservative mainstream readers? Could they be persuaded to accept that black juvenile delinquents deserved the same psychologically sensitive care their white counterparts received?

To sell Wiltwyck's psychiatric mission to a wider audience, the board would have to challenge the public's perception of Harlem and its children. The racialist assumption that African Americans were natural troublemakers was not the only conceptual hurdle.[19] Even if audiences became convinced that this rural reform school had found a way to understand and treat the black psyche, questions would remain about that treatment's long-term practicality. Would this valuable work unravel once children returned to the streets of central Harlem, a region that had become nearly synonymous in the 1940s with the worst that urban living had to offer—poverty, slums, crime?[20] Why would anyone donate money to help those who, according to conventional wisdom, were beyond saving?

Wiltwyck's board needed to convince the charitable public that blacks were innately capable of benefiting from psychiatric care. To do that, these antiracist New Yorkers had to learn how to articulate their own largely unstated assumptions regarding the color-blind nature of the human psyche. In one sense, "changing images and representations of race" was new territory for these racial liberals.[21] This does not mean that their ongoing battle against racial inequality in the New York child-welfare system had never been a fight against racist ideas. On the contrary, their opposition to institutional racism had been made possible by a shift in the way they imagined that race mattered. If Polier and her cohort of civil servants and philanthropists did not all share the same color-blind understanding of the black psyche they would not have insisted on equal access to public mental health services. Until now, Polier and her allies never really had to unpack, theorize, and explain their position on race and psychology. For them, the proposition that the human psyche was an unraced space was intuited and taken for granted. It had never been discussed. Now they saw a need to translate their powerful yet inchoate feelings about race into a concrete and persuasive position for the unconverted.

"The Negro Patient": The Color-Blind Approach in the Psychiatric Literature

Between 1941 and 1950 a small but growing universalist strain in the psychiatric literature provided Wiltwyck's backers with a model for explicating their own racial assumptions.[22] Several articles and books had been published characterizing the "Negro patient" in race-neutral terms. These sympathetic representations of the African American psyche emerged in the midst of a wartime and postwar shift toward outpatient care, psychotherapy, and the treatment of emotional disorders. Prior to the war, white Southern asylum doctors working with the severely mentally ill had written much of the literature on black patients. Most of it was racialist. It was not always psychodynamic either. In contrast, psychiatrists toiling on World War II battlefields, in Veteran's Administration clinics, or in private outpatient facilities penned the new work on the "Negro patient." The patients they studied suffered from anxiety and stress, not severe mental illness.[23] The new authors took pains to illustrate how representative these patients were and how treatable their conditions were with minimal psychotherapy.

Although the new authors tended to examine adults rather than children, they still shared the Wiltwyck administrators' interest in representing the black patient's psyche in a race-neutral way. The authors were either black themselves or associates of Wiltwyck's board. For instance, the African Americans Walter Adams and Laynard Holloman worked at Chicago's black proprietary Provident Hospital. The black psychiatrist Dr. Rutherford Stevens and the white psychoanalyst Dr. Helen McLean of Chicago's Institute for Psychoanalysis were two of Bernard's colleagues on the Group for Advancement of Psychiatry's Committee on Social Issues in 1946.[24]

These new articles and monographs set the early standard for how antiracist psychiatrists should write about the black psyche. They shared much in common, and two patterns of presentation emerged that proved relevant to the Wiltwyck administration's goals. First, rather than disguise their patients' races, the writers emphasized that biological race did not clinically matter in psychiatric cases. Consequently, their publications boldly declared that the black psyche was neither racially inferior nor racially unique. In Dr. Adams's words, for the "mentally sick Negro patient . . . the core of his hidden problems . . . are the same kinds that haunt, enslave, torture, and degrade men of all races."[25] His fellow Chicagoan Dr. McLean went either further, dismissing racialism altogether. At the time, the psychiatric literature still abounded with statements that the black body was hardwired to respond to emotional stimuli in race-specific ways.[26] McLean and others explicitly repudiated that possibility, offering a color-blind style of psychiatry as the only acceptable approach to race. According to McLean, since "[biologically] the Negro differs, as far as we know, in no important attribute from other human beings," then "the Negro's fundamental human needs and . . . inherent [psychological] potentialities" must not be any different from those of whites.[27]

The second pattern, the one most central to Wiltwyck's mission, involved a reconceptualization of the relationship between race, gender, and the human psyche.[28] By insisting that psychiatric principles should describe the black psyche without reference to race, antiracist psychiatrists ascribed full humanity to blacks. To take color-blind analysis to its logical extension—to fully depict African Americans as universally human in their emotional makeup—meant that antiracists had to rethink how gender and race interacted in the development of the black psyche. Since gender was assumed to be the most natural of all social categories, the psychological nature of African Americans could not truly be thought of as racially indistinct from that of whites until psychiatrists presented black men and women as fundamentally male and female in nature.

"Boys Are Really the Same": (En)gendering the Black Psyche

The act of depicting the black psyche in a stark, gender-bifurcated manner was an essential stage in the development of a more color-blind psychiatry. American psychiatry had long been rooted in the assumption that male and female psyches were fundamentally different by nature. Such sexual binarism in affect was supposed to be an evolutionary advancement, further evidence of humanity's superiority.[29] Psychiatrists generally regarded blacks as an exception to this rule. Racial determinists recognized much less difference between the emotional makeup of black men and black women. Racialists deemed them equally oversexed and overwrought emotionally. This marked the black race as intrinsically less advanced and thus less human than the white race.[30]

Antiracist authors indicated that the gender gap between the psyches of black men and women was much wider and thus less exceptional than the psychiatric literature indicated. For example, when the psychoanalyst Helen McLean suggested that "men and women are not equal, they are different," she included her African American patients in this race-neutral declaration.[31] Expecting to see stark psychological differences between black men and black women, color-blind psychiatrists reified the alleged universality of their profession's gendered assumptions.[32] The discursive effect was clear: the more that black men and women appeared to differ from each other, the less the black race seemed to differ from the white race.

Yet psychiatrists did not regender the psychological color line by plugging African Americans into timeless gender categories. Gender constructions are mutable and historically specific phenomena. During and immediately after

World War II, tensions within the United States led many Americans to revitalize a rigid set of assumptions about the innate behavioral and emotional differences between men and women. Despite the increasing numbers of women engaged in the wartime and postwar workforce, for some this was also a period of renewed commitment to the idea that the heterosexual, nuclear family was our species' natural social unit.[33] Within such a climate, many recommitted themselves to the concomitant belief that men and women had fundamentally different yet complimentary natures—as breadwinners and homemakers.[34]

In the antiracist psychiatric literature of the 1940s, this renewed American gender conservatism[35] culturally mediated the race-neutral recasting of black men and women's essential natures.[36] In these writings, psychiatrists presented African American men and women as respectively driven by tendencies deemed universally masculine and feminine. Each gender was innately different. These differences made psychologically normal men and women compatible and it drove them toward the same goal: the formation of nuclear families. The authors agreed that black males and white males are all born with identical "strong aggressive drives." As adults they try to channel this innate masculine drive toward the manly goal of "security for himself and his family."[37] Black women and white women were depicted as having a maternal nature and an intrinsically female desire for men to take care of them.[38] Hence, the nuclear family, the centerpiece of the postwar American dream, was uniquely suited to serve the gender-specific needs and drives of all men and women, regardless of race.

Similarly, Wiltwyck's backers portrayed their school as uniquely suited to meet the universally masculine needs of its predominantly black student body. In Maeder's glowing account of Wiltwyck: "Boys are really the same, wherever we find them, [no matter] if they are now of another color or another creed."[39] Throughout the 1940s, Wiltwyck and its allies actively deployed this sentiment in their promotional material.[40] As a means for generating sympathy and potential support for the largely black student body, Wiltwyck boosters emphasized that these children only succumbed to delinquency in Harlem because they were boys rather than girls. What set Wiltwyck boys apart from well-behaved boys was that central Harlem had been unable to meet the Wiltwyck boys' masculine emotional needs. According to Wiltwyck's boosters, those psychological needs could best be met in the Catskill Mountains.

Juvenile Delinquents and Unmanageable Girls

Even the 1947 report of the Harlem Project—an effort organized and run by many of Wiltwyck's directors—argued that a stay in the country could do wonders for central Harlem's disruptive boys. Yet owing to its color-blind approach to gender norms, the report's writers, including Polier and Bernard, considered the treatment of disruptive girls to be another matter entirely. All troublemaking children were not created equal. Males were dubbed "juvenile delinquents." Females were labeled "unmanageable girls."[41] This was an important distinction, given that the Harlem Project's analysts asserted that even Harlem's "most 'unmanageable' girls could be adjusted within the regular school."[42]

Viola Bernard and the Harlem Project's Research Committee contended that female personalities were easier for Harlem's public schools to contain and treat. According to their line of reasoning, the well-adjusted female personality was largely the product of domestic spaces. Warm, close relationships forged in an intimate setting with a maternal figure, preferably the mother, enabled girls to become well-adjusted women. Reflecting the Harlem Project's condescending class bias, the Research Committee claimed that most unmanageable girls misbehaved because their working-class mothers did not give them enough love or attention. Still, a disruptive junior high girl could be set straight within Harlem if the school became the new locus of her emotional maturation.[43] Home, the site where a girl's emotional development was forged, could be replaced by another intimate setting such as a counselor's office. In private sessions conducted in these proxy domestic spaces, female psychiatrists, counselors, caseworkers, and teachers served as "mother substitutes" for these young women.[44] Given enough on-one-one attention, a Harlem school could redirect a troubled girl's emotional center away from both her home and her "inadequate mother."[45]

In contrast, the Harlem Project report warned that central Harlem's public schools could not offer similar therapeutic benefits to some African American male "juvenile delinquents." Misbehaved boys were more than simply the products of bad mothering and insufficient homes. Instead, the report presented the most emotionally disturbed male junior high students as products of Harlem's total environment. Mothers could not confine boys from fatherless homes to the domestic sphere the way they could daughters. Without a strong male presence, peer influence was expected to affect the development of boys more than it would girls. Seeking causes for male delinquency at J.H.S. 120, for example, the Research Committee drew attention to the "negative impact of these boys' deprivation, economically, socially, emotionally: their chaotic, poverty-burdened, overcrowded homes; their encirclement by gang warfare in the streets; their search for substitute parental interest and affection"—especially from a paternal role model.[46] Judging from this catalog of influences, the researchers determined that the private and public sides of Harlem had influenced the boys' emotional development. Yet they also made it clear that the male-dominated street was the primary bad influence.

Given the ubiquitous temptation that the public domain presented troubled boys, the Harlem Project report suggested that it was harder to help them cope with life in Harlem. Whereas a mother substitute might save even the most recalcitrant girl, the report intimated that more drastic changes were called for in the case of males. Driven by masculine impulses to seek out personal space, camaraderie, mentors, and outlets for aggression, fatherless boys met these needs in Harlem's gangs and underground economy. With insufficient classrooms, a dearth of male teachers, and scant after-school activities, the research committee deemed Harlem's public schools incapable of substantially altering these boys' life patterns.

Wiltwyck's supporters thus argued that the most intransigent Harlem boys needed more than mother substitutes: they required a substantial change of environment, a removal from Harlem to a new milieu. In 1942, Viola Bernard of the Special Child Guidance Harlem Unit recommended that one of P.S. 139's most troublesome boys would be unlikely to improve if he remained in Harlem: "I am acquainted with the Wiltwyck set-up and tried to weigh the boy's needs and what Wiltwyck offers. . . . It was my conclusion that the boy's best opportunity for improvement would be through several years of exposure to environmental and re-educational treatment in an atmosphere of mental-hygiene understanding, such as is offered at Wiltwyck."[47]

The Quiet One: Wiltwyck at the Movies

This image of Wiltwyck as a therapeutic last chance for Harlem's hard-to-reach African American boys eventually attracted the attention of filmmakers in 1946. Following World War II, the film industry became so interested in medical matters that a distinct "medical film genre" emerged.[48] Exploiting this trend, two aspiring Jewish American film auteurs, Janice Loeb and Helen Levitt, proposed to make a motion picture about Wiltwyck. The two young women were neighbors on New York City's Upper East Side and active in the modern art scene. Loeb was a researcher for the Museum of Modern Art (MOMA)[49] and Levitt an up-and-coming street photographer associated with the New York School of gritty, neorealist photography.[50] The two were initially attracted to Wiltwyck because Levitt's subjects, including those for her 1943 MOMA exhibition, hailed from the same neighborhoods as Wiltwyck boys.[51] According to Loeb, the duo's "interest in Wiltwyck ties in with the work we did and are doing, recording life in the streets of Negro and Porto-Rican [sic] Harlem."[52]

Levitt typically took photos of children playing in their own neighborhoods, demonstrating that an individual could only be understood in reference to his or her environment.[53] Similarly, Levitt and Loeb hoped their film would explain how Wiltwyck could rehabilitate a boy from Harlem's mean streets. As a street photographer, Levitt believed she could capture the human self's complexities on camera. Art collectors and critics agreed. MOMA's James Thrall Soby claimed that Levitt's art had "thrown a great deal of light on the psychology of city children in the poorer neighborhoods."[54] For Levitt and other New York School photographers, this psychology was the product of both nature and nurture: an assemblage of environmental conditioning, personal tendencies, and a basic capacity for emotional depth that all humans shared—regardless of race.[55] Levitt and Loeb wanted film audiences to see how a change of place could emotionally transform a child, in this case a black child from central Harlem.[56] To this end, the film would initially show how Harlem slum life could drive boys to engage in "symptomatic acts of delinquency." It would conclude by presenting Wiltwyck as a place of "therapy" and adjustment, where "the minimal needs of the child in terms of understanding, care, love, and attention" could be met.[57]

An employee of a private institution herself, Loeb was aware that bad publicity could jeopardize Wiltwyck's future. Given that the American Cancer Society and other health charities had successfully used film to raise funds, she had the same expectations for her Wiltwyck film.[58] So in her initial pitch, she repeatedly assured the school's Board of Directors that she and Levitt were humanist sympathizers whose "approach to the subject should stimulate support for Wiltwyck, support for the ideas of child care and treatment, and imply the need for other agencies like it." Loeb promised that the "basic philosophy of child care embodied in the film would be that of the Wiltwyck staff."[59]

Eager for good promotional material, the board agreed to Levitt and Loeb's plan to promote Wiltwyck's therapeutic reputation. It allowed production to commence, with the stipulation that their members retain control over the product. Such an arrangement was fairly common within the medical film genre.[60] Indeed, the two women had approached Wiltwyck because they wanted to make a medically accurate film.[61] As neorealists intent on creating "a great sense of reality and authenticity," they wanted to shoot on location with actual staff and students.[62] As was often the case, the filmmaker's "desire for accuracy matched [the] medical desire for control and led to close relationships" between the film industry and medical professionals.[63] In exchange for the right to use Wiltwyck's site, staff, and clients in the film, Film Documents Inc. agreed to allow the board to shape how the school and its population were depicted.[64]

Bernard served as the project's psychiatric adviser. She was intimately involved in brainstorming and script development.[65] Bernard met repeatedly with the producers and reviewed drafts of the final script. In the film's early stages, she spent time teaching the auteurs the "basic principles of interpersonal relations" and psychodynamics.[66] The psychiatrist became intimately involved in both character development and plotting the script. According to Bernard, "I met rather continuously with them in relation to what the people portrayed were like, how they felt, and what made them tick, while they knew a lot about that side too and were able to translate this into the film medium."[67] As psychiatric adviser, she helped "create the individual characters as valid human beings," meaning ones that emoted and behaved in ways she deemed "technically accurate from the standpoint of psychodynamics,"[68] and even convinced Levitt and Loeb to change scenes when they did not reflect the characters' profiles.[69]

Bernard spent most of her time helping Loeb and Levitt cast the protagonist Donald Peters as victim rather than villain. The film, directed by the Jewish American filmmaker Sidney Meyers, depicts Donald, an African American boy from Harlem whose chronic misbehavior lands him in Wiltwyck.[70] "Donald the victim" was not an easy sell. Traditionally, white Americans had been inclined to see such children as either racially predisposed to misbehavior or the products of weak discipline. To get a largely white audience to feel sorry for Donald, Bernard hoped that moviegoers would identify with the internal suffering that drove him to commit antisocial actions. Bernard urged the filmmakers to downplay what marked Donald as alien: his race and place of residence.

The entreaty to minimize certain social factors when explicating the protagonist's misbehavior may have come as a bit of a shock to Levitt and Loeb.[71] Consider that in their initial pitch, the filmmakers wanted "a major portion of the film to show the economic, social, and emotional conditions which produce the damaged child."[72] In their 1946 film treatment, Levitt and Loeb described Harlem as a land of "hostile street[s]" that "continue . . . to spawn [delinquents] by the thousands."[73] Bernard opposed the depiction of Harlem as a unique breeding ground for delinquents. She agreed that masculine street life helped cause delinquency. But other influences in a Harlem male's environment—including "cold and meaningless classrooms"—were also causal factors. So in her copy of the script, Bernard crossed out "spawn" and urged the filmmakers to minimize the role of Harlem's social conditions in emotionally wounding Donald. If the film too strongly suggested that Harlem, already popularly identified as a black, crime-ridden slum, was responsible for Donald's problems, a white audience might then be inclined to assume that his race and place of residence explained his behavior.[74]

Instead, Bernard urged the filmmakers to attribute the cause of Donald's emotional conflict and delinquency to two universally human factors, the first being gender difference. For the filmmakers to depict Donald as a "valid human being," they needed to frame his motivations and emotional states as typically male. If Film Documents Inc. presented Donald's actions on-screen as the natural, gender-specific reactions of a troubled young man, Bernard imagined that white audiences could then learn to see his race as a psychologically inconsequential trait. Throughout the project Bernard generally approved of the way the scripts handled the relationship between his gender, his affect, and his actions. In an early film treatment, Levitt and Loeb described the protagonist lashing out through violence and breaking windows. Bernard agreed with this characterization because child guidance experts generally considered acting-out behavior to be a typically masculine way of expressing frustration. Apparently Donald behaved the way Bernard expected an emotionally deprived boy of any race would act.[75]

Bernard also encouraged Levitt and Loeb to create a neglectful family as the primary cause of his problems. Wiltwyck board members believed that outside influences, including peers, shaped the psyches of boys more than they did girls. Yet these child guidance experts also expected families to exert a greater influence over any child's emotional development, regardless of gender. Polier and her fellow racial liberals assumed that a stable, two-parent family could meet a child's need for security better than other arrangements. So from the project's inception, Bernard supported the filmmakers' decision to make an unstable, emotionally cold, single-parent home the ultimate cause of Donald's descent into delinquency.[76] In the film's final cut, Meyers used home-centered scenes from the boy's past to visually demonstrate his family's neglect.

Bernard also backed the filmmakers' decision to make a father figure the source of Donald's emotional transformation in the Catskills. In the script, Levitt and Loeb detailed Wiltwyck's success in turning around boys from neglectful homes by providing a "stable and consistent environment" staffed with equally stable male role models.[77] Thus in *The Quiet One*, Donald develops an attachment to an African American counselor named Clarence,[78] a relationship described by the film narrator Gary Merrill as nothing short of an "important miracle." Donald becomes more affectionate, friendlier, and even improves his schoolwork. "Donald has come a long way with us," Merrill intones, "thanks largely to his friendship with Clarence."[79]

Bernard supported the characterization of Wiltwyck's male personnel as the school's best therapeutic tool for several reasons. First, Bernard wanted the audience to realize that Donald's removal from Harlem to upstate New York was not the only reason his life improved. A simple change in locale was "not enough without the human element involving warmth, kindness and interest."[80] The film should emphasize that Wiltwyck offered Donald and other boys the chance to develop healing relationships with well-adjusted men. In her estimation, Donald would be likely to seek out a male counselor as a paternal figure. He would want a relationship with Clarence. According to Bernard, "Donald, at a certain stage would try and emulate a grown man he could like and admire."[81] Their bond could "slowly help straighten him out." She expected that a male role model would meet his gender-specific "healthy growth needs" much better than his female-heavy family and school back home.[82]

To visually demonstrate Clarence's—and Wiltwyck's—healthy masculine influence, the film shows Donald actively emulating his counselor. Bernard strongly suggested to Levitt and Loeb that mimesis would be a healthy phase of Donald's adjustment, and "the film-makers, with their skills and control of the medium, devised the specific form of Donald's positive identification with Clarence."[83] The director Meyers presents Donald's imitation of Clarence as healthy and manly. Donald watches Clarence smoke, lights his cigarettes for him, and tries on Clarence's blazer. In the most memorable scene, Donald watches Clarence shave and then mimes this quintessential modern adult male ritual. The narrator Merrill remarks that Donald not only sees himself in the shaving mirror but also sees in Clarence the "man he hopes to be like."[84]

Bernard was confident that this characterization presented Donald's blackness as if it had no bearing on his emotions or behavior. In a letter to a colleague, she noted that "at no place in the film is there any direct mention of Donald's being Negro."[85] *The Quiet One* was never intended to be a film about black youth, Harlem, or the psychological problems affecting blacks. Instead, the film's deracialized dialogue, provided by James Agee, universalized Donald's subjectivity, presenting his internal world as human and male rather than intrinsically Negro. If the movie achieved this color-blind effect, Bernard imagined that white audiences would "emotionally identify" with Donald, recognizing his shared humanity in the cinematic representation of his emotional pain.[86] The board hoped that sympathy for Donald would translate into increased financial support for Wiltwyck, a place uniquely equipped to save boys like him.

When the film debuted in 1948, Bernard and her fellow Wiltwyck administrators used the film as a public-relations vehicle. They promoted the school's therapeutic image, sponsoring screenings of *The Quiet One* in 1950–51 for "publicity and fund-raising purposes, in private homes, schools, and churches."[87] Wiltwyck's boosters hoped the film's powerful visuals and jargon-free narration would help potential donors understand how the campus rehabilitated Harlem's black delinquents. Bernard especially wanted the public to learn that Wiltwyck's therapy worked with those students because of the universality of the principles on which the treatment was based.[88] Wiltwyck could handle troubled black boys because boys were essentially all the same—regardless of race.

Some critics and moviegoers did watch *The Quiet One* as a race-neutral story. Judging from film reviews and letters to Wiltwyck administrators, some audiences understood that the film should not be read as a movie about blacks only. From 1948 to 1949, fellow psychiatrists, film critics, medical societies, schools, and a wide range of health professionals and colleagues of Bernard hailed *The Quiet One* as an exemplary mental hygiene film. By this they meant that the film succeeded in communicating general, race-blind psychiatric principles in an easy-to-understand fashion.[89]

By treating juvenile delinquency as largely a psychological matter, *The Quiet One* effectively transformed central Harlem's African American juvenile delinquents into objects of sympathy for some viewers. Film critics, including those at *The New Republic* and *The Nation*, saw the movie as a lesson on how delinquents, black or white, were really emotionally deprived boys who needed Wiltwyck's help.[90] *New York Times* critic Bowsley Crowther agreed. He suggested that "the race of the boy is a circumstance. For this is essentially the story of any child who has hungered for love. . . . It is also a clear illumination of the psychology of such a child and of the delicate handling and patience required to help him find some heart and strength."[91] As Bernard intended, Crowther and other cosmopolitan critics read Donald's race and place of residence as inconsequential details in a story about the very real suffering poor parenting could cause.

Criticizing *The Quiet One*: Color-Blind Psychiatry Divided in New York City

Still, not all racially progressive psychiatrists in New York approved of *The Quiet One's* portrayal of Harlem's black juvenile delinquents. Hilde Mosse, a German Jewish psychiatrist, was one of the film's toughest critics. Employed with Queens General Hospital and Quaker Emergency Medical Center, she was not affiliated with Polier or any of her colleagues. Nonetheless, Mosse and some of her coworkers also practiced both race-blind universalism and social psychiatry—and in Harlem no less.

There was a good reason why Mosse was so interested in making sure the public understood what made a Harlem delinquent tick. After her clinical hours were over in Queens on Tuesday and Thursday nights, Mosse regularly volunteered at central Harlem's Lafargue Mental Hygiene Clinic, a facility she had cofounded in March 1946. Located in the basement of St. Philip's Protestant

Episcopal Church, this facility offered free outpatient psychiatric care on 133rd Street and St. Nicholas Avenue. Similar to Wiltwyck, the little clinic was also run by antiracists who believed that race did not determine an individual's psychology. The biggest difference was that the Lafargue Clinic's staff was composed entirely of unpaid volunteers. In contrast to any program that Polier or Bernard had established, this clinic did not primarily treat black children. Catering mostly to black adults, Lafargue volunteers also served the poor, the middle class, whites, Latinos, war veterans, the elderly, and children.[92]

Despite these facilities' shared commitment to Harlem, no alliance developed between the Wiltwyck School and Lafargue Clinic. Apparently it was not for lack of trying on the part of Lafargue founders, one of whom was Fredric Wertham, a colleague of Mosse's at Queens General Hospital. He and Mosse served as the clinic's primary physicians. Wertham claimed that he had repeatedly asked the La Guardia administration to open a public mental hygiene clinic in Harlem. His requests fell on deaf ears.[93] Before the Lafargue Clinic opened in 1946, Wertham had made an attempt to win the financial support of Wiltwyck's benefactors. He had contacted Louis Weiss, a lawyer and adviser to the Wiltwyck board member Marshall Field III and his philanthropic Field Foundation. Despite getting some initial interest, neither Field nor any other Wiltwyck benefactor provided the Lafargue Clinic with financial assistance.[94]

Mosse, Wertham, and his wife, the sculptor Florence Hesketh, suspected that Justine Wise Polier's "La Guardia Liberals" had sabotaged their efforts to secure Field's support.[95] All three never publicly disclosed their resentment of Polier and Wiltwyck's board. But their interactions with other Lafargue associates reveal just how much they reviled and distrusted the Domestic Relations Court judge. After attending a dinner at Louis Weiss's in 1945, Wertham came away with the impression that the Harlem Project and Wiltwyck School did more harm than good for "children in Harlem." In his private correspondence, Wertham wrote: "A woman like Judge Polier is really like a mass-murderer of children," doing little but incarcerating them or keeping them under the watch of government authorities, leaving them "really crushed so that they can never come back again."[96] Hesketh claimed that "Judge Polier . . . walks around the 70 Wiltwyck reformatory kids as proof that Harlem is well looked after! Uses that as a stick to prevent anything else."[97] All three were convinced that Polier disapproved of their clinic. They firmly believed that "the liberals have not helped us" because Polier had blackballed them.[98] Mosse and Wertham latched on to any gossip they could get regarding Wiltwyck, Polier, Bernard, and the Harlem Project.[99] Wertham even devoted an entire Lafargue staff conference to the failings of the 1947 Harlem Project report.[100]

It is not exactly clear why this rift developed between the Lafargue Clinic and the Wiltwyck board members they maligned as "La Guardia liberals."[101] Some commentators blamed Wertham. Among psychiatrists, he had a reputation for being overbearing, dictatorial, and prone to conspiracy theories. Even so, political differences must have played a role in the rift. Wertham and Mosse did not consider themselves racial liberals. They were more left of center than

Polier and Bernard. That should not come as a surprise, given that Wertham and Mosse named their clinic after Karl Marx's son-in-law, Paul Lafargue—the founder of France's Communist Party. Mosse and Wertham were not Communist Party members, however. Both were influenced by Marxist theory, believing that many of the emotional ills plaguing Harlem's black community were structural in origin. Although she never publicly disclosed her ideological leanings, Mosse was privately a Trotskyist. She felt that "socialism can be made to work" and considered juvenile delinquency one of the "capitalist diseases."[102] Wertham and Mosse regarded racial liberalism with skepticism. Both thought it unlikely that racial inequality would diminish because bureaucrats included more African Americans within New York's social services. Wertham argued that the "hostile world" in which that system of services operated needed restructuring before racial inequality could ever decline.[103]

Without the patronage of the Field or Rosenwald fortunes, Lafargue Clinic was dependent on private donations and charity from individuals.[104] Fortunately, the Lafargue Clinic's founders understood the value of good publicity.[105] They actively positioned the clinic in both the national and local press.[106] Indeed, four founders were already established writers: the Harlem-based novelists Richard Wright and Ralph Ellison, the journalist Earl Brown, and Fredric Wertham—a public intellectual who had published some of the first books on forensic psychiatry.[107] All of the Lafargue staffers, including the head psychiatrist Wertham, were very careful about what they said to the press. Wertham was a masterful publicist. In most press accounts, he served as the chief source of information about the clinic, promoting its mission in each interview.[108]

Lafargue's founders used promotional media to elicit sympathy for the people they initially sought to help: Harlem's black delinquents. Even though most of the patients were adults, the men and women who started the clinic had originally intended to address juvenile delinquency.[109] Two of the founders, Wright and Wertham, were deeply invested in the matter, having already contributed substantially to the ongoing public discourse on the subject. Wright's 1940 best-selling novel, *Native Son*, was an exploration of the mind of the young black murderer Bigger Thomas. Wertham's 1946 nonfiction work, *Dark Legend*, was one of the first psychiatric case studies of a teenage killer written for a mainstream audience.[110] Not surprisingly, then, Lafargue's founders thought they knew how to get the public to see Harlem's delinquents in the most sympathetic light.

Clearly Lafargue administrators would have preferred that *The Quiet One* tell its audience that Donald's race and place of residence *did* matter. Both the Lafargue Clinic's media coverage between 1946 and 1948 and Mosse's review of the film reveal this stance. Were Lafargue's staff, then, racial determinists? No. As Wertham claimed: "We're simply here to treat [blacks] like other human beings."[111] Moreover, Wertham, influenced by the anthropologist Ashley Montagu and by Marxism, was one of the few within the wartime medical community to publicly declare that biological race was not "real," it was a social construct.[112] As social psychiatrists, Wiltwyck and Lafargue's clinicians both believed that structural inequalities facing an African American in Harlem helped make the experience of delinquency there different from that of a white child living elsewhere.[113] What set Mosse and her Lafargue colleagues apart was the conviction that *The Quiet One* had a moral obligation to let the movie audience know that.

Mosse criticized *The Quiet One* for failing to inform its predominantly white audience that juvenile delinquency was an acute problem in Harlem. Neither the film's scenes nor the narration indicated how many "Donalds" there were. As a result, it was possible—but not likely—for an uninformed moviegoer to fail to appreciate the scope of the problem. Presumably few moviegoers were unfamiliar with Harlem's growing postwar reputation in the media and popular culture as a crime-ridden, gang-infested slum. Although *The Quiet One* sidestepped that perception, contemporary media coverage of Lafargue addressed it. In press accounts of Lafargue published between 1946 and 1948, youth crime was depicted as nearly rampant in Harlem.[114] What is more, Mosse also claimed in her film review that juvenile delinquents there were much more dangerous and violent than lonely Donald with his penchant for breaking windows. "Children in Harlem," she opined, "are subject to much more violence" and pervasive gang intimidation "than is portrayed in the film."[115]

The Lafargue Clinic's promoters also realized that potential donors would want to know *why* Harlem's African American population apparently had such a problem with juvenile delinquency. Thus they stressed that socioeconomic forces beyond the average African American family's control were ultimately responsible for Harlem's high rate of youth arrests. Mosse's biggest criticism of *The Quiet One* was that it offered up the African American family as the sole cause for juvenile delinquency in Harlem. Mosse lambasted the film for blaming Donald's maladjustment on his family without providing audiences some structural reason why his family became so unstable. Consequently, family members are reduced to little more than one-dimensional villains "whose actions appear vicious and senseless." Because the film "points the finger at the individual where society is the dynamic factor," Mosse worried that audiences would come away convinced that Harlem was prone to juvenile delinquency because African Americans did not know how to raise children properly.[116]

Instead, Mosse and her colleagues insisted that the public should be made aware that the "social implications of racial discrimination" were chiefly responsible for the prevalence of juvenile delinquency in Harlem. Donald's family members, the film's apparent villains, were not solely responsible for the boy's troubles because they themselves were the "victims of social, economic, and racial discrimination."[117] For Lafargue, racial injustice had transformed central Harlem into a place where it was difficult for black families to fulfill the emotional needs of their children.[118] In contrast to *The Quiet One*, Lafargue's news accounts do not blame the parents. Rather, these stories are sympathetic and explain how these parents' racially segmented housing options, unfulfilling menial jobs, and long work hours did not make for happy homes.[119]

Mosse also criticized the film for failing to indicate that Donald's emotional problems had gone unnoticed because racism left Harlem with little psychiatric care. In both Mosse's review and the Lafargue coverage, readers learn that Harlem lacked the resources needed to fight juvenile delinquency.[120] According to Richard Wright, "Harlem's high rate of juvenile delinquency . . . stem[s] not from biological predilection toward crime existing in Negroes, but from an almost total lack of community services to cope with the problems of Harlem's individuals."[121] From this vantage point, Film Documents Inc. ignored racial inequality, giving audiences no reason to believe that Donald's immediate environment was devoid of medical care they took for granted.

Whereas *The Quiet One*'s creators worked to get white audiences to identify with a single black individual, the Lafargue Clinic wanted that public to feel that same sympathy for Harlem's broader black population. As the image of the black delinquent was becoming a synecdoche for black Harlem in popular culture, Mosse and her colleagues did not challenge this metaphorical link. Instead, they sought to influence the meaning of this imagined linkage and generate support for both Harlem and Lafargue's efforts to serve that maligned community. Lafargue's media coverage presents the emotional suffering of the black male delinquent as an example of racism's wholesale impact on Harlem. As a stand-in for collective black emotional pain, the suffering black delinquent was intended to serve as a signpost alerting readers to Harlem's unnoticed mental health needs. Lafargue's promoters hoped these portrayals would replace the public's scorn for Harlem with feelings of sympathy and charity.

In this postwar contest over the power of imagery, Mosse and Bernard disagreed as to the best way mass media could be used to convince whites to identify with the emotional suffering of urban African Americans. To forge this emotional connection, Bernard assumed that image makers would have to work hard to get audiences to overlook on-screen differences of race and place. Mosse countered that audiences needed to be made aware that differences of race and place did matter. She claimed that a responsible public depiction of Donald would have explained the complex social relationship between his race, his place of residence, and his fragile psyche. She even implied that they might feel more sympathy for black Harlem youth if they learned that their emotional problems were caused by injustices whites did not have to face.

Bernard did not share Mosse's hope that US audiences in 1949 were ready for such a controversial message about racial injustice. Racial stereotypes about the black mind were still prevalent. More so than Mosse, Bernard imagined that too much focus on the differences between black and white lives might only reinforce beliefs in black racial exceptionalism. Bernard envisioned *The Quiet One* as a way to sell white moviegoers on the proposition that the psyches of white men and black men were not intrinsically different. In Bernard's estimation, for blacks to appear more sympathetic to whites, whites first would have to be convinced that black suffering was just as real and deep as white suffering. Although that was an assumption antiracists held, most Americans did not. Bernard saw this film as an opportunity to close that gap.

Fighting Scientific Racism in the Psychiatric Literature

New York City's antiracist psychiatrists did not all agree on what laypersons should be told about the emotional life of African Americans. But they did agree that the "racist approach to variation in human behavior" did not deserve a place in psychiatric discourse.[122] By the early 1950s, clinicians associated with either Wiltwyck or the Lafargue Clinic attempted to police the racial etiquette of the psychiatric literature and promote a more color-blind racial orthodoxy. Both camps argued that the appearance of racist ideas in print potentially posed clinical harm to black patients. One way for universalist clinicians to ensure that black patients were treated properly was to influence how their colleagues nationwide wrote about them in journals and monographs. If they could change what other psychiatrists read about patients of color, maybe they might also change how they interacted with those patients.

Thus New York universalists sought to expunge racialism from the current literature. One way they attempted to do so was by branding a writer's ideas "racist," a charge usually accompanied by the related accusation that the author was unscientific. Such a claim sent the clear message that biological determinism did not belong in medical science. The new literature disputed the notion that a patient's biological race might determine how his or her mind worked. It also urged psychiatrists to abandon the custom of citing older racialists as race experts.[123] Bernard's colleagues at Northside Testing and Consultation Center, Harlem's newly opened child-guidance clinic, claimed that the old racialists' experience did not constitute expertise. Their racist ideas and observations were "pseudo-scientific" and patently invalid.[124] The only proper way for a responsible clinician to deal with such ideas was to purge them from his or her mental toolkit. According to universalists, Lauretta Bender's older provisional approach to racialism was equally untenable. Clinicians should either declare their adherence to an "outmoded" approach or, preferably, embrace the newer tenets of psychiatric antiracism.[125]

Race-blind psychiatrists also condemned ethnopsychiatry. Ethnopsychiatrists such as Columbia University's Abram Kardiner did not believe that biological race produced psychological differences. Rather, they claimed that cultural differences could cause a race to develop its own group psyche. According to those employing the "cultural approach to personality," each culture imprinted itself on the natural process of human psychological development.[126] So even though all humans were born with the same basic potential, each culture encouraged the growth of personality traits that best fit its values and circumstances. If a race was socially isolated enough to possess its own culture, ethnopsychiatrists believed that group could develop its own "basic personality" type.[127]

Although most universalists did not outright discredit ethnopsychiatry as racist in the same way they did racialism, Wertham and Mosse—as well as black psychiatrists in the National Medical Association—strongly objected to any claim that African Americans shared a distinct psychological type. They found it hard to believe that ontogenesis, the development of individual personality traits, could really differ that much between cultures let alone between segments of a single society.[128] More important, they regarded the very idea of a psychological color line between black and white minds to be incongruous with universalism. In a 1952 National Medical Association roundtable of leading black psychiatrists, the Veterans Administration clinician Prince Barker rejected ethnopsychiatry because it jeopardized the universalist claim "that Negroes act as individuals."[129] Strict universalists such as Barker assumed that the Western concept of human "selfhood" (the autonomous individual) was not a culturally relative one. For them, the discretely bounded, autonomous self was a natural, universally *human* phenomenon. To suggest otherwise was to deny the full humanity of African Americans.

By contrast, the racial liberals affiliated with the Wiltwyck School did not entirely discount the possibility that cultural differences might cause African Americans and white Americans to develop group-specific personality traits. Between 1947 and 1953, Bernard and some of her colleagues evinced doubts about the universality of the Freudian laws of psychodynamics and ontogenesis, given their origination in clinical encounters conducted exclusively with whites. They believed that "transcultural analyses"[130] of American patients would eventually provide "an objective and realistic theory of the relation between culture and personality,"[131] helping to parse the "ways in which derivatives of the patient's specific cultural experience—of which his being a Negro is a part—have become integrated, as basic formative ingredients of the personality, into the deepest layers of his being."[132] Ultimately, they hoped that conclusions drawn from "work with patients whose social environments differed sharply from those of the white middle class groups who have provided the dominant source for psychiatric studies" could help them discover what was natural and universal about the human psyche.[133]

Bernard and the Lafargue group agreed that if a "Negro personality" existed, it would be neither pathological nor the result of racism. As universalists, they all refused to believe that America's culture of institutional racism and Jim Crow had really embedded itself into every aspect and stage of black psychological development. Bernard openly derided clinicians with a "tendency to overemphasize the effects of being Negro on their patient's personality difficulties."[134] She refused to believe that racism was so powerful a force that it prevented all African Americans from developing a normal, adult human psyche. Indeed, even to consider that it had that power could have undercut the proposition that African Americans deserved equal access to psychiatric care.

Nevertheless, between the 1940s and 1952, some psychiatrists did argue that racism had fundamentally altered and damaged the black psyche.[135] From this perspective, racism was the most significant cultural influence on African Americans. It was the thing that had made black life so different from white life. It logically followed, then, that Jim Crow laws, structures, and customs, imprinted on black psyches since infancy, were principally responsible for molding the raw human potential of African Americans into a unique "Negro personality" type—one that was as pathological as the racism that produced it.[136]

Even though some historians claim that antiracists did not object to the damaged "Negro personality" thesis until the 1960s,[137] a number were outraged by such ideas as early as 1951.[138] These clinicians even accused the proponents of this thesis with justifying "the continuation of discrimination," especially in the distribution of mental health resources.[139] Much of the backlash targeted one 1951 monograph by the New York psychoanalysts Abram Kardiner and Lionel Ovesey—*The Mark of Oppression*. In this best-selling book, Kardiner examined twenty-five Harlemites. He concluded that they all shared a "basic Negro Personality" type. According to him, this type developed because American society restricted opportunities for blacks and yet paradoxically blamed them for their lack of success. Consequently, the black psyche was wracked by a deep-seeded mistrust of others, self-hatred, aggression, low self-esteem, and mind-numbing anxiety over both success and failure.[140] In a racially unjust society, whites were the only people who could develop normal, healthy personalities. Kardiner characterized African Americans as thwarted white Americans, people whose "wretched internal life" could never be anything more than "a caricature of the corresponding white personality."[141] The psychological end product of oppression was a psyche too sick to ever rise above it.[142]

Some antiracist clinicians in New York bitterly assailed both Kardiner and his imitators for disseminating a dangerous new "psychoanalytic stereotype" rooted in cultural determinism. Bernard and her Wiltwyck colleagues were also interested in uncovering what was "culturally determined" about the African American psyche, but they believed that Kardiner had gone too far, reinvigorating racialism.[143] Although Kardiner's emotionally crippled "basic Negro personality" was the product of cultural rather than biological determinism, Bernard panned him for creating an equally reified portrait of the black psyche: "Negroes, struggling against the standard racial stereotypes are understandably alarmed by the threat of such a sophisticated new version of racial stereotypy, under the aegis of psychodynamics."[144]

What most alarmed Mosse was Kardiner's contention that psychotherapy could not help African Americans. According to Kardiner: "Obviously, Negro self-esteem cannot be retrieved, nor Negro self-hatred destroyed as long as the status is quo. . . . There is only one way that the products of oppression can be dissolved, and that is to stop the oppression."[145] As long as racism remained, psychiatry would be of no use to black patients. By emphasizing the intractability of the mark of oppression, Kardiner's work seemed to question the universalist underpinnings of the Lafargue Clinic and Wiltwyck School. Representatives of those institutions attacked Kardiner for failing to see that blacks could overcome the alleged psychological scars of racism, even with the aid of psychiatry. In Mosse's view, *The Mark of Oppression*'s therapeutic nihilism threatened Harlem's access to psychiatric care. She feared that policymakers might use his argument to justify the continued neglect of Harlem's mental health needs.[146]

Some race-blind New York clinicians were not only disturbed by Kardiner's therapeutic nihilism, but they also found his call to end racism disingenuous. Although Kardiner offered no viable plan to end racism, his book intimated that black Americans themselves could play no active role in its dismantling. People that emotionally damaged could not be expected to organize protests.[147] For citizens who had been involved in New York's interracial civil-rights movement since the 1930s, Kardiner's claim was patently ridiculous. Given their shared conviction that no society could irrevocably stunt an entire group's psychological development, they saw no reason why African Americans would lack the emotional stability needed to resist oppression.[148] To argue the point, Charles W. Collins, one of the Lafargue Clinic's black therapists, recommended that Kardiner recall the struggles of the Jews, Irish, and Native Americans. A true universalist, Collins rhapsodized: "American Negroes share with the people of the Earth an identity of response to oppression. This response to oppression is a human characteristic, not a 'racial' one. And the response is definitely not associated with a loss of self-esteem."[149] For race-blind clinicians, African Americans were fundamentally human. As humans they psychologically respond to persecution with healthy resistance—the very quality psychotherapy was supposed to stimulate in any patient population, including Harlem.[150]

Conclusion

Entering the 1950s, New York's race-blind psychotherapists resisted racist ideas in both print and film. Although such efforts might not seem directly relevant to the movement to improve the black community's access to psychiatric care, they were. In the struggle against institutional racism in mental health care delivery, attempts to convince white Americans to identify with the emotional suffering of African Americans were crucial. By actively promoting a new color-blind understanding of the black psyche in both popular culture and in the psychiatric literature, racial liberals made it more likely that Harlemites would eventually gain greater access to quality psychiatric care.

Ever since Northern civil-rights activism began in the 1930s, public servants in New York's Domestic Relations Court and Bureau of Child Guidance struggled to make psychiatric universalism the racial commonsense of their workplaces. By World War II's end, more and more of the staff at those public institutions and the Wiltwyck School had come to assume that blacks and whites were psychological equals. Once that began to happen, those spaces became less tolerant of racism in mental health care delivery. Through film and print media, racial liberals helped to accelerate the pace of institutional change. By 1962, the "institutional patterns of cultural value" within New York City's health care apparatus had changed enough that Harlem Hospital finally opened its own full-time psychiatric division.[151]

Chapter Six

Psychiatry Comes to Harlem Hospital

Community Psychiatry, Aftercare, and Columbia University, 1947–62

In 1955 Hubert T. Delany lost his position as Children's Court Justice. One of Polier's trusted colleagues, Delany was also one of the New York civil-rights movement's most outspoken leaders. A member of the NAACP Board of Directors, he was associated with the National Lawyers Guild, which the House Un-American Activities Committee (HUAC) suspected was a Communist front. Yet even at the height of the postwar Red scare, Delany refused to pull his punches. In the early fifties, he routinely condemned police brutality against African Americans and declared that New York's housing and public schools were racially segregated. Some saw the antiracist causes he championed as subversive. Still he persisted. He openly criticized politicians and Roman Catholic leaders who brandished anticommunist rhetoric in defense of racial segregation and racism. When the State Department alleged that the NAACP founder W. E. B. DuBois was a Communist and revoked his passport in 1951, Delany defended him. Delany's courage proved to be his undoing.[1] When his term came up for renewal, Mayor Robert F. Wagner Jr.—a liberal Democrat—did not reappoint him, claiming that Delany's "left-wing views" disqualified him from the job.[2]

One of Delany's liberal African American allies, Dr. Kenneth B. Clark, wrote the former judge in September, expressing his sympathy. A fellow member of the Urban League's committee on education,[3] Clark was a City College of New York psychologist and cofounder of Harlem's Northside Center for Child Development. The Clarks founded this private child-guidance facility on Harlem's West 150th Street with the support of Delany and many of the same judges, psychiatrists, racial-justice activists, and philanthropists behind the Harlem Project and the Wiltwyck School for Boys.[4] And in 1954 Clark had helped secure a major victory for the national civil-rights movement through his participation in the landmark *Brown v. Board of Education* Supreme Court case.[5] Clark lamented the sacrifice of this "eminently qualified and humane judge" on the altar of anticommunism, informing Justice Delany that "I have admired your courage and insistence upon the fundamental rights of equality and democracy." Despite Clark's admiration for Delany, this was the end of their association. Certainly by the 1950s activists identified as too left-leaning had become a liability to those seeking to both combat racism and shield themselves from accusations of Communist alliance.[6]

It is within that political climate that the courts and schools' efforts to improve mental health care within the black community stalled. Since the late 1930s the Domestic Relations Court had been at the center of such efforts. Collaboration along the left-liberal spectrum made it possible for civil servants in the Domestic Relations Court and the Bureau of Child Guidance to offer some psychiatric services to select African American children. Yet with "New York an epicenter of anticommunism"[7] in the 1950s, Delany and fellow antiracists in the Children's Court found themselves under attack as possible subversives, unable to use their public posts to create anything like the defunct Harlem Project and Domestic Relations Court treatment clinic.

Although their influence within the public sector seemed to be in decline, racial liberals did not abandon black Harlem's emotionally ill residents. As this chapter will show, Dr. Bernard and others continued to sustain color-blind psychiatry on a more limited scale through the voluntary sector and academia. From 1946 through the late 1950s, Bernard in particular found a home for antiracist clinicians at Dr. Kenneth Cark's Northside Center, the Wiltwyck School for Boys, and Columbia University's schools of medicine and public health. As Bernard developed community psychiatry and its local model of care at Columbia, Wiltwyck's board began to see the school's Catskills location as a major drawback. To help black Harlemites maintain therapeutic gains made at Wiltwyck, its board searched for a Manhattan facility that could provide black clients with aftercare. The pickings were slim in the late 1950s. In 1960 ideological divisions between Dr. Clark and Wiltwyck's board ruled out Northside as an option. But in 1962 Wiltwyck's quest ended when Harlem Hospital's psychiatric division opened.

The last half of the chapter examines how New York's municipal hospital system managed to bring psychiatry to Harlem Hospital in 1962. A convergence of factors helped make this historically significant policy shift possible. First, Columbia University's Community Psychiatry Program and School of Public Health had become home to Viola Bernard, Ray Trussell, Lawrence Kolb, and other racial liberals who actively supported the expansion of psychiatry into black communities. Second, in 1960 the Harlem Neighborhoods Association—a local civil-rights organization—began making calls for Mayor Richard Wagner Jr. to provide Harlem Hospital with full psychiatric care. And third, Wagner appointed Columbia University's Ray Trussell as Commissioner of the Department of Hospitals. With a racial liberal at the helm of the public hospital system, Columbia's School of Medicine developed a formal affiliation with Harlem Hospital in 1961. For our story, the most significant outcome of this affiliation was the creation of Harlem Hospital's first full-time psychiatric department in 1962, Ward 9-K.

Harlem Psychiatry without the Lafargue Clinic

It is unlikely that Harlem Hospital's psychiatric division could have opened in the 1950s. The political scientist Richard Iton described the early fifties as "a moment in which civil rights and communism were conflated in the American mind."[8] Since the 1940s, the black freedom struggle had reflected the interests of a wide range of groups along the left-liberal political spectrum. Within New York, the ranks of the wartime black freedom movement contained black trade unionists such as the CIO's Eleanor Goding and Ewart Guinier, racial liberals such as the NAACP's Walter White and Earl Brown, Communist Party members including Ben Davis, and even suspected fellow travelers such as Du Bois. Given its homogeneity, the agenda of this antiracist coalition was wide-ranging. It was not yet focused on the Jim Crow South and procedural rights. Instead, it was transnational and included opposition to Jim Crow in the military, European colonialism, apartheid, US segregation, police brutality, and institutional racism in employment, unions, housing, education, and heath care.[9] Yet entering the McCarthy era, the black freedom struggle's inclusion of leftists became suspect. Consequently, the civil-rights movement began to narrow its scope in response to accusations that anyone calling for the redistribution of wealth, advocating the humanization of capitalism, or criticizing colonial empires was anti-American.[10]

Even in New York City, which had been a primary staging area for the wartime racial-justice coalition of liberals and leftists, retrenchment had set in by the 1950s. Racial liberalism was transformed during the mayoral tenures of Republicans William O'Dwyer (1946–50) and Vincent Impelliteri (1950–53), and the first term of Democrat Robert F. Wagner Jr. (1954–65), son of the pro-labor New Deal senator. According to Martha Biondi, New York's racial liberals typically responded to the anticommunist crusades of the early 1950s by ending collaborations they had established during World War II with trade unionists, socialists, and advocates of economic justice. The organized labor movement and mainstream civil-rights organizations such as the NAACP and the American Jewish Congress began purging their rolls. Members named names before public hearings and publicly disavowed any prior leftist allegiances.[11]

Even Justice Polier found it necessary to actively identify herself as anticommunist and break off contact with more progressive activists. In 1952, the House of Representatives Cox Committee Investigation looked into Polier's past association with the labor movement and social justice organizations, probing for evidence of communist sympathies. In her affidavit before this House Committee, Polier condemned communism and denied that she had ever belonged to any "subversive" group. As evidence, she even revealed that she had actively been working with other racial liberals to oust Communists from their organizations. As vice president of the American Jewish Congress she led a campaign between 1949 and 1951 to identify and officially cut all ties with leftist Jewish groups who "follow the Communist line."[12]

Not surprisingly, anticommunism's impact on racial liberals such as Polier derailed the New York Domestic Relations Court's fight against racial inequality in public mental health policy. Opportunities to create programs similar to the Harlem Project or the Domestic Relations Court treatment clinic never materialized—not even during the first term of Mayor Wagner's free-spending administration. Both of those programs had been the result of collaboration between Domestic Relations Court justices and members of the Field Foundation, an organization HUAC considered subversive.[13] In the postwar era, New York's public sector had become much less welcoming to left-of-center ideas and influences. Between 1948 and 1956, the Welfare Department, the public schools, and other municipal agencies even subjected employees to anticommunist loyalty oaths and background checks, discouraging active collaboration between liberals and leftists.[14]

Although the Domestic Relations Court did not entirely stop serving as a force for antiracist change, the relative power of its antiracist personnel declined precipitously in the 1950s.[15] The court's wartime battle against institutional racism in mental health care had been waged by four judges: Polier, Delany, Jane Bolin, and Dudley F. Sicher. In the 1950s, their broad-based antiracist activism aroused suspicion. The resulting scrutiny limited their ability to take a united stand against racism. As had many other racial liberals, Polier chose to limit her range of antiracist action to the pursuit of formal equality under the law. This put her in good stead with the mainstream civil-rights movement as it began to focus on the legal battle against de jure segregation in education.[16] In 1950 Bolin alienated herself from those same racial liberals when she criticized the mainstream civil-rights agenda as increasingly "sterile and barren," resigning from the NAACP Board of Directors.[17] Combined with Sicher's retirement in 1953 and Delany's ouster in 1955, the Domestic Relations Court's antiracist cohort had been depleted and neutralized.[18]

Polier had difficulty keeping color-blind psychiatry alive within the Domestic Relations Court. After its treatment clinic closed in 1945, the diagnostic clinic was all that remained of its psychiatric apparatus. Throughout the 1950s the quality of the overworked clinicians assigned to that clinic declined. Only a few psychiatrists, such as Dr. Joseph King, still shared Polier's interest in racial justice, taking time to carefully evaluate the court's African American charges. Most did not. Polier also criticized court clinicians for relying too heavily on IQ tests as a diagnostic tool. She felt that the use of such a culturally biased test in the cases of poor black children fostered misdiagnoses and inadequate treatment. Polier found that some private agencies used the lower IQ scores of blacks, Puerto Ricans, and even white ethnics to deny them access to psychiatry. Before the 1960s, many mental health professionals believed that a low score signified that a patient had difficulty thinking and communicating, thus rendering psychotherapy useless. Without enough court psychiatrists committed to racial justice, the Domestic Relations Court no longer led the New York drive to eliminate racial disparities in mental health care.[19]

Elsewhere in the United States, especially in the South, African American access to medical treatment increased through federally subsidized hospital building. Between 1947 and 1971, the 1946 Hill-Burton Act provided close to $13 billion in federal aid and matching grants to build hospitals all across the country—half of them in the South. Dispersing Hill-Burton funds below the Mason-Dixon Line resulted in the construction of segregated, "deluxe Jim Crow" hospitals. Despite their racially bifurcated structure, the historian Karen Kruse Thomas found that the proliferation of these biracial facilities improved African American access to both general and state mental hospital care so much that Hill-Burton "materially benefited black southerners as a group more than any other Roosevelt-era program."[20]

Hill-Burton did not help provide Harlemites with local psychiatric care. Manhattan's African Americans already had access to state mental hospitals and Hill-Burton did not fund local psychiatric services during the 1950s. In the absence of a supportive public sector, Northern racial liberals increasingly looked to civil society to help them meet the mental health needs of African Americans.[21] For most emotionally ill African Americans, children and adults alike, local inpatient psychiatric services simply did not exist. For outpatient care, activists such as Polier and Bernard lent their support to a number of over-burdened private mental hygiene clinics and child-guidance centers serving Harlemites. These voluntary, racially integrated agencies included the Lafargue Mental Hygiene Clinic, Edmund Gordon's Harriet Tubman Mental Hygiene Clinic, the Morningside Heights Mental Hygiene Clinic, and Kenneth and Mamie Clark's Northside Center. With many of these outpatient facilities dependent on outside support and charity for resources, the private sector could not be counted on to adequately meet Harlem's mental health needs.

Especially for adults, the availability of outpatient services was precarious at best in Harlem. When 1958 ended, the Lafargue Mental Hygiene Clinic closed. Given the low-cost facility's left-wing political origins, it is a wonder it survived the early Cold War years as long as it had. When the New York City Community Mental Health Board failed to renew the clinic's license, the cofounder Fredric Wertham even speculated that "the Lafargue Clinic is on the blacklist."[22] For a variety of reasons, this improbable little clinic located in the parish-house basement of St. Philip's Protestant Episcopal Church finally shut down after Rev. Shelton Hale Bishop retired. As the rector who had initially provided the clinic rent-free space in 1946, Bishop believed that central Harlem was badly in need of expanded psychiatric services. His daughter Elizabeth B. Davis, partly inspired by her father, even earned a degree in psychiatry from Columbia University. Nonetheless, the clinic did not figure into the long-term plans of the next rector, Rev. M. Moran Weston. Lafargue's closing meant that emotionally ill African American adults had lost their primary source of outpatient care.[23]

Rev. Weston did not close the Lafargue Clinic because he opposed psychiatry. A social activist himself, Weston was actively involved in helping black children secure some mental health services in Harlem. He simply may not have viewed the Lafargue Clinic as necessary, given his close ties to both the Northside Center and its financial backers.[24] Ordained a Protestant Episcopal minister in 1951, Weston was a social scientist and activist with a doctorate in history from Columbia. Before his rectorship, he had been an active participant in the wartime civil-rights movement. He was even a board member on several Harlem church and social organizations, including the CWCCH.[25] During this early phase of the black freedom struggle, Weston befriended Kenneth and Mamie Clark, becoming a founding board member of their Northside Center.[26]

Rev. Weston helped make the Northside Center a financially viable venture. He connected the Clarks with New Yorkers who had backed the Harlem Project and the Wiltwyck School for Boys. In its first year of operation, Weston had helped persuade Julius Rosewald's heiresses, Marion Ascoli and her sister Adele Levy, to fund the Northside Center, brokering a relationship that lasted until 1960. Linking the Clarks with Rosenwald money, Weston inserted Northside into a circle of liberal Jewish philanthropists and activists that included the Wiltwyck directors Bernard and Polier.[27]

Up until 1960, Bernard exerted some control over Northside's clinical operations. As a condition of Ascoli's financial aid, the Clarks allowed Bernard, Polier, and several other Wiltwyck board members to join Northside's Board of Directors. Bernard also chaired Northside's Professional Advisory Commitee, involving herself in its day-to-day operations. Not surprisingly, Bernard envisioned that psychiatry would have a central role to play at Northside. The Clarks had wanted their Northside to be a multidisciplinary agency. It would offer children a wide range of services ranging from psychological testing to remedial education. No one approach or discipline was supposed to dominate. Yet through her influence over the Professional Advisory Committee, Bernard and her clinical team treated Northside as though it were a child-guidance clinic. Installing the Columbia University psychoanalyst Dr. Albert Bryt as the center's clinical director, Bernard pushed a strict medical focus and a psychiatrist-centered model of authority.[28]

Wiltwyck's Plans for Harlem: The Continuous-Care Model

One year after Lafargue Clinic's closing, the Northside Center broke ties with Dr. Bernard and the Wiltwyck School's leadership. This break was the culmination of a power struggle between the Clarks and Ascoli's contacts on the Wiltwyck board. Throughout the Ascoli-Northside partnership, tension existed between Dr. Bernard's vision of increased psychiatric authority and the Clarks' less doctrinaire approach. Some of Northside's clinicians wanted a relatively greater clinical focus on social factors than the psychoanalysts offered. These tensions finally came to a head in 1960. Almost all of Northside's staff, including the Clarks, threatened to resign if Ascoli's Board of Directors did not remove the authoritarian psychoanalyst Albert Bryt from his position as clinical director. Ascoli resigned as board president in March, taking her sizable charitable donation with her. Without Ascoli, Bernard and psychiatry lost their tenuous hold over the Northside Center. In April, Bernard and Polier resigned their positions on Northside's board, essentially ending Wiltwyck's connection to the Clarks' Harlem facility.[29]

Had the closing of Lafargue Clinic and the demise of the Wiltwyck-Northside alliance sealed the fate of universalist psychiatry in Harlem? As far as Bernard was concerned, it had not. Throughout the 1950s and the early 1960s, she and other veterans of the Harlem Project and the CWCCH still sought to make psychiatric treatment more available to Harlemites. And not all of those therapeutic options were located in Manhattan.

Well into the 1960s, the Wiltwyck School for Boys in the Catskill Mountains still provided the Domestic Relations Court with one of its only reliable placement options for troubled prepubescent black males. Polier and her colleagues still encountered real difficulty placing black children in either local private agencies or foster care. Backlogs were common. In August 1953, 193 of the 203 children sitting in detention at New York City's Children Center, unable to be placed, were African American. In 1956 Mayor Wagner's administration finally constructed the Hillcrest facility, a final public-placement option for children the private agencies rejected.[30] Yet even after Hillcrest opened, Wiltwyck still provided space for quite a few young black men—especially those with psychiatric needs. As Wiltwyck board members, judges Polier and Bolin steered eligible black children to their institution. By 1963, 65 percent of Wiltwyck's Manhattan referrals were black.[31]

As early as 1949, Wiltwyck's increasingly pro-psychiatry Board of Directors decided to transform the largely custodial school into a residential treatment center. The board created a Professional Advisory Committee with Bernard at the head.[32] That same year the board chose the Austrian-born Ernst Papanek as the new executive director. Both Papanek and the former director Robert L. Cooper had been social workers. But the board considered Papanek much more of a devotee of modern psychology. Papanek's term at Wiltwyck lasted from 1949 to 1958. During that period, Papanek became Wiltwyck's strongest promoter of the compassionate, therapeutic image the board wanted for its school.[33] Papanek encouraged his staff to be much more sensitive to their charges' emotional needs. Most significantly, Papanek prevented counselors from using corporal punishment, an accomplishment that had eluded Cooper.[34]

Some of the Wiltwyck boys noticed the difference. Claude Brown recalled that as a Wiltwyck student he believed that "[Papanek] was probably the smartest and deepest cat I had ever met." Brown was particularly impressed by Papanek's understanding of emotions, which struck young Claude as a mysterious special talent only Papanek possessed.[35] In 1950, the hiring of more psychodynamically oriented staff, including the world-renowned art therapist Edith Kramer, enhanced the school's reputation.[36] By 1952 the Child Welfare League of America reported: "Wiltwyck has made definite progress in developing a treatment program, and it would no longer be true to say that it is mainly a custodial institution. Its direction, purpose and philosophy is definitely treatment-oriented."[37] Wiltwyck's changes convinced city officials that it was finally a residential treatment center worthy of public investment.[38]

Nevertheless, the Board of Directors received reliable evidence in 1954 that Wiltwyck's reputed therapeutic effects wore off once children returned to

Harlem. That year Papanek asked the New York School of Social Work to analyze fifteen years of Wiltwyck case files. Papanek wanted to see if rates of recovery for a variety of mental ills had improved during his therapeutic regime.
Sophia Robison, a former Harlem Project researcher and student of Marion
Kenworthy, studied the case records. The results were discouraging. Robison
found that the recidivism rate for Wiltwyck graduates had plateaued at a constant 50 percent since the school's inception. Apparently no matter what the
school did, half the children fell back into their old destructive patterns upon
release. Robison analyzed her findings and concluded: "The explanation for
the failure of half of the boys to maintain the gains registered in the institution is no doubt related to the conditions in the Harlem ghetto to which most
of them must return. . . . To be sure, there were some boys who required and
received intensive psychiatric therapy. This did not, however, compensate for
the deprivation in the home community."[39]

To some degree, the Board of Directors agreed that Harlem's slums caused
recidivism. The 1954 study only confirmed what many of them had already suspected: personality adjustments made on Wiltwyck's sylvan campus could be
undone on Harlem's streets. Two years earlier, the Child Welfare League of
America had drawn a similar conclusion. It reported that the "sociological environment surrounding Wiltwyck" was so geographically and culturally removed
from Harlem that "it does not permit an easy 'testing-out' of the child's adjustment at Wiltwyck, in the community from which he comes and to which he will
return." The solution called for Wiltwyck to provide treatment services in New
York City. If the school could not be relocated closer to the city, the League
urged, Wiltwyck's board needed to provide former students with aftercare
services within one of the five boroughs. For the remainder of Papanek's tenure, the board tried to implement these suggestions. Between 1954 and 1958,
Wiltwyck set up its first aftercare facility in St. Alban's, Queens, and increased
the size of the staff at both its main campus and its city office.[40]

As Wiltwyck sought to create continuous care, Bernard pressed for greater
psychiatric control of the school's treatment program. Papanek's resignation
in 1958 opened the door for Bernard to give psychiatrists more authority over
Wiltwyck's therapeutic activities. In anticipation of psychiatry's greater role at
the school, Bernard renamed the Wiltwyck Professional Advisory Committee the
Advisory Committee on the Treatment Program. Bernard also successfully proposed that the Board of Directors subdivide Papanek's vacated position as executive director into two new directorships. One director would be administrative.
The other would be a clinical and medical director. After appointing Nathan
Levine as the administrator, the board spent much of 1958 and 1959 searching
for a psychiatrist to serve as clinical director.[41]

Psychiatry's expanded role constituted a major institutional shift at
Wiltwyck.[42] Bernard and her allies on the board pursued this change because
they still believed in psychiatry's power to help the school's clientele.[43] Bernard's
faith had not been shaken by Robison's study, the Northside Center's growing
resistance to psychiatric control, or the persistent conflicts between the Wiltwyck

board and its staff over "policy, philosophy, and future plans."[44] On August 1959, the Wiltwyck board promoted Dr. Edward Auerswald, a staff psychiatrist, to clinical director.[45] In April 1960 he declared that he shared "the Board's commitment to run Wiltwyck as a residential treatment center for children with 'emotional disturbances.'" Two more part-time psychiatrists were hired, forming what the executive assistant George Haskins called "the nucleus of a very promising psychiatric team."[46]

Bernard and the Wiltwyck board also believed that a mere increase in psychiatric services was not enough to guarantee that Wiltwyck's new "continued-care program" would work with Harlem children.[47] To ensure that a program of combined residential and aftercare therapy could preserve the therapeutic gains Harlemites had made at Wiltwyck, the board determined that a new psychiatric approach was in order. Formerly, child guidance had been the primary method social psychiatrists had used with working-class children from Harlem. But the child-guidance model, in which the child was the sole therapeutic subject, had not produced lasting results with a majority of Wiltwyck boys. Yet another survey conducted in the late 1950s revealed that the recidivism rate had not improved since Robison's report came out in 1954. In 1959, the board president Sylvia Liese worried that "we have not been receiving maximum benefit from the large proportion of our funds which we have been expending on psychiatry." Subsequently, the board tried to reap that maximum benefit. In 1960 Wiltwyck latched onto a new therapeutic modality, one it hoped could counter some of the negative social forces within Harlem.[48]

Family therapy, as a formal therapeutic approach, is generally thought to have developed in the early 1950s. As a new technique, it certainly was a bold deviation from the standard one-on-one therapeutic model. Group therapy had already been in use since World War II, primarily as a way to reduce time, cost, patient isolation, and the negative effects of patient-to-clinician transference. The Cold War-era clinicians who employed the technique believed, as did most social psychiatrists, that the human self was primarily a social entity, not a solitary one. Accordingly, family therapists contended that treatment would be more effective if the clinician structured the session to reflect the social nature of the self. In 1951 John Elderkin Bell made the first attempt to do this, conducting sessions with members of his patients' primary social unit, their families. Soon others began experimenting with family therapy. One of New York's pioneers was Nathan Ackerman, a psychiatrist and colleague of Bernard who worked with Jewish Family Services. Much of this experimentation was still rooted in the Freudian assumption that the family relationship was the primary social force in a child's life. If the family could be altered, made more conducive to mental health, then any clinical gains made with the child could be preserved. By the 1960s, family therapy had become an integral part of Wiltwyck's psychiatric program.[49]

The psychiatrist who developed the family-therapy model for Wiltwyck's continuous-care program was Salvador Minuchin. Wiltwyck hired Minuchin in 1960. He was a thirty-nine-year-old Argentinean Jew with psychoanalytic training.

Minuchin had worked in New York clinics and agencies since 1950. After less than a full year at Wiltwyck, he and the clinical director Auerswald agreed that they would achieve more in therapy at Esopus if they could observe and even change how a Wiltwyck child and his Harlem family interacted as a unit.[50]

Both clinicians had experience with family therapy. Minuchin, Auerswald, and the social worker Charles King had studied family dynamics at other institutions.[51] Minuchin and Auerswald sought a "better understanding of the forces within the families that contributed to the development of pathology in our children." They felt that new family-therapy techniques were required to help them acquire this understanding. Up until then, Wiltwyck followed "the traditional manner of treating the child individually and parallel to treatment of the family members," usually only the mother.[52]

In 1960 Minuchin devised a new program whereby multiple therapists conducted individual and group sessions with a child and all of his family members. This psychiatric program began with an intake at Wiltwyck's city offices. Wiltwyck provided the boy with therapy on campus. The family received treatment in the city. In aftercare, Wiltwyck's aftercare team conducted further sessions for the client and his family. Throughout this continuous care, Minuchin and his staff attempted to uncover a boy's family dynamic, determining how its unhealthy features had produced his personal problems. What is more, they also aimed to determine how the family's relationship could be improved to promote a healthier social milieu for a recovering delinquent.[53]

The Wiltwyck School's adoption of family therapy helped attract funding for its continuous-care program. Between 1959 and 1960, Wiltwyck secured the necessary funding thanks to a grant from the newly formed Taconic Foundation. The Taconic Foundation was a charity that initially promoted racial integration, civil-rights activism, and efforts to reduce racial disparities within underserved black communities—especially in Harlem.[54] The Taconic Foundation dollars were earmarked only for psychiatric treatment.[55] By 1961, Minuchin and Auerswald decided that effective therapy with the families of Harlem delinquents ("acting-out" boys, as they were then known in the psychiatric literature) required a more formal investigation of those families. Not much was known about their internal dynamics. Many on Wiltwyck's staff assumed that the "slum family" would be pathological, but they had no evidence. Desiring proof, Minuchin and his colleagues devised a grant proposal for a "research project to further study these families and to test the efficacy of our interview technique as a therapeutic tool."[56]

In December 1961, Minuchin's Wiltwyck team received a three-year grant from the National Institutes of Mental Health (NIMH). The NIMH had been looking to promote this sort of community-based approach. In 1965 Minuchin and his team received a supplementary NIMH grant to continue their "action research project," the then-fashionable term for a psychiatric program combining investigation, clinical treatment, and policy advocacy. With this new funding, Wiltwyck created a continuous-care model that met the state and city's requirements for a residential treatment center.[57]

To reintegrate Wiltwyck boys back into New York City, the school officially opened the new halfway house on 18th Street in February 1962. Beyond Minuchin's experimental program, the Wiltwyck administration had high hopes for its halfway house, named for celebrity benefactor Floyd Patterson, the former boxing champion.[58] First, the downtown Floyd Patterson House was the closest link Wiltwyck's board had made with their Harlem students' neighborhoods. For the children of Harlem, the Bronx, and other Manhattan neighborhoods, this aftercare facility was closer to their old stomping grounds than either the "relatively isolated residential treatment center" in Esopus or the Queens aftercare facility. Second, the new institution gave Wiltwyck staff the chance to exercise more control over the process of reintegration. According to Auerswald, the facility allowed Minuchin's team to "move the ingredients of residential treatment with the child as he is gradually introduced into the community." The children lived at the new facility rather than in their old homes. They went to public school. They saw the staff child psychiatrist Hugh F. Butts[59] and received the outreach programs of the Boys Club, Bank Street College, and other social agencies.[60]

The Wiltwyck board also sought an affiliation with a Harlem facility offering psychiatric services to teens. Realizing that Wiltwyck was unable to provide aftercare services for former students over the age of thirteen, the board worried that Harlemites would suffer relapses during their critical teen years. So in 1959 Bernard encouraged the board to seek out an aftercare liaison with a psychiatric facility in Harlem. She hoped it might create a web of private psychiatric care for Harlem's troubled families that extended from residential treatment in the Catskills, to the halfway house, and ultimately to the local clinic.

In early 1959 when this plan was initiated, Wiltwyck's administration had considered the Northside Center the most promising possibility for this Harlem liaison. The fit seemed natural at the time. The directorial boards of both institutions contained many of the same people. So before her falling-out with the Clarks, Bernard proposed that the Wiltwyck board ought to cultivate a formal relationship with Harlem's Northside Center. At its February 5, 1959, meeting, Wiltwyck's board authorized Bernard to offer Northside a partnership of some kind. Northside appealed to Wiltwyck's board for four reasons: it was "interracial at all levels," it was then still moving in a psychiatric direction, the two institutions shared "a number of mutual Board members, and Bernard was the head of both facilities' Professional Advisory Committees. Given the involvement at both places, Northside appeared to a sure bet.[61]

Sure enough, Bernard and her allies at both institutions began working on this proposed partnership in April 1959. A Joint Committee of Wiltwyck and Northside, including members common to both boards, agreed to create "some type of preferential intake and referral service . . . between the two agencies. Thus a child being treated at Northside would be given first consideration at Wiltwyck and a child returning to the community from Wiltwyck and requiring Northside's type of program would receive the same priority." Although the Joint Committee's work continued, the partnership never occurred. Bernard had been such an influential Wiltwyck administrator that her 1960 break with the Northside Center put an end to such an affiliation.[62]

Community Psychiatry, Racial Liberalism, and the Creation of the Harlem Hospital Psychiatric Ward

The collapse of Northside and Wiltwyck's proposed partnership did not end the drive to link Wiltwyck with a Harlem clinic. In fact, a partnership did develop between the school and a facility not yet in existence in 1959. Although some racial liberals supported Wiltwyck, Northside, Lafargue, and other voluntary attempts to reduce Harlem's mental health disparities, they still considered the elimination of racial inequality the city government's responsibility. In the 1940s when Bernard, Polier, Winsor, and several other colleagues worked with the CWCCH, they had identified a publicly funded psychiatric clinic as a critical Harlem need. In 1962 that wish came true. Harlem Hospital got its own psychiatric department.

In the late 1950s, civil-rights activists helped put that goal back onto the racial-liberal radar. After the Lafargue Clinic closed in 1959, some local Harlemites started pushing for a full-time psychiatric department at Harlem Hospital. The Harlem Neighborhoods Association (HANA) led this charge. HANA was a largely black, middle-class "independent community organization" established in December 1958.[63] In 1959 HANA established a mental health committee to create "an active program for improving the treatment and preventive aspects of mental health in Harlem."[64] Alluding to the Lafargue Clinic's recent closure, the committee asserted in June 1960 that "financial pressures" had made "less services available through voluntary mental health clinics in Harlem." HANA then proposed that Mayor Robert F. Wagner Jr. ought to remedy this lack.[65]

In May 1961, HANA determined that Harlem's "dominant [mental health] need is for the development of an expanded psychiatric program at Harlem Hospital in keeping with modern knowledge." HANA's mental health committee, led by the Children's Court psychiatrist Dr. Joseph King, criticized Harlem Hospital's existing outpatient psychiatric services as inferior, overcrowded, understaffed, and lacking "adequate professional leadership." Among other things, HANA called for Harlem Hospital to develop a full-time department with a director, medical school affiliation, inpatient care, emergency services, consultations, and a "strong social service staff."[66]

Heading into the election year 1961, Mayor Wagner and his political secretary, the "Harlem Fox" J. Raymond Jones, were courting the black vote in Harlem. Since Mayor Wagner's tenure had begun in 1954, civil-rights leaders including Kenneth Clark had recommended that he do more to integrate city services and end racial inequality in the distribution of public resources. Unwilling to desegregate the public schools, Wagner looked for other less politically charged ways to demonstrate support for racial integration and equal opportunity.[67] Given this need, Wagner embraced HANA's proposal. With the active intervention of well-placed racial liberals in Wagner's administration and political circle, Harlem Hospital would have a new department by year's end.

Among the historical factors that help explain the creation of Harlem Hospital's psychiatric department, none is perhaps more pivotal than the community psychiatry movement. Intended as an alternative to state hospital care, this movement melded social psychiatry and mental hygiene with epidemiology.[68] In community psychiatry, clinicians treated patients within their own neighborhoods, offering services tailored to a local population's aggregate psychological needs. To administer this decentralized model of care, major cities created community mental health centers. These were fully equipped psychiatric clinics located within a local hospital. In the 1960s, the federal government subsidized the development of mental health centers. The endorsements of the 1961 Joint Commission for Mental Health, the National Institutes of Mental Health, and President John F. Kennedy convinced legislators. In 1963, Congress passed the Mental Retardation and Community Mental Health Centers Construction Act, subsidizing the construction of mental health centers. With this new aid available through state grants, public hospitals lacking a psychiatric wing could no longer claim that money was unavailable.[69]

Bernard had been seeking support for community psychiatry since the early 1950s. New York was receptive. Long before the Kennedy administration promoted the decentralization of psychiatric care, New York had been the nation's leader in community psychiatry. In 1954 the New York state legislature passed the first Community Mental Health Services Act in the United States. That same year New York created its own Community Mental Health Board.[70] Academia also threw its support behind this retreat from the state hospital model of care. In 1955 Bernard founded Columbia University's new Division of Community Psychiatry. Its first director, she aimed to train administrators to run the nation's new locally based psychiatric units.[71]

Bernard argued that the proliferation of new local clinics necessitated a new breed of administrator—one cut from the same cloth as her mentors Kenworthy and Max Winsor. Social psychiatry had been a discipline Bernard learned on the job, by observing Winsor. He taught her how to recognize a community's specific needs by using a race-blind lens. Through trial and error, she figured out how to communicate that vision to staff, supervisors, policymakers, and the public. Although she had learned all of this on the job, Bernard believed these skills and sensibilities could also be taught in a more formal way. To create the ideal clinical administrator, she crafted a curriculum rooted in public health, mental hygiene, and a race-neutral approach to psychodynamic theory. Bernard explained that "the social psychiatrist's therapeutic influence is transmitted indirectly and at a distance, as through consultation and administration."[72] Bernard expected her future community psychiatry administrators to transmit this therapeutic influence by forging an antiracist, institutional culture within their clinics. That is what she felt Winsor had done in the Harlem Unit and she hoped it could be replicated in the nation's new community mental health centers.[73]

Bernard would not have been able to create this experimental community psychiatry program had racial liberals failed to make inroads within the Columbia University College of Physicians and Surgeons. Fortunately for Bernard, Columbia was home to two kindred spirits with political pull: Lawrence Kolb, the chair of the Department of Psychiatry, and Ray E. Trussell, Dean of the Columbia School of Public Health and Administrative Medicine. Her program's success depended on their support. Kolb and Trussell were converts to the community mental health movement. Just as important, these two shared Bernard's liberal faith in the psychological equality of the races. Like Bernard, Trussell and Kolb believed that the mental health needs of the black communities surrounding both Columbia's main campus and Columbia-Presbyterian Hospital had been severely neglected. In 1957, both men, along with Bernard, had undertaken a long-term study of the psychiatric needs of the largely black and Puerto Rican neighborhoods of Washington Heights—the Columbia-Washington Heights Community Mental Health Project.[74]

Most significantly, Trussell's interest in both community psychiatry and the fight against racial inequality helped sell the Wagner administration on a race-blind assessment of central Harlem's psychiatric needs. In the late fifties, Trussell immersed himself in health care politics. He first served as the executive director of a mayoral commission studying the city's hospital care. Trussell argued that a stronger partnership between the public sector and academic medicine would make health care more efficient. He persuaded Mayor Wagner and gained his confidence.[75] A direct heir to the New Deal liberalism of his senator father, Wagner and his Democratic administration actively promoted union rights, public schools, and public housing. As his most lasting legacy, Wagner proved willing to stem capital flight through massive subsidies to industry and academia.[76] Public investment in the city's medical schools made sense to an administration eager to use municipal funds to enhance the private sector. In 1961, Wagner's favor earned Trussell an appointment as New York City's Commissioner of Hospitals.[77]

Trussell's presence at the very top of the metropolitan health care system afforded him the opportunity to make wide changes within the racial distribution of medical resources. With the assent of Mayor Wagner, Trussell overhauled New York's hospitals in the 1960s. He increased funding, expanded services, and created more coordination between the underfunded municipal hospitals and the higher quality voluntary hospitals. More than any previous public health official, Trussell paid particular attention to the city's psychiatric care facilities. By 1962, Trussell found that seventeen of the twenty-one municipal hospitals lacked psychiatric care. Harlem Hospital still had only a small mental hygiene clinic, and the hospital's "other major psychiatric function there was to sedate and restrain psychotic patients for transfer to Bellevue." Without a university affiliation, the clinic had difficulty retaining staff and providing consistent care for the indigent. Owing to the recent demise of the Lafargue Clinic, overcrowded Bellevue was filling up with Harlem patients that Harlem Hospital could not handle.[78]

To convince Mayor Wagner to establish full psychiatric services at Harlem Hospital, Trussell called on his Columbia colleague Lawrence Kolb. In 1961 Trussell appointed his fellow community psychiatry advocate as the head of a Special Advisory Committee on Psychiatric Services. Trussell instructed Kolb's committee to investigate and propose solutions to the city's mental health care problems.[79] Both Trussell and Kolb, in the committee's September "Kolb Report," recommended the community psychiatry approach. The Kolb report advised the city to forge "patterns of affiliation" between "municipal hospitals, university hospitals, medical schools and teaching hospitals." The effect would be to "improve the quality of care in municipal hospitals," spreading inpatient psychiatric services throughout the city's hospitals.[80] Although the academic health center model was only in its infancy in the 1960s, the provision of municipal services through private-sector arrangements had a long tradition in the history of American public welfare.[81] Since the 1930s, New York's racial liberals had not been averse to such partnerships—just as long as resources were distributed equally to all deserving citizens.[82]

In response to Trussell and Kolb's full-court press, Wagner agreed to fund "comprehensive psychiatric services" in the municipal hospital system, starting with Harlem.[83] Apparently the mayor relented only after Kolb and Trussell took him on a guided tour of Bellevue's psychiatric ward. The visit gave Wagner a better sense of both Bellevue's overcrowding and the insufficiency of Harlem's reliance on a facility nearly six miles south of 110th Street.[84] In any event, Trussell and Kolb won mayoral approval for a proposed psychiatric unit at Harlem Hospital that did not seem all that different from what HANA had urged Wagner to build.[85] In the public promotion of Harlem Hospital's redevelopment, the Department of Hospitals carefully avoided framing it as a remedy for racial inequality in the delivery of mental health services. Instead, Trussell couched the project within the Wagner administration's rhetoric of universal entitlement. In a press release, Trussell urged the public to regard its investment in Harlem Hospital as part of a larger effort to improve the entire municipal hospital system. According to the commissioner, the city was doing little more than fulfilling its responsibility to provide neighborhood hospitals for the poor. With so many financially needy people in Harlem reliant on the municipal hospital system, fairness dictated that the facility designated for that population be equipped to meet all of its medical needs.[86]

Concerned as they were with increasing the quantity of care available to African Americans, racial liberals were just as adamant that such care should be high quality. To give Harlem Hospital a top-flight psychiatric department, Trussell entrusted that mission to his other employer, Columbia University. As Commissioner of the Department of Hospitals, Trussell cleared the way for the development of a new psychiatric department by forging a formal affiliation between Harlem Hospital and Columbia University's College of Physicians and Surgeons. Trussell first championed this proposed affiliation in 1959 while heading a mayoral commission on hospitals. A plan had been on the table since 1960, but the affiliation did not become official until October 1964. The process of redeveloping Harlem

Hospital's departments began in April 1961 when Commissioner Trussell finally secured the public funds and political will needed to build a "working arrangement" with Columbia.[87] Dr. Aubre L. Maynard, the Harlem Hospital surgeon who claimed to have saved Dr. King's life in 1958, was impressed with Trussell's "relentless drive" in pursuit of this affiliation. In the late seventies, he remarked that "one could not recall a Commissioner who had gone to such lengths on behalf of this ghetto institution." What Trussell pursued was not business as usual within New York City's system of health and public welfare. Racial liberals had gained a foothold within the commissioner's office and changes appeared to be on the way for Harlem Hospital—especially in mental health care.[88]

At Trussell's request, Kolb and the Columbia University Department of Psychiatry were tasked with developing Harlem Hospital's new psychiatric department.[89] According to Department of Hospital rules, affiliated medical schools staffed their municipal teaching hospitals. This meant that Harlem Hospital's full-time staff members had to be Columbia faculty. As a result, many of Harlem Hospital's physicians—especially the most senior clinicians, the majority of them white—lost their positions.[90] Although Trussell tried to involve Harlem Hospital's existing medical program in the process of hiring new staff, he wanted little more than a rubber stamp for Columbia's handpicked candidates. For the most part, Harlem Hospital's old guard did not stand in the way of the drastic changes Lawrence Kolb had in store.[91]

As the affiliation developed, a race-neutral model of community psychiatry continued to gain ground within the New York Department of Hospitals. Enjoying unprecedented freedom to reduce racial inequality within health care, Kolb took full advantage of his policymaking opportunities, creating an innovative community psychiatry program at Harlem Hospital. Kolb himself took over the duty of overseeing the development and budgeting of the new psychiatric department. Kolb provided Columbia faculty, graduate students, interns, residents, administrators, and psychiatric consultants to staff, assist, and operate the new psychiatric ward.

On the first of July 1962, Harlem Hospital officially established its psychiatric department. In its first year, outpatient services for both children and adults were revamped and expanded, new emergency room services were created, follow-up procedures were established with outside agencies, and the Psychiatric Day Hospital opened. In 1963 the new department opened its first inpatient service—the crown jewel of the revamped psychiatric program. Thanks to an NIMH grant in 1964, the hospital even opened an aftercare facility, the Harlem Rehabilitation Center. In 1965 Harlem Hospital opened a child psychiatry division. Community psychiatry had come to Harlem.[92]

The Harlem Hospital psychiatric clinic was the sort of facility the City-Wide Citizens Committee for Harlem had called for during World War II. In contrast to the Northside Center, there was no question that Harlem Hospital's new department was psychiatric in orientation. The clinic was designed, administered, staffed, and advised by Bernard's Columbia colleagues. As a result, Harlem Hospital's psychiatric division met her strict standards of psychiatric care. Many of the first clinicians on the interracial staff of the new psychiatric "Ward 9-K" were people Bernard knew.[93] The first chief of inpatient services was Hugh F. Butts, a black psychiatry professor at Columbia and the clinical director of Wiltwyck's new Floyd Patterson halfway house. The first chief of Harlem Hospital's consultation services and emergency room services was Hagop [Jack] Mashikian. Mashikian was a white psychiatrist who had been a fellow in Bernard's community psychiatry training program and a Wiltwyck staff psychiatrist. June Jackson Christmas, a black clinician and the first head of Harlem Hospital's Rehabilitation Center and Group Therapy Program, was also a Columbia staff psychiatrist, a contact of Bernard's early in her career, and an associate of both the Northside Center and the Lafargue Clinic.[94]

Probably no one on Harlem Hospital's staff met Bernard's approval more than Margaret Morgan Lawrence and Elizabeth B. Davis. Lawrence joined as the head of the Developmental Psychiatry Service in 1963 and Davis became the psychiatric department's first director. Lawrence and Davis had been two of Bernard's first black female recruits. At Columbia, Bernard had trained both of them. Davis (who would later marry Ray Trussell) even joined Columbia's faculty. She served as a staff psychiatrist at Columbia-Presbyterian's Vanderbilt Psychiatric Clinic in 1959 when Bernard and Kolb were conducting the Washington Heights Project. Davis and Lawrence had lived and worked in Harlem, developing the kind of hands-on familiarity with postwar Harlem that few clinicians possessed. Not only had Lawrence and Davis both served at the Northside Center, but they also interned at Harlem Hospital, with Davis working in its mental hygiene clinic for almost five years during the late 1950s. Davis also worked with Harlemites through the James Weldon Johnson Mental Health Center and the Social Service Society. A daughter of Shelton Hale Bishop, Davis had even volunteered at the Lafargue Clinic while she was in medical school. Regarding her as a clinical and social expert on central Harlem, Kolb consulted with Davis before he agreed to help Trussell develop Harlem Hospital's first psychiatric division.[95] Just as important for Bernard, both women generally subscribed to her model of community psychiatry.[96] With her training, Harlem connections, and liberal proclivities, Davis seemed ready to become the administrator Bernard hoped her community psychiatry program would produce. From Bernard's vantage point, the future of psychiatry at Harlem Hospital was in capable hands.

Harlem and the Hudson Valley: The Harlem Hospital-Wiltwyck Partnership

Elizabeth Davis's new division was peopled with like-minded psychiatrists committed to ending racial disparities in mental health care. As June Jackson Christmas recounted, the clinicians who came on board with Davis shared an "esprit de corps," a feeling that they were working for a much "bigger cause" than simply the creation of a new psychiatric unit. She and her fellow clinicians, many of them African American, had given up financially lucrative positions to serve central Harlem's black community. What motivated her colleagues to accept these positions was a shared desire to help people whose human needs had been either ignored or disavowed by both psychiatry and the public sector. According to Christmas, the mission that she and some of her fellow black colleagues seemed to share was born of a "sixties"-era sense of "social responsibility for others that we as black people have to have."[97]

Harlem Hospital's new psychiatrists framed this concern with the "linked fate" of the black community in psychological terms.[98] Drs. Davis, Christmas, Butts, and their new colleagues had rejected the old racialist rationales for the neglect of black mental health, namely, that African Americans were naturally "better able to cope" with stress and strain. Many of these new hires were antiracists who recognized that in central Harlem "black people have all these range of problems" found in predominantly white communities, but lacked the psychiatric facilities to adequately diagnose and treat them. Color-blind racial liberalism found a welcome home within Ward 9-K.[99]

Given that a pocket of racial liberals seemed to be forming within Harlem Hospital's newest division, the Wiltwyck School made overtures to Dr. Davis almost immediately.[100] Beyond its racial politics, Harlem Hospital also appealed to the board because it now offered inpatient and day treatment services that Wiltwyck could not provide its clients and aftercare residents.[101] After Davis informed Bernard that Harlem Hospital planned to open its child psychiatry division in early 1963, an effort was made to formally link the two institutions.[102] Between November and April, representatives from the two facilities agreed to a four-pronged relationship: "staff interchanges" so that representatives from one institution could serve as consultants for the other, collaboration on cases where clientele overlapped, demonstrations of Minuchin's family therapy for the Harlem Hospital staff, and a preferred referral system.[103]

In the proposal for the Harlem-Wiltwyck liaison, Bernard and her fellow authors chose to present the linkage as "part of a community psychiatry design." Bernard cited a then-unreleased study she was working on for the Department of Hospitals. This paper, known as the Abbate report, stressed that the public sector could promote community psychiatry by linking private children's agencies with affiliated municipal psychiatric departments. The authors of the Wiltwyck-Harlem proposal argued that a "relationship of Wiltwyck with the Departments of Psychiatry at Harlem Hospital and Columbia University will carry out the intent of this recommendation," enmeshing Wiltwyck's boys within a web of care extending from the Catskills back to their neighborhoods.[104] Trussell confirmed the plan in October 1963, creating an official link between Wiltwyck, its halfway house, and Harlem Hospital's new Department of Psychiatry.[105]

Conclusion

When the Lafargue Clinic first opened in 1946, its cofounder and booster Richard Wright announced in the international humanist press the headline

"Psychiatry Comes to Harlem."[106] Yet in 1962, three years after the clinic closed its doors, analogous headlines might have read: "Psychiatry Comes to Harlem Hospital." Although the opening of an independent facility almost two decades earlier might seem unrelated to the creation of the publicly funded Ward 9-K in 1962, the two events are very much related.

The activists and professionals who founded and supported small, independent facilities such as Wiltwyck, Northside, and Lafargue had not given up hope that New York's government agencies would someday invest more equitably in the emotional health of black Harlem. Facing a hostile Cold War political climate within the public sector of the 1950s, color-blind psychiatrists found support for their ideas and practice within both Columbia University and the Harlem Neighborhoods Association. Public policy, civil society, and academic medicine were not discretely bounded domains, especially at the municipal level. Mayor Wagner's administration provided an opportunity for racial liberals to devote public resources to the race-neutral brand of community psychiatry they had patiently nurtured within both academia and the voluntary sector. Making the most of new connections between the Department of Hospitals, Columbia, HANA, and the Wiltwyck School, Trussell and Kolb finally found color-blind psychiatry a home at Harlem Hospital. Nevertheless, what that would mean for central Harlem's black population would not be as simple as racial liberals naively expected.

Chapter Seven

The Limits of Racial Liberalism

Harlem Hospital and the Black Community, 1963–68

In a 1983 interview, Elizabeth Davis recalled a public forum held at 135th Street's Countee Cullen Library in the late 1960s. At the event, citizens reacted to a controversial new Harlem Hospital program. The psychiatric department had been prescribing elective tubal ligation as a treatment for poor mothers diagnosed with postpartum psychosis. Some locals strongly opposed this therapy. Black Power advocates—whom Davis remembered as "no-doubt sincere community leaders"—called sterilization a genocidal white plot. These "leaders" did not trust the hospital authorities. Instead, they regarded them as conspirators. One man, directing his venom at Davis, accused this Harlem-raised African American of being a Jewish outsider preying on the black community.[1]

What had happened? The opening of Harlem Hospital's psychiatric department in 1962 seemed to have been a success story. Nevertheless, the vignette indicates that it would be misleading to end this book on a note of uncomplicated triumphalism. Certainly racial liberals expected that racial inequality would decline as African Americans received greater access to public resources. Historical outcomes often defy expectations, however. Ward 9-K and its race-neutral standard of care had not eliminated the mental health disparities facing the black community. In some ways, color-blind psychiatrists even exacerbated those inequalities.

This chapter examines Dr. Davis's first five years of community psychiatry in Harlem, taking stock of its successes and its failures. First, it will investigate how universalism became widely accepted among antiracist psychiatrists even as they became divided over the best way to implement it. Second, it will explore the consequences of color-blind psychiatry's own built-in contradictions. The drive to understand a black patient's social circumstances without reference to race actually blinded Davis and her associates to racism. In place of race, community psychiatrists at Columbia, Wiltwyck, and Harlem Hospital framed their patients' problems as a class issue. These clinicians were drawn to the ostensibly race-neutral "culture of poverty" and "cultural deprivation" theories, both of which blamed Harlem's ills on the behavior of its poorest families.

Third, this chapter examines the relationship between Harlem Hospital and the community it served. Throughout the 1960s, central Harlem had become more racially segregated, economically disinvested, and radicalized. Yet in assessing the community's needs, the Department of Psychiatry staff generally worked with people who supported racial liberalism. Davis relied on informants in the Harlem Neighborhoods Association (HANA), an organization of liberals and moderates. Yet Davis was not opposed to fresher ideas. In 1964, she allowed the psychiatrist and civil-rights activist Dr. June Jackson Christmas to create the Rehabilitation Center. That exciting program empowered Harlem residents to help state hospital patients readjust to life. But even that program's participants shared the racial liberals' faith in the power of equal opportunity, expecting racial inequality to abate when motivated individuals gained inclusion within the public sector.

Fourth, the chapter concludes with an analysis of Harlem Hospital's sterilization controversy. Not everyone in Harlem believed Ward 9-K had their best interests at heart. Despite Davis's good intentions, she and her psychiatrists continued to overdiagnose psychosis among African Americans. This racial disparity did not persist because the staff suffered a lapse in race neutrality. Rather, their color-blind approach is what allowed it to endure. Analyzing the psychology of poor black mothers, Davis and her staff unintentionally reified old racial stereotypes, uncritically deploying psychodynamic theory loaded with racialized assumptions about black primitivity. Harlem Hospital's local reputation was further tarnished by its association with Columbia University, one of upper Manhattan's most unpopular landlords. Local dissatisfaction with psychiatry reveals that Ward 9-K's early history was not a story of unqualified success. Instead that dissatisfaction illuminates racial liberalism's limitations in the fight against racial inequality, raising questions as to how much psychiatry had really broken free of its racist foundations.

Universality of the Human Psyche

By the 1960s, color-blind and environmental explanations of clinical differences between races had become almost axiomatic in the psychiatric literature. When the prominent antiracist psychiatrist Benjamin Pasamanick posited in 1963 that "most Negro-white differences had been traced to their environmental sources," he was not alone. Much of the new work on race and psychology confirmed his claim. Published articles with a racialist slant had substantially declined. In their survey of the literature, the psychologists Ralph Mason Dreger and Kent S. Miller noted a marked decrease between 1959 and 1965 in the number of "naive papers . . . attempting racial comparisons" in print.[2]

As racialism declined within the psychiatric literature, some writers finally felt comfortable enough to openly declare that blacks and whites shared the same basic emotional makeup. That assumption had been at the root of most antiracialist thought on psychology since the 1930s. Yet before the 1960s, antiracist psychiatrists had not developed that unstated assumption into a clearly articulated statement of faith. Compared with other professions—including psychology and anthropology—psychiatry had been relatively slow to abandon scientific racism. Bolstered by the new postwar discourse of human rights, leading scholars in the social sciences had already proclaimed their color-blind convictions, most famously in the 1950 UNESCO Statement on Race. Still, a belief in the psychological equality of the races had not reached that level of acceptance within psychiatry early in the Cold War.[3] Entering the 1960s, antiracists exerted more influence within the profession. Psychiatrists even changed the way they wrote about race. As Anne C. Rose has ably documented, the literature witnessed a rise in books touting the psychological "unity of the species."[4] Universalism's emergence as a clearly articulated position indicated that psychiatry had entered a new historical moment.

In 1964 Harlem Hospital's director, Elizabeth B. Davis, unpacked her race-neutral assumptions in a symposium on the "Negro Family." At the outset of her paper on personality formation among African Americans, Davis explicitly stated that for "all human infants . . . we can assume" that "most" were born with "more or less the same limited capacities . . . the same physiological and emotional reactions, and the same potential for individuation and socialization." Biological race did not determine one's psychological destiny. She acknowledged the existence of "real differences among individuals in the limits of these capacities and potentials." But the "distribution" of those differences "is similar if not identical for all racial and national groups." Davis had not offered any new ideas. What was new was Davis's presentation of taken-for-granted, unspoken assumptions as hard facts. She boldly asserted that "most reliable evidence" now supported the psychological equality of black and whites.[5] Racial liberals had consigned racialism to the dustbin of medical history, openly replacing it with a race-neutral understanding of psychiatry's truths.

Despite universalism's seeming triumph over racialism, questions remained as to the precise relationship between race and psychology. Obviously, race neutrality presupposed that race did not determine psychology. Nature lacked the power to generate a black personality type. But did nurture lack that power? According to community psychiatrists such as Dr. Davis, the children of all races matured along similar lines when raised in comparable environments. So was it possible that black children and white children grew up in contexts so dissimilar from one another that black life had generated a uniquely black psyche?

In the early sixties, some clinicians—especially racial liberals—refused to consider the possibility that black culture nurtured a black psychological type. According to the historians Mark Brilliant and Lorrin Thomas, postwar racial liberals tended to shy away from open discussions of black cultural difference.[6] Since the early 1940s, they had urged the public to equate equality with homogeneity. Too much attention paid to the uniqueness of African American life threatened to undermine psychological arguments made in defense of racial integration. Racial liberals promised that desegregation would work precisely because blacks and whites were so fundamentally similar, both culturally and psychologically. But *The Mark of Oppression* and other early studies of racism's impact on African Americans tended to depict black culture and the black psyche as distinctive and damaged. Racial liberals feared such studies implied that black life produced individuals too maladjusted for racial integration to succeed. In reaction, some psychiatrists took a stricter race-neutral position, shying away from questions of cultural differences between the races.[7]

Some critics recognized that a number of liberals had taken this hard line on race neutrality as a defense against conservatives. The Northside Center psychiatrist Alexander Thomas acknowledged that most racial liberals believed that blacks faced unique social pressures. But, he noted, those same "color-blind" clinicians denied that the black experience with racism was formative enough to produce a black personality type.[8] Even when color-blind psychiatrists analyzed racism, they regarded it as merely a superficial "triggering mechanism" for deeper, more fundamentally human emotional conflicts. According to Thomas, those clinicians took this position out of fear that racists might use evidence of deep psychological differences between the races to justify the exclusion of African Americans.[9]

Nevertheless, some antiracist psychiatrists recognized that "blindness to black cultural patterns" might be just as dehumanizing as racialism. Echoing a criticism Bernard had made as early as 1947, Thomas claimed that some naïve but well-intentioned psychiatrists were doing little but scrutinizing black patients for signs of "universal personality trends" drawn from studies of neurotic middle-class whites. According to him, color-blind clinicians never seriously examined whether these allegedly "universal" patterns of development were culturally specific to whites. Thomas's criticism was representative of the cultural interactionists—antiracist psychiatrists interested in the "dynamic interaction between the human organism and its culture."[10]

Cultural interactionists warned that a continued blind eye to race could have dire consequences for black patients. According to the young black San Francisco psychiatrists Drs. William H. Grier and Price Cobbs, white clinicians unaware of the cultural "black norm" would misinterpret the culturally specific meaning of a black patient's behavior, making misdiagnosis likely.[11] Thomas agreed, opining that a strict color-blind approach dehumanized the black patient, ignoring that "as with any other human being, what he is as an individual involves his specific social experiences."[12] Cultural interactionists urged clinicians to stop reifying white patterns of personality development as though they were a "universal" human condition. Instead, they encouraged them to study how the black experience could impact emotional development.[13]

In the 1960s, cultural interactionists insisted that the black experience had generated a unique psychological type. It was healthy, strong, and adaptive. Black personality development deviated from the unmistakably middle-class "white norm" naturalized in seminars and textbooks. These developmental differences were not congenital. Rather, they were the product of the specific social forces impinging on the lives of African Americans from cradle to grave.[14] Inspired in part by the anticolonial psychiatrist Frantz Fanon and other Black Diasporan critics of racism's psychological impact, young social scientists, intellectuals, and black nationalists imagined the internal life of African Americans in new ways during the 1960s. On the one hand, thinkers in the Association of Black Psychologists (formed in 1968) and the Black Psychiatrists of America (1969) considered the black psyche a gauge of the harm white supremacy had inflicted on people of color. They also regarded it as a fertile seedbed for the growth of a black revolutionary consciousness.[15] Historians have noted that "what distinguished the thought of these leftist social scientists was their rejection of images of pathology and victimhood, their embrace of black pride, and their reading of the African American past as characterized by cultural resistance."[16]

Grier and Cobbs's 1968 *Black Rage* was representative of these new studies. These two African American clinicians argued that black culture had produced a healthy black psychological type. The black community was a strong, resilient force steeling individuals against racism. They claimed that black culture imprinted on emotional development during infancy, generating a personality equipped to survive the stress of racism. According to the authors, racism caused emotional pain for all blacks. Pent up over time, they warned, this pain could explode into "rage—black rage, apocalyptic and final."[17] The black community, however, helped individuals develop an inner life capable of safely sublimating this rage, preventing racism's toll from becoming individually debilitating. Grier and Cobbs implored clinicians to recognize that black culture enabled blacks to thrive in the United States, arguing that it endowed the black psyche with a "'healthy' cultural paranoia," meaning a state of vigilance against racism.[18]

While *Black Rage* certainly presented the black psyche as distinctive, its authors also wanted readers to be aware that nature had nothing to do with it. Grier and Cobbs asserted that the psyches of all races worked in the same way:

> There is nothing reported in the literature or in the experience of any clinician known to the authors that suggests that black people *function* differently psychologically from anyone else. Black men's mental functioning is governed by the same *rules* as that of any other group of men. Psychological principles understood first in the study of white men are true no matter what the man's color. . . . [So] while the *experiences* of black people in this country are unique, the *principles* of psychological functioning are by definition universal.[19]

In reassuring readers that they supported universalism, Grier and Cobbs shielded themselves from the accusations of racism that greeted Kardiner and Ovesey's study of the black psyche in the 1950s.[20] Grier and Cobbs argued that nurture had produced the black psychological type. Yet they also acknowledged that nature endowed blacks and whites with the same psychological potential and capacities.[21] That shared assumption—that blacks and whites were psychologically similar from birth—set all antiracist psychiatrists apart from racialists. Nonetheless, the cultural interactionists split from racial liberals in insisting that black culture helped generate deep psychological differences between blacks and whites as early as childhood.[22]

Psychiatrists involved in the Southern civil-rights movement were also convinced that black culture promoted emotional stability. Since the 1930s, racial liberals demonstrated a tendency to "locate the human in a universal capacity to suffer." As early as 1949, James Baldwin, one of America's most perceptive critics of racism, warned that "associating the human with suffering actually limits the human to a mode of absolute passivity."[23] By the mid-1960s, Baldwin's view gained wider adherence as activists found the rural towns on the black freedom struggle's frontlines to be sources of psychological strength.[24] Between 1965 and 1966, the young East Harlem-raised Alvin Poussaint served as the "first southern field director" for the Medical Committee on Human Rights (MCHR), a group of physicians who provided protestors with first aid.[25] As a member of Harvard's medical faculty, Poussaint accused psychiatrists of being "too quick to find only pathology in the black experience in America." Fearing that such an approach might only reinforce "racist attitudes," he urged clinicians to locate "the many strengths of the black community."[26] The psychiatrist Robert Coles, a white racial liberal and Poussaint's Harvard colleague, also discovered "that alongside suffering I have encountered resilience and an incredible capacity for survival" in the South's black communities.[27] In 1968, a pair of researchers wrote: "There have been few, if any attempts, to find more sources of strength. . . . Yet such sources must exist."[28]

The Culture of Poverty and Its Discontents

Bernard and Davis did not search for sources of cultural strength within Harlem. Their community psychiatry focused on the treatment and prevention of group pathology.[29] Yet when studying African American patients, racial liberals resisted identifying race as the social category that bound them together as a group.[30] Instead they searched for a race-neutral way to talk about the specific social issues affecting African American neighborhoods. How could clinicians make sense of the particularities of black life without racializing them as exclusively black problems?[31]

According to color-blind clinicians, what bound their black patients together was class—an ostensibly race-neutral category. Harlem Hospital's and Wiltwyck's staff were strongly influenced by psychological studies of poverty. During the late 1950s and early 1960s, researchers claimed that poverty forced the poor to generate their own unique culture.[32] They urged middle-class therapists to learn the way impoverished Americans thought, acted, and expressed themselves. According to these studies, the circumstances and "values" of the poor conditioned their emotional development. If clinicians remained ignorant of the ways poverty imprinted on a patient's psyche, a communication gap might form, making diagnosis and treatment difficult.[33]

Davis and Bernard drew intellectual inspiration from this new work on the social psyche of the poor.[34] Davis relied on that literature when comparing the psychological impact of poverty and racial discrimination on her patients. By the mid-1960s, both she and Bernard thought that poverty, more than racism, explained any apparent differences between the personality development of blacks and whites. Davis, a product of the black middle class, was convinced that economic differentiation within the "'American Negro' subculture" mediated and determined how individuals emotionally handled the socioeconomic dislocations racism had forced on them. "The way in which any American Negro deals with these problems will depend on" his or her class. For Bernard and Davis, the black lower class was more than a status. It was a pathological "subculture" with its own "values, patterns of behavior and satisfactions."[35]

Bernard's and Davis's focus on the pathology of the black poor placed their research and publications in the 1960s in line with the "culture of poverty thesis" and "cultural deprivation theory."[36] According to these new theories—which enjoyed popularity between 1959 and the late 1960s—poverty was a deficient lifestyle rather than an economic circumstance.[37] Poverty perpetuated itself as the poor passed on this inferior culture to the next generation. Daniel P. Moynihan's much-maligned report of 1964, *The Negro Family*, echoed this sentiment, arguing that the black family's allegedly matriarchal culture had stunted black social progress. Although many researchers working in this vein did tend to study poor African Americans, they generally wrote about them using ostensibly race-neutral terms such as "culturally deprived," "disadvantaged," "disorganized," and "underprivileged."[38]

Although Salvador Minuchin was not a pioneer in this short-lived era of cultural-deprivation studies, his clinical work with former Wiltwyck students enjoyed the support of Dr. Bernard and Davis's Harlem Hospital staff. Having followed Minuchin's ongoing study of lower-class families with multiple delinquents since 1961, Bernard and Davis regularly cited the Wiltwyck psychiatrist when situating their professional thinking within the cultural-deprivation discourse.[39] With sessions conducted in Wiltwyck's Manhattan aftercare facilities, Minuchin's treatment study focused on twelve lower-class, non-Anglo families from "the most disadvantaged ghetto areas of New York City."[40] Eight of the families were African American and the remaining four were either Puerto Rican or Italian in origin. The end product of Minuchin's family-therapy experiment was the 1967 monograph *Families of the Slums*.[41] Informing the Wiltwyck study was the claim that families systematically transmitted "social rules and regulations to the growing child and provid[ed] blueprints for his cognitive and emotional development."[42] According to Minuchin, family was the primary mechanism by which culture molded a child's psyche.[43] Starting from that premise, Minuchin argued that his study's slum families shared the same parenting style. This childrearing style was the foundation of an emotionally unhealthy "subculture of poverty."[44] Minuchin argued that clinicians needed to become aware of these "disorganized pathological families" since they were likely to produce children with emotional problems, learning disabilities, and delinquency.[45]

According to Minuchin, the children of slum families could not function in mainstream society. Minuchin asserted that Wiltwyck's delinquents typically grew up in poor, disorderly homes with an overwhelmed single mother. Allegedly, this mother imposed arbitrary discipline, providing no fixed rules for her children to internalize. She failed to teach them how to regulate their own behavior or to take stock of the effect they had on anyone else.[46] These children found it hard to control their impulses, learn and apply rules, process abstract ideas, express themselves clearly, or develop empathy.[47] Minuchin concluded that these "children are equipped neither to meet a culture with demands different from those of their own nor to use the ensuing clash with that different culture to refashion their coping patterns." The study insinuated that these families would produce adults lacking the healthy, autonomous self that racial liberals expected color-blind psychiatry to promote. If slum families proliferated and central Harlem teemed with maladapted adults, Minuchin feared that the community's precarious mental health would only worsen.[48]

Nevertheless, Minuchin did not write off these families as therapeutically "unreachable."[49] Since the 1930s, antiracist psychiatrists had been confident that the capacity to benefit from psychotherapy was evenly distributed across the color line.[50] In an effort to help slum youth reach their full potential, Minuchin devised family-therapy techniques intended to help clinicians overcome "the specific limitations in the introspective and communicative abilities of these parents and children."[51] Minuchin called for therapists to spend time altering the family's style of interaction, which would, it was hoped, create a dynamic closer to the normative middle-class model. Without active interventions in the family unit, Minuchin warned that such children were likely to do poorly in school, fail to hold a job, fall prey to the lure of crime, and pass on this lifestyle to their children.[52]

Heavily influenced by Minuchin's Wiltwyck team, Davis and Bernard also depicted the culture of poor black families as pathological. Both reinforced his claim that slum family culture could arrest a child's emotional development. Davis and Bernard incorporated Minuchin's insights into their own explorations of the culture-personality interaction. Davis theorized that the "effect of poverty on ego development" and "learning ability" left lower-class blacks emotionally and cognitively "incompetent," unable to compete with other Americans.[53] Like Minuchin, they were confident that the slum family was not "only a possible source for the etiology or reinforcement of mental illness, but . . . a major focal point for its prevention and treatment."[54]

The culture of poverty thesis was controversial. Social scientists, civil-rights activists, and mental health professionals attacked it for treating the poor as an undifferentiated mass of broken people incapable of improving their lot.[55] Bernard, Minuchin, and Davis were aware of the critique, asserting that the culture of lower-class Harlemites was merely one of a number of possible group responses to poverty. Both Minuchin and Davis relied on the sociologist Herbert Gans's division of the poor into two types: a stable working-class family able to thrive despite destitution and an unstable lower-class family.[56] Apparently the culture of poverty thesis pertained only to this latter type of family. Similarly, in 1965 Bernard warned psychiatrists that "certain catch-all terms—for instance, the 'culture of poverty,'" led to the "error of over-simplified psychiatric generalizations about 'the underprivileged,' as if they were a single category."[57]

Still, some civil-rights activists and black intellectuals criticized psychiatrists for disproportionately applying these catch-all terms to the black poor. In 1968 the authors of a survey on race in the mental health literature complained: "For the most part, published research during this period has continued to focus on family *disorganization* among Negroes."[58] Quite a few black social scientists, including the Northside Center psychologist Kenneth B. Clark, recognized that ostensibly race-neutral phrases such as "culturally deprived" referred to African Americans and Puerto Ricans more than whites. These racially loaded terms were weighed down by "unspoken assumptions" about the behavior and inner lives of the nonwhite poor.[59] When clinicians such as Bernard and Davis analyzed black communities using cultural-deprivation theory or the culture of poverty thesis, they did not treat class and poverty as the product of social forces and economic structures. Instead, poverty was taken to be the result of bad behavior, inferior childrearing, and psychological illness. Alexander Thomas, Kenneth Clark's colleague, noted: "The concept of 'cultural deprivation' places the emphasis on the psychological characteristics of the poor individual himself—his language use, perceptual level, cognitive style, emotional attributes."[60] Replacing race with class in liberal analyses did little to reduce the public perception that Harlem's residents had blighted their own communities.

HANA: Assessing the Community in Community Psychiatry

Nevertheless, Davis and her new department sincerely believed that they understood these low-income residents and their social circumstances. In a 1967 workshop on "The Inner City," Davis argued that "we inner city psychiatrists can still identify and make known those aspects of poverty which are specifically pathogenic and specifically remediable within the context of existing social institutions."[61] A former Harlemite herself, Davis felt that she had an insider's knowledge of Harlem's "terrible deprivations." Growing up around her father's parish on 133rd Street and St. Nicholas Avenue, she had gotten to know central Harlem. She had also worked in several local clinics before taking the Harlem Hospital post. But Davis no longer lived in Harlem. She was even financially secure enough to send her daughter Liberty to the exclusive Walden High School on East 89th Street. Nonetheless, Dr. Davis claimed that her "experience in all the Harlem communities had prepared me to see their needs."[62]

Still, the Harlem of the 1960s was not the one of Davis's youth. What had happened in Harlem was part of a larger historical shift within the racial geography of postwar United States. In the prewar era, when housing discrimination was legal, segregated black communities displayed a high level of economic differentiation. Nationwide, urban living spaces such as central Harlem, Bedford-Stuyvesant, and Watts had long been home to African Americans of all classes. In the postwar era, urban renewal, slum clearance, race-based public-housing construction, the Second Great Southern Migration, capital flight, and fair-housing legislation coincided, reducing the number of businesses and upper-income blacks within the inner cities.[63] These older inner-ring urban spaces became almost entirely nonwhite spaces with high poverty levels. By 1970 Harlem and other black-identified neighborhoods were more than twice as racially homogenous as they had been in 1930.[64]

A host of problems beset central Harlem during this demographic shift. Residents endured declining access to opportunities for mobility, increasing poverty, overcrowded schools, onerous tax burdens, disinvestment, and police brutality.[65] The Harlem riot that took place between July 18 and July 20, 1964, dramatized the community's frustration. The trigger for these nightly uprisings was fifteen-year-old James Powell's shooting death at the hands of the off-duty white police officer Thomas Gilligan. Protests against police brutality filled Harlem's streets the next two days. On July 18, the police overreacted to the political demonstrations. In frustration, crowds of Harlemites resisted. Some fought back against the police. Others destroyed property and looted businesses for three nights.[66]

In the popular imagination, postriot Harlem was no longer an economically diverse black cultural mecca with just a few slum neighborhoods. As the news of the Harlem riot reached the national news, more and more Americans came to think of Harlem as an entirely black slum or "ghetto."[67] The white sports journalist Robert Lipsyte's popular 1967 young adult novel, *The Contender*, depicts a bleak, garbage-strewn wasteland inhabited by heroin addicts, gangs, layabouts, politically naïve young people, a few remaining Jewish-owned stores, and "raggedy and skinny" children.[68] Harlem appeared in the media as a sinking ship with abandonment the most rational response to it.

Many white Americans believed that African Americans themselves had brought about Harlem's decline. In a 1969 survey reported in *Science News*, a majority of the respondents agreed that individual "lack of motivation" accounted for any racial gap in education and economic achievement.[69] Urban spaces such as Harlem teemed with poor African Americans because its residents had not pulled themselves up by their own bootstraps and moved to more desirable locations. Of course this perspective ignored the role racism played in the shaping of America's racial geography. Explaining this gap in perception, the sociologist George Lipsitz argued that the postwar era's white middle class quickly normalized suburbia as a reward for individual success. For them, Harlem's image as a slum populated by society's failures served as proof that African Americans caused their own socioeconomic woes, thus dooming any efforts to ameliorate their living conditions.[70]

Despite what others believed, central Harlem of the late 1960s was still home to successful politicians and activists, each with their own assessment of the collective needs, talents, and *strengths* of its black residents.[71] Rather than abandon Harlem, these folks sought to sustain and improve it. Racial liberals advocated equal inclusion within government social programs.[72] Moderate civil-rights organizations sought public-school reforms, including racial desegregation, increased appropriations, and greater neighborhood say over school policy.[73] After Malcolm X's assassination in 1965 however, Black Power activists became a stronger presence, calling for greater community control of West and Central Harlem.[74] Locals tried taking the reins of their economy, launching new black-owned theaters, art studios, dance studios, consumer cooperatives, and Afrocentric lifestyle shops.[75]

Although Davis was confident in her own knowledge of Harlem, local activists helped her identify the region's mental health needs. Across the country more and more racial liberals chose to engage with the some of the more militant political voices as the 1960s drew to a close.[76] Davis, however, still preferred to work with groups loathe to antagonize "the white power structure." Davis sought an amiable working arrangement with powerful mainstream institutions, not unlike the links Polier forged within the La Guardia administration during the late 1930s. Davis hoped that strong relationships with city officials would help increase Harlem's access to quality mental health care.[77]

Since World War II, racial liberals had fought institutional racism from the inside. They attempted to acquire positions within New York's public sector, changing its internal culture enough that they could actually craft policies that restored racial fairness. Davis's presence within Harlem Hospital's psychiatric department fit this historical model. As department head, she could actively shape the kind of mental health care African Americans received.[78] Yet Davis had only just become such an institutional insider. Her department was brand new. As a black female administrator she had little political leverage within New York's health-policy machine. And the stakes were high. She was tasked with ensuring that her underserved population *retained* the mental health care services that had long been denied them. Maintaining the good will of the city's powerbrokers became a priority for her as she sought to achieve that goal.

Given her cautious avoidance of Harlem's more contentious voices, Davis turned to liberal and even socially conservative ones when assessing the "true needs of people in the Harlem community for medical care."[79] Mostly formal organizations, these included local churches, the YMCA, the United Block Association, the Urban League, and HANA.[80] Davis maintained an open dialogue with these middle-class agencies. Her staff served as liaisons or consultants with them, all in an effort to design programs "which are actually wanted and needed by the community as well as satisfying the clinician's need to use himself in ways which are relevant to his specific training."[81]

Early on, HANA helped provide Harlem Hospital with one gauge of black mental health needs. At times, HANA's growing support for self-determination and confrontational community action strategies put the group at odds with Davis's more cautious approach. But for the most part, Davis and HANA's leaders shared many of the same sensibilities and goals. HANA's leadership was an interracial cadre of middle-class liberals who had called for Harlem Hospital to expand its psychiatric services since 1960. HANA members such as Joseph King and Milton Yale considered mental health care such a critical unmet need in Harlem that the organization formed its own mental health committee in 1961. Well after Ward 9-K opened, the mental health committee "sustained its on-going role of exploring areas of needs and gaps in mental health services in Harlem."[82]

In the early 1960s, HANA held conferences in which hospital representatives heard the mental health concerns of Harlem activists. At one such event held on June 17, 1963, on the "Mental Health Needs of Harlem Youth," community activists alerted Harlem Hospital's child psychiatrist Virginia Wilking to the needs of unmarried mothers, teens, drug addicts, alcoholics, and children whom the public schools could not handle.[83] When HANA's mental health committee members identified a potentially significant mental health issue within central Harlem, they brought it to the hospital's attention. Between 1965 and 1968, HANA helped organize Harlem parents who opposed the public school system's suspension policy.[84] In late 1965 HANA's James Soler set up the Ad Hoc Committee on School Suspensions. It examined the problem from a variety of angles, including the possibility that the current policy psychologically harmed suspended children.[85]

Harlem Hospital had not previously identified school suspensions as a psychiatric issue. Nonetheless, HANA's James Soler succeeded in convincing Virginia Wilking to permit "the cooperation of Harlem Hospital in this venture."[86] To this end, the psychiatrist Cesarina Paoli served as liaison to HANA's Ad Hoc Committee. With Paoli's assistance, the committee relied on the psychiatric point of view to form its critique of the school suspension policy.[87] She helped them design a workshop where participants were encouraged to judge the policy's effectiveness at meeting the "special emotional and social needs of the suspended child."[88]

Out of such dialogue, Davis's staff designed programs to meet local needs. In some cases, Harlem Hospital sought the assistance of local agencies.[89] With the help of Associated Community Teams, the Domestic Peace Corps, the YMCA, and eventually the Board of Education, Harlem Hospital found space and a teaching staff for the new Harlem Child Study Center. The Center was a special all-day school for "emotionally disturbed" boys who were not yet ready for public school.[90] Similarly, in 1965 the Division of Child Psychiatry partnered with St. Philip's Community Youth Center, creating the Harlem Nursery for Child Development. This was a small "therapeutic nursery program" designed to prepare preschool children with severe developmental problems.[91] St. Philip's Episcopal Church pastor M. Moran Weston provided the Youth Center's "nursery school room to house the program."[92] This was not an unprecedented act. In 1946, Rev. Shelton Hale Bishop, Dr. Davis's father, allowed the Lafargue Clinic to open rent free in St. Philip's parish house basement. In forging similar local links, Davis was confident her department was doing its best to fill the gap in care left by Lafargue's closure.[93]

Deinstitutionalization, Community Empowerment, and Racial Liberalism

This relationship—racial liberals reliant on the black community for support— was not uncommon with the civil-rights era. Under Davis's watch, some laymen even received the chance to help provide their own neighbors with mental health care. Despite Davis's own circumspect policy approach, she permitted one of her most progressive staff members to create a pioneering experiment in community empowerment. In 1964, the Harlem Hospital psychiatric department opened its most ambitious project: Dr. June Jackson Christmas's Harlem Rehabilitation Center.

A product of Boston University's School of Medicine, Christmas was a multitalented, politically active African American woman. She believed that physicians ought to advocate for their patients' communities. Her strong sense of social responsibility for Harlem Hospital's population was born of the black freedom struggle. She had been active in the civil-rights movement since her high-school days organizing with the NAACP Youth Council. As with many Northern black activists in the sixties, her politics defied easy categorization. Christmas had been a member of the Student Nonviolent Coordinating Committee, a volunteer with the Lafargue Clinic, an MCHR member, and a proponent of public-school decentralization who counted David Dinkins and other rising Harlem Democrat as allies. She was familiar with the tokenism and paternalism of white "surface liberalism." Throughout her career as a municipal employee, Christmas remained suspicious of racial liberals even as she worked within the limited spaces for progressive change they had opened up within the public sector.[94]

Despite Christmas's own well-founded doubts about racial liberals, she developed a program that fit their mental health agenda. Harlem Hospital's Rehabilitation Center addressed a racial health disparity just emerging within Harlem, one produced by the historical convergence of deinstitutionalization and the postwar racialization of space. With the greater use of tranquilizers, antipsychotic drugs, and the passage of the US Community Mental Health Act, the deinstitutionalization of the state mental hospital population had just begun.[95] Since African Americans had long been overrepresented in state hospitals, black communities stood to receive a disproportionate share of the nation's discharged mental patients.[96]

Anticipating deinstitutionalization's local impact, Harlem Hospital developed one of the nation's first psychiatric aftercare facilities in 1964.[97] Though Davis may have been wary of political radicals, she was not opposed to leftist ideas. Given the space to innovate within Harlem Hospital's pocket of racial liberals, Dr. Christmas crafted a unique new program that was a fusion of liberal and leftist health-care trends. It combined community psychiatry and the community health center model of social medicine that the MCHR cofounder Dr. H. Jack Geiger spearheaded in Boston and Mississippi between 1965 and 1967.[98] Dubbing her approach "sociopsychiatric rehabilitation," Christmas crafted a program in which "group support was a critical change factor."[99] It provided clients with drug treatment and limited psychotherapy in group settings. Christmas hoped such an approach could return African Americans to productive and independent lives in central Harlem.[100]

Perhaps the most innovative aspect of the aftercare program was its reliance on local paraprofessionals. In the early 1960s, Saul Alinsky and other activists theorized that social programs would work better if locals ran them. The federal government's War on Poverty encouraged the "maximum feasible participation" of aid recipients.[101] With the help of the Domestic Peace Corps, Harlem's own Associated Community Teams, and other antipoverty groups, Christmas recruited three local women. They lacked formal training in either social work or medicine.[102] But as emotionally stable residents of the neighborhoods Harlem Hospital served, they were ideally suited for the job.[103] Given their "experience in, knowledge of, and identification with the lifestyle of the Harlem community,"[104] these locals had been hired to help the deinstitutionalized readjust to life across 110th street. In recruiting laypersons, Christmas conceded that residents knew more about day-to-day survival in central Harlem. Hiring those who "can speak the language of patients," she validated their community-situated knowledge.[105] Christmas imagined that Harlem contained well-adjusted individuals who had learned to manage life there. She looked for them. She found them.[106]

The Harlem Rehabilitation Center's lay workers served as cultural brokers in the broadest possible sense. The first lay workers, Viola Washington, Harriet Carter, and Hilda Wallace, were hardworking middle-aged women with children. As the program expanded, the profile of Christmas' recruits changed as well. The workers eventually included single men, young people, and even individuals struggling with their own social and emotional stability.[107] Owing to the "cross-class affinities" African Americans developed in segregated living spaces, these upwardly mobile workers helped patients from the lower end of the class spectrum find employment, job training, and recreation, and gave advice on where to live, shop, and eat in Harlem.[108] They relied on their knowledge about what "it took to cope in the community," assisting patients as they negotiated social services and the new Medicare and Medicaid programs created in 1963.[109] As Christmas explained: "We recruited persons in Harlem who had successfully used survival strategies—an honest day's work, hustling, dealing with 'the man,' breaking the law or abiding by it, or getting the most out of a demeaning welfare system."[110] What is more, Christmas provided her staff with enough mental hygiene training to serve as the clinic's cultural "expediters." In this role, the lay workers relied on their familiarity with local slang, cultural references, as well as West Indian patois and Southern rural idioms to help clients and clinicians understand one another better.[111]

Antipoverty activists hoped that greater citizen empowerment could restructure American society. The Rehabilitation Center's first paraprofessionals may not have shared that same expectation. These women were recruited because they understood how to negotiate within the structure of America's health care and welfare institutions. When describing their positions, Washington, Wallace, and Carter expressed little interest in replacing "the system" with something else. Instead they seemed to share a perspective closer to racial liberals.[112] Racial liberals understood that communities were enmeshed within a complex web of overlapping governmental systems, each with their own rules, bureaucracies, and resources. They presumed that racial disparities would decline when individuals from neglected communities finally gained access to those systems.[113] For local lay workers, Christmas's program offered an opportunity for fuller inclusion in established systems, the chance to redistribute resources to their underserved neighborhoods.

Christmas's hires also shared another value in common with racial liberals: individual responsibility. Once resources became available to formerly disenfranchised groups, racial liberals expected individuals to take the initiative and make use of them. The first lay workers agreed. They were go-getters with middle-class aspirations. Employment at Harlem Hospital offered Washington, Carter, and Wallace a chance for personal advancement. As they were surely aware, federal and state subsidies made health care the fastest growing industry of the 1960s. In addition, the 1964 Civil Rights Act outlawed racial discrimination in the public sector, offering African Americans a white-collar path to the middle class. In New York, some lay workers forged careers at Harlem Hospital. A few participants even became medical professionals.[114]

Statistics and Sterilization: The Racialization of Color-Blind Psychiatry

Despite their growing influence over urban policy in the 1960s, racial liberals did not eradicate black health disparities. In their new positions of public authority, they faced embedded policy constraints, political pressures, and institutional prerogatives that made it hard to reverse racial inequality. Even more distressing, some even served as unwitting agents of racial injustice, which earned them the scorn of the black community's radicals. Taking a color-blind stance, administrators failed to address the racialist logic encoded within psychiatry. Through the enforcement of racially loaded but ostensibly race-neutral practices, racial liberals helped reproduce and even create new health care disparities.[115] At Harlem Hospital, color-blind psychiatry unintentionally reified race as a medically salient category. In particular, its sterilization program for women with postpartum psychosis reveals how allegedly race-neutral medical care could reproduce and even create substantial racial differences in clinical outcomes.

Although Davis and her staff had rejected racialism outright, they still overdiagnosed African Americans as psychotics. Black rates of schizophrenia and postpartum psychosis were disproportionately high in the 1960s.[116] In fact, clinicians only began to diagnose and treat black men with schizophrenia during that decade. In this era of increasing civil-rights action, schizophrenia was redefined as a disease of violence, anger, and hostility. According to Jonathan Metzl, US psychiatry "positioned itself as an authority that made sense of the crisis posed by angry, protesting black men during the civil rights era." Psychiatrists began overdiagnosing black males as schizophrenics, framing this "epidemic" as somehow related to the rise in civil-rights agitation.[117]

Historians have not yet paid the same attention to racial patterns in the diagnosis of postpartum psychosis. But they were just as real. Between 1962 and

1964, Harlem Hospital diagnosed a disproportionate number of black women as having postpartum psychosis. As early as the 1920s, psychiatrists had normalized the so-called childbirth blues as a relatively harmless part of the puerperal experience. In the 1960s many clinicians still believed that "psychoses in the time immediately after childbirth did not represent a specific form of illness."[118] Harlem Hospital's staff, however, did not evince this same reticence to diagnose postpartum psychosis. According to Davis, in 1968 the "Harlem Hospital rate was about 200 percent above the national rate."[119]

Dr. Davis and her staff were not racialists. But they unwittingly reproduced the racialized evolutionary logic long engrained within Freudianism. Psychoanalytic theory had been articulated in allegorical terms. Freud had likened individual human development to the "evolution" of races and civilizations. Healthy personality development was analogous to the advancement of white Victorian civilization and the superiority of the bourgeois family. Conversely, Freud and other psychoanalytic theorists imagined madness and psychosis as arrested development akin to the immaturity of childhood, the backwardness of working-class family life, and the primitivity of nonwhites. By the 1960s psychodynamic theory appeared to be race neutral. Nevertheless, its racialist-evolutionary logic continued to suffuse the diagnostic thinking of even antiracist clinicians. And most of them were not aware of their profession's continued entanglement with the racialist past.

Informed by a psychodynamic theory embedded with disturbing assumptions about race and class, Harlem Hospital's community psychiatrists expected to find psychosis within the black community's poor families. Although color-blind clinicians framed class as a race-neutral category, it certainly did not operate free of racial meaning. Encoded within the community-psychiatry approach to class were many of the same racialized assumptions that had informed blatantly racist understandings of the black psyche. Dr. Davis defined psychosis as a severe developmental deficit characterized by disorganized and immature thinking, emotional volatility, and an inability to apprehend reality. Racialists had long described the black psyche in similar terms. In the 1960s, racial liberals described the psychology of the poor in those same terms. A paper Davis presented before the National Medical Association's annual meeting in 1967 is instructive here. Relying heavily on Minuchin's *Families of the Slum*, Davis's description of the lower-class child's psyche eerily echoes well-worn racialist claims about the allegedly primitive Negro psyche. Immature, erratic, and a poor fit for the Space Age's "constantly expanding world," lower-class children developed personalities that tended toward the psychotic. Although Davis deliberately deracialized her class analysis, cautioning her audience that such arrested development could happen to the "child of any family at the lowest end of the socio-economic scale," the racialized lineage of her lower-class psychological type is still unmistakable.[120]

Certainly the liberal pathologization of poverty helped perpetuate the overdiagnosis of psychosis among African Americans. Davis and her colleagues recognized that psychoses were overrepresented on Harlem Hospital's wards.

But they were convinced that this apparent racial disparity was actually a class disparity. In 1967 Davis explained that African Americans disproportionately suffered from severe mental illnesses because their poverty rate was so high. Harlem Hospital's community psychiatrists believed that poverty bred psychosis. So to Davis and her staff, it made sense that the race with the highest incidence of poverty would be more prone to psychotic states. According to Davis: "It comes, therefore, as no surprise to discover that the incidence of all the grosser forms of mental illness including psychosis, disorganized delinquent behavior and addiction, as well as the incidence of multiple physical and social disabilities is higher for Negroes than for other groups."[121] Clearly, deploying class in place of race did nothing to reduce a diagnostic pattern that extended perhaps as far as back as the 1890s. Instead, class renewed it, transforming a racial disparity into a seemingly nonracial side effect of slum life. As long as liberal psychiatrists remained unaware of the racial logic still underwriting their analysis of poverty, they could not see they were making class do the work of race. Lacking that awareness, color-blind clinicians were unable to make a clean break with the legacy of racial determinism.

Consequently, Harlem Hospital's race-tainted understanding of poverty's emotional impact informed its solutions to Harlem's high rates of postpartum psychosis. Davis and her colleagues worried that Harlem's rising concentration of poverty might produce more disorganized slum families and more psychosis, leaving fewer Harlemites prepared to handle mainstream American life. Since the 1930s, racial liberals expected that racial inequality would subside once equal access to opportunity stimulated black class mobility. But by 1965, some clinicians feared that long-standing poverty left some blacks psychologically incapable of climbing the economic ladder—even when given a fair chance. To break this cycle of poverty and psychosis, Davis imagined a new way to help impoverished families suffer less mental illness. Intent on keeping postpartum psychosis from reducing upward mobility in Harlem, she turned to a drastic intervention: the sterilization of poor black mothers with large families.

In conjunction with the obstetrics department, Davis established a formal program of elective sterilization for poor women with large families in 1965. Donald P. Swartz was the hospital's young white Canadian director of obstetrics and gynecology. As Davis and Swartz searched for ways to address "emotional and psychiatric problems around reproduction," they hit on this interdepartmental sterilization effort.[122] Dr. Davis believed that central Harlem's rising levels of slum poverty had begun to produce an epidemic of postpartum psychosis. She argued, as did Bernard before her, that women from "socially disadvantaged" families were more likely to become pregnant out of psychological compulsion rather than careful planning.[123] As a temporary emotional fix for what ailed them, the one pregnancy was never enough. Multiple unplanned pregnancies often followed. Davis observed that these indigent mothers could not cope with the large families they had created. Even when the father was present in the household, the mother was stretched too thin. Owing to the "extra effort" it took for slum mothers to help their children "avoid the pathological consequences of ghetto living," each additional child simply made life all the more stressful. As a poor mother's family grew, so did her risk of psychosis.[124]

It was not only the mother's emotional state that worried Davis. She was also concerned that psychotic mothers would unintentionally compromise their children's mental health. Reviewing recent cases in 1968, Davis stated that mentally ill mothers could not be expected to "provide adequate maternal care." Consequently their children might be emotionally insecure and neurotic. What is more, Davis warned that the daughters of psychotic mothers were likely to form the large, disorderly families in which they had been raised. To prevent postpartum psychosis and reduce the risk that Harlem's future would be dominated by Minuchin's slum families, she advocated that poor women with several children voluntarily submit to tubal ligation.[125]

After three years of voluntary sterilizations, Davis concluded that her program had dramatically reduced Harlem's rate of postpartum psychosis. Davis's colleague Dr. Hugh F. Butts performed the psychiatric examinations and Swartz's surgeons in obstetrics performed the tubal ligations—a reversible procedure. In all, Davis's program sterilized 250 Harlem patients between 1965 and 1968. In 1968, Davis reported that the program brought Harlem's rate of postpartum psychosis down to parity with the national average. According to Davis, it had been a textbook example of community psychiatry. Harlem Hospital had helped poor black women stave off future outbreaks of an illness that had disproportionately afflicted their neighborhoods.[126]

Still, not everyone in Harlem thought the sterilization program had been good community psychiatry. The Harlemites who disapproved had not criticized the hospital for operating on emotionally unstable women who may have lacked the capacity to grant full consent. That no one offered this as an objection to Harlem Hospital's controversial policy is somewhat surprising. The 1960s saw increased activism and legislation on behalf of both women's reproductive rights and the rights of the mentally ill.[127] Davis's critics were radical black men with a different agenda. According to them, performing tubal ligations on black women was genocide.

In the late 1960s, it was not uncommon for Black Power advocates to oppose sterilization. African Americans hotly debated these surgical procedures. Authorities had long subjected nonwhites to forced sterilizations and even more drastic forms of genital mutilation for either punitive or eugenic reasons. This history extends as far back as the antebellum era. Unwanted surgical tampering with black reproductive capacities had even increased in the 1960s, especially in the South. Since the 1930s, state legislatures had ordered physicians to take select black prisoners, mental patients, and welfare recipients and render them infertile. With full government support, white doctors regularly sterilized black women—including the prominent Mississippi civil-rights activist Fannie Lou Hamer—without their consent. As the number of black women forced to undergo irreversible hysterectomies rose in the 1960s, black nationalists became even more pro-natalist. In Harlem, the Nation of Islam, the New York Black Panther Party, and the Nation of Gods and Earths strongly opposed the use of sterilization and other forms of birth control. These pro-natalist Black Power advocates believed that sterilization in a largely black community was tantamount to genocide.[128]

Davis's showdown with a Black Power activist notwithstanding, the sterilization issue did not split central Harlem's black community along lines of class and political ideology. A majority of African American women—regardless of class—supported birth control as long as they retained the right of refusal.[129] HANA's middle-class leaders publicly supported the hospital's efforts to expand access to birth control and tubal ligations. And 16,056 women, most of them poor or working class, chose to make use of its Family Planning Services in 1967.[130] Although the Black Power males who opposed Davis were vocal, they did not speak for all Harlemites. The sterilization program continued and racial liberals retained their medical authority to determine Harlem's mental health needs.

Nevertheless, Davis's confrontation with an irate man at a public forum for elective tubal ligation, recounted at the start of this chapter, exposed the limitations of the color-blind approach to community psychiatry. Davis did not recall her accuser's name, the organization he represented, or the date of their encounter. But she vividly remembered the jarring fact of his accusation that she was a Jewish outsider preying on the black community. Yes, his conspiratorial assertions were incorrect. His diatribe did not produce policy change. Nonetheless, this lay critic had hurled an indictment so startling that Davis recalled it long after the details of the incident had faded away: he had charged racial liberals with racism. Even the most vocal professional critics of color-blind psychiatry had not done that. In alleging that Harlem Hospital had acted as the agent of a genocidal white power plot, this vociferous activist had *racialized* what was supposed to have been a race-neutral exercise in community psychiatry. His outburst signaled that color-blind psychiatry had not negated race and the operation of racism within Harlem. Instead it highlighted how ignoring race could perpetuate racism.

The accusation that Harlem Hospital constituted an outside force, a tool of the white establishment, raised the specter of racial liberalism's complicity with institutional racism and the structural forces disrupting urban black communities in the 1960s. Racial liberals had become a fixture within public-health policy and psychiatry. But in the process, they unintentionally reified race as a clinically significant factor, reinforcing mental health disparities through the uncritical deployment of racially loaded assumptions. What is more, the very existence of the Harlem Hospital psychiatric department depended on a partnership with one of Harlem's largest and most despised white-identified institutions: Columbia University.

For many black residents, Columbia University was the most tangible symbol of the dramatic changes central Harlem underwent in the postwar period. Between 1957 and 1968, Columbia, long one of Harlem's primary landlords, amassed even more properties. It demolished homes, displaced residents, and acquired a reputation as a slumlord. Resentment against Columbia ran high in Harlem, culminating in a student-led protest of a proposed gym in nearby Morningside Heights in 1968.[131] Harlem Hospital's future had been a source of concern for some residents ever since the Columbia affiliation began in 1963. For these black Harlemites, Columbia's relationship with their municipal hospital was further proof that local government had sacrificed them to rapacious outside capital.[132]

Given Harlem Hospital's partnership with Columbia, the locals' distrust of their venerable medical institution grew. For many Harlemites, Columbia was the face of the destructive white establishment.[133] Some community-action organizations such as Harlem Teams for Self-Help, Inc., Harlem's CORE chapter, and the Harlem Health Council openly criticized and opposed the affiliation, questioning whether the hospital served Columbia's or Harlem's best interests.[134] In 1968, after the Morningside Heights protest, the Harlem rumor mill had it that Columbia was bent on completely privatizing Harlem Hospital, potentially jeopardizing this municipal hospital's duty to serve the poor. At the time of the sterilization controversy, Davis probably knew of such rumors and was aware of the community's distrust of both Columbia and Harlem Hospital.[135] Those racially inflected town-gown tensions supplied the historical context that had animated the exchange between Davis and the unknown Black Power advocate who defamed her. Davis felt some sympathy for this speaker and those she imagined he represented. Perhaps this sympathy was born out of a sense of her own complicity and collusion with institutions whose interests and prerogatives were often antithetical to those of Harlem's black residents.

Conclusion

Dr. Davis's memory of the sterilization controversy speaks to the conflicted paternalism that informed both community psychiatry and racial liberalism in Harlem. In her 1983 interview, Davis evinced some disappointment in her controversial program's failure to satisfy members of the very community she was trying to help. As racial liberals gained a firmer hold within New York's system of health care, some of them acknowledged that not all of their beneficiaries recognized their "good intentions."[136] Perhaps what was most unsettling for Davis was the revelation that black Harlemites—across lines of class, gender, and political affiliation—did not necessarily see her professional interests as aligned with their own. Racial liberals presumed that they knew what was best for the black poor. But to some African Americans, the color blind were not working to pry open the white power structure. Instead, they seemed to be in collusion with the establishment, further exposing already vulnerable black communities to noxious social forces. Despite all that Harlem Hospital's Department of Psychiatry provided emotionally and mentally ill African Americans, its commitment to the problematic project of color-blind personhood left a complicated legacy.

Conclusion

Health, Race, and the Color-Blind Legacy of the Long Civil-Rights Era

To think is to forget a difference, to generalize, to abstract.

—Jorge Luis Borges, *Ficciones*

That the practice of medicine reflects the values of a particular time and place has become conventional wisdom for many historians. Clearly, this book supports that point of view. It also demonstrates that modern medicine has the power to change the way race matters in American life. The historian and psychiatrist Jonathan Metzl argued in 2009 that psychiatry has not just mirrored changing ideas about race, but it has also helped shape the meaning and practice of race in the twentieth century.[1] The story told here confirms Metzl's argument. In tracing the efforts of the civil servants and psychiatrists who extended psychiatry's reach across 110th Street in Harlem, the preceding chapters demonstrated how these individuals altered psychiatry and its allied professions. More important, the institutional changes they made affected the lives of ordinary African Americans in practical ways, increasing their access to a medical specialty whose practitioners once doubted whether blacks were even human enough for them to help.[2]

Between 1936 and 1968, racial liberals came to understand racial equality as equal black potential for mental health and stability, transforming the African American psyche into a site worthy of public investment and civil-rights activism. They expected that all races would be fully capable of benefiting from the latest developments in psychiatric theory and practice. Although racial liberals were never a majority, enough of them did gain positions of power within New York's systems of justice, medicine, and education. As they institutionalized their race-neutral understanding of the human psyche within their workplaces, more opportunities for African Americans to experience psychiatry emerged in schools, courts, and hospitals.

Thanks to Justine Wise Polier and the support of Mayor Fiorello La Guardia, this racial change began in New York's system of juvenile justice and corrections in 1936. Given overlapping personnel and interdepartmental networking between the courts and schools, psychiatrists such as Max Winsor, Viola

Bernard, and Marion Kenworthy extended this process into the public schools' Bureau of Child Guidance and the private Wiltwyck School for Boys in 1940. After the battle against mental health disparities intersected with the wartime civil-rights movement in 1942, it suffered a slight retrenchment in the early Cold War. In the 1950s, the psychiatrists Viola Bernard and Lawrence Kolb, and the future Commissioner of Hospitals Ray Trussell, helped keep that fight alive at the Columbia University School of Public Health and Administrative Medicine. With Trussell's appointment to the Department of Hospitals in 1961, psychiatry's expansion into Harlem's black neighborhoods received its most substantial policy support yet. By 1962, Harlem Hospital's psychiatric division opened under the direction of Trussell's wife, the longtime Harlem resident Elizabeth B. Davis.

Yes, the story is one of racial change. But those changes were limited. The meaning and practice of race changed only partially during the so-called long civil-rights era. Pockets of racial liberals coalesced within hospitals, schools, courts, reform schools, and other public sites. Yet this did not mean that most people necessarily shared the egalitarian assumptions held by Polier, Bernard, and Davis. As select niches within the public sector became more racially inclusive, other institutions such as churches and families had not. Instead, they continued to serve as vehicles for the perpetuation of regressive racial attitudes. Despite the conservative political analyst Karl Rove's assertion that twenty-first-century America entered a postracial era with the presidential election of Barack Obama in 2008, plenty of citizens still think that biological race shapes who and what we are.[3]

One of the reasons why racial change was so limited in scope was that racial liberals did not tamper with the nature of American thinking about race. In its felt certainty and dogmatic resistance to counterevidence and constructive dialogue with opponents, most thinking about race resembles faith. The activists and policymakers in this story assumed that biological race had no effect on the human psyche. When Polier, Bernard, Winsor, and Davis rooted out racialism from courts, schools, and hospitals, they simply replaced one faith about race with another. None of those racial liberals claimed that race was a social construct.[4] Race was as biologically real to them as it had been to white supremacists. Yet while it may have been a biological reality for these well-meaning activists and clinicians, they also believed it had no bearing on personality development and the contraction of mental illness. Although racial liberals believed that race shaped the way one's body looked, they did not claim it determined how one would feel or think.

The major deficit of color blindness stems from the fact that racial stereotypes can be fostered even without racial categories. In concert with other categories of social identity, racial categories help place us in time and place. They mark each of us as certain types of people. Over time, racialized meanings get reinscribed or mapped onto other forms of identity. They then become imperceptibly bound up with allegedly race-neutral categories. If these race-entangled concepts remain in place, without any effort to unpack them, other social identities can act in place of race even when racial categories are not directly invoked. Although the clinicians and civil servants who combated racial dispari-ties in midcentury New York rejected racialism, they still left many other perni-cious assumptions about class, gender, culture, and sexuality virtually intact. In the contemporary era of official color blindness, these ostensibly race-free cat-egories are still primed and ready to do the work of racial stereotypes, perpetu-ating and even creating racial inequalities, not just within health care but also within all arenas of twenty-first century-life.

Color-Blind Care or Cultural Competency?

Between the late 1930s and the 1960s, racial liberals were certain that the full and equal inclusion of African Americans in modern life would eliminate racial disparities. It was one thing to simply include someone without reference to color in order to remove racial barriers. But once he or she was included, it was another thing entirely to treat or care for that individual without reference to color. By the time Harlem Hospital had opened its psychiatric wing, another antiracialist approach to black patients had developed alongside race neutrality. Like the racial liberals, some of these new critics—including the black psycholo-gists Reginald L. Jones, William Cross, and Joseph White—assumed that blacks and whites were psychological equals. Yet they also believed that a color-blind approach to diagnosis and therapy was not the best way to deploy that assump-tion within a clinical setting. According to the political scientist Uday Mehta, liberals drew a "distinction between universal capacities and the conditions for their actualization."[5] In New York community-psychiatry circles, racial liberals such as Columbia University's Viola Bernard and Harlem Hospital's Elizabeth Davis enacted this distinction by identifying class rather than race as the condi-tion for the human psyche's actualization in Harlem. Their critics recognized that they had unintentionally reified race as a salient marker of clinical differ-ence. The racial liberals' substitution of class for race had not erased racial dis-parities in patient care. Instead, their analyses of poverty and slum life continued to justify the overdiagnosis of psychoses among African Americans and reinforce claims that the black community was fundamentally flawed.

Starting in the mid-1960s, a generation of young African American psychia-trists offered an antiracist alternative to such demeaning portrayals of black life. Their formulation seemed much better suited to an era when some activists and scholars framed racial justice as the recognition of black culture's uniqueness.[6] With the emergence of the Black Psychology movement in 1966 and the Black Psychiatrists of America in 1969, black mental health professionals led the way in promoting what would become known in twenty-first-century health discourse as "cultural competency" or "racial sensitivity."[7] These critics of color-blind psy-chiatry underscored that a color-blind approach did not eliminate the operation of racial assumptions within the clinical encounter. Instead, the cloak of race neutrality forced clinicians to fall back on popular stereotypes of blackness when diagnosing an African American patient. Some black mental health experts argued that clinical interactions between white psychiatrists and black patients might improve if clinicians became more familiar with black cultural idioms and styles of personal interaction. They argued that black culture modified a patient's expression of basic human psychology in distinct yet healthy ways. Starting in the 1970s, noted black mental health professionals even began publishing child-rearing manuals, relationship guides, and other pieces of advice literature written expressly about and for people of color.[8]

"Natch!!"

At least one white racial liberal regarded psychiatric advice for black parents with more than a dash of skepticism. Viola W. Bernard's archives contains a January 1971 *Redbook* article entitled "The Question Every Black Parent Asks: What Shall I Tell My Child?" The talented young black psychiatrists Alvin F. Poussaint and James P. Comer cowrote this contribution to the burgeoning field of African American childrearing literature. The piece was an early version of material they later published in 1975 and updated in 1992 as *Raising Black Children*. When looking over Bernard's personal copy, I noticed a written annotation in the margins written in response to the following line in the article: "the abundance of child-rearing information directed to the white parent is of little use to black families." Responding with caustic irony to this understatement, Bernard scribbled: "But the rest of their advice is based on it—Natch!!"[9]

Bernard's annotation can be interpreted in a myriad of ways, opening up new questions about the legacy of racial liberalism. It is possible that Bernard had merely recognized that she and the writers shared the same faith in the psychological equality of the races. Yes, Poussaint and Comer contended that African Americans required psychological advice that addressed the particularities of the black experience. This did not mean, however, that the African American psyche was the product of biological race. Instead, both psychiatrists acknowledged in *Raising Black Children* that "the basic needs of children are universal" and that "there is no distinct black or white psychology."[10] With few exceptions besides the controversial Frances Cress Welsing and other proponents of black essentialism, most black mental health professionals tended to accept that individuals from all races were endowed with the same psychological potential.[11]

Was that all Bernard had noted in the margins, then—that the psychiatrists' analysis of African American life was grounded in fundamental principles of human psychology? Perhaps. But that interpretation does not adequately explain her emphatic and rather critical use of the colloquial "natch." In the Vietnam War era, "natch" was short for "naturally." This little bit of slang carried the same dismissive and ironic connotation that the phrase "of course" can often have when trailed by one exclamation point, let alone two. She certainly found irony in the statement she highlighted. Yet it was not because Poussaint and Comer had relied on basic principles of psychology to explain how African

Americans had been forced to cope with social stressors white people never had to face. Instead, it was because the white creators of those basic principles never intended for them to describe anything more than the psychology of white people. And here were two black clinicians uncritically deploying theories about the white experience as though they were universal human truths that could reveal the black experience. To Bernard, nothing could be more ironic.

What Bernard recognized within Poussaint and Comer's piece was a problem intrinsic to any race-neutral approach to psychiatry. As early as 1947, Bernard worried that a color-blind application of psychodynamic principles with African Americans might not be able to provide accurate readings of the black psyche. The problem was that modern psychoanalytic theory's claims to universality were specious. She had long realized that most psychodynamic theory had been constructed by white middle-class men and women conducting clinical encounters with other white middle-class men and women. She feared that there was no way to be sure that psychodynamic theories crafted to describe whites could be applied in a one-size-fits-all manner. Could psychoanalytic concepts and principles really illuminate the inner worlds of all men and women?

When Bernard began recruiting potential black psychiatrists in the 1940s, she assumed that African Americans would be better positioned to solve this problem. For one thing, she expected that their experiences as people of color might enable them to better apprehend how the black psyche operated. More important, in the process of comparing what they learned about black psychology with established principles, black clinicians might finally uncover whether psychodynamic theory contained any universal truths.[12] Perhaps her disapproving reaction to the 1971 *Redbook* article reflects the exasperation she may have felt upon learning that two leading black psychiatrists had—in her estimation at least—simply recapitulated the psychiatric profession's racially loaded assumptions about human selfhood. That she saw this alleged failure as a pattern others were doomed to repeat best explains her dismissive "Natch!!"

Race and Deracialization

Bernard recognized that psychiatry could not fully deracialize if the profession failed to reassess its basic assumptions about what it meant to be a person. She seemed to understand that the color-blind acceptance of psychiatry's basic assumptions about human nature could not remove race from psychiatry. Instead, she was asking for a more thoroughgoing deconstruction, unpacking, and even unmaking of modern psychiatry's conception of selfhood. If Americans clinicians wanted more certainty as to whether psychodynamic theory really described the human psyche that everyone shared, or if culture really did modify the expression of our basic human capacities, they had to start from the premise that we did not yet know what those basic capacities even were.

Nevertheless, most of the racial liberals in this account—including Bernard—were not able to do that. Their understanding of what race was held them back from making that cognitive leap. For them, race was a biological condition, a category marked by perceived differences in skin color and physiognomy. By contrast, scholars today in a variety of disciplines understand race to be a culturally specific and historically changing system for assigning meaning culturally not just to bodies but also to places, objects, ideas, and even other categories of identity.

By continuing to conceive of race as biological difference, the well-meaning activists and clinicians documented here were unable to fully appreciate the difficulties involved in deracializing mental health care. Fundamental assumptions about race, gender, sexuality, and class are so inextricably woven within both psychiatry's and mainstream culture's ideas about human selfhood that a thorough removal of race from those systems of meaning would necessarily entail fundamental reassessments about what it means to be male or female, rich or poor, heterosexual or homosexual. Even today, psychiatry's diagnostic categories, drug-marketing campaigns, and gendered patterns of diagnosis and treatment have become imperceptibly entangled with race in ways that neither color blindness nor cultural competency can dislodge.[13] Whether Bernard recognized it or not, attempts to understand African American patients through a class-based community psychiatry failed to deracialize black patients. Instead, these efforts activated and mobilized the racist metaphors deeply sedimented within psychodynamic thinking in new ways.[14] Simply replacing race with another category of analysis without stopping to unpack the racial meanings imbedded in the new category did little to neutralize the concept of "race" within either psychiatry or American life.

Failure of a Color-Blind Public Sector

Ultimately, racial liberals' midcentury engagement with psychiatry reveals the limits of color-blind state inclusion as a solution to racial inequality. Liberal color blindness was initially supposed to ensure individual equality of access to all available public opportunities and resources. Yet as scholars in a variety of fields, from the sociologists Howard Winant and Eduardo Bonilla-Silva to the historian Daniel HoSang and the civil-rights advocate Michelle Alexander, have routinely demonstrated, color-blind state policies and political discourse have done very little to eradicate racial inequality. Today, the color-blind avoidance of race talk has morphed into little more than a conservative political pose. Simply asserting that race no longer shapes our lives is somehow supposed to make white Americans feel not only unaccountable but even comfortable living in a nation where racial inequality persists.[15]

Nevertheless, color blindness initially emerged from a place of discomfort with the existence of racial inequality. In the historical development of that early liberal stage, color blindness involved more than the removal of racial language from laws and official policies. It was a new way of imagining, seeing, thinking, and acting. At its core, the color blind assumed that all humans were equally endowed with the same psychological capacities. Americans who shared this assumption believed that the potential for exercising law-abiding citizenship, regulating emotions, forming stable relationships, and achieving happiness and success as adults was equally distributed across the color line. Within those institutions where this faith in the psychological equality of the races had become an embedded assumption, policymakers and administrators expected that mental health disparities would decline once the races received equal treatment. Yet over time, the adoption of race-neutral individualism as public policy has allowed conservatives and liberals alike to ignore structural inequalities facing the black community. This new era of colorblind individualism within both public policy and mental health care has even generated new racial disparities in mental health.

Despite racialism's official retrenchment within mental health care, the emotional life of African Americans still remains a site for the creation and perpetuation of institutional racism. Greater inclusion within the state's system of mental health care did not generate a widespread liberating effect. What it did produce was more institutionalization and incarceration. This greater inclusion did not rejuvenate postindustrial black ghettos. Nor did central Harlem's streets suddenly teem with people that policymakers, police patrolmen, teachers, judges, and probation officers would regard as law-abiding individuals. Simply including African Americans on an ostensibly color-blind basis—without unpacking how race continues to regulate our ideas about citizenship and selfhood—did not eliminate racial inequality.

Within mental health care, racial disparities continued and even worsened from the 1960s onward. Entering the twenty-first century, the era of biopsychiatry and deinstitutionalization, the rate at which blacks were diagnosed with psychoses had not declined. It increased. Studies conducted between 2003 and 2009 showed that African Americans had been diagnosed with schizophrenia and other psychotic disorders at a rate that was three times higher than for whites. Blacks were far more likely to have their mental health needs met in public institutions and emergency-care units than in private outpatient care facilities. And whereas black children within the juvenile-justice system had been denied access to mental health care before the 1960s, efforts to end this inequity eventually produced an overabundance of institutionalized black youth offenders receiving some mental health attention. The US justice system's steadily increasing tendency to assign black children's cases a psychological dimension coincided with historically unprecedented rates of black male incarceration in the late twentieth and early twenty-first centuries. Consequently, the African American experience with psychiatry retained a coercive element. A racially disproportionate number of black males within the correctional system have been diagnosed with psychotic disorders.[16] In hindsight, young Claude Brown's fear and distrust of the well-meaning Judge Jane Bolin's courtroom now seems to border on the prescient.

Admittedly, this is a bleak picture of psychiatry's relationship to both racial liberalism and the perpetuation of racial inequality. It gets even bleaker once we consider that racial liberalism took hold only in limited pockets within American life, failing to substantially strike out at racism within the culture as a whole. For one thing, these pockets of racial liberalism necessarily operated in an era when plenty of institutions still supported white privileges. The necessity of working within these structures of domination hindered racial liberals' ability to implement progressive change, even in New York. Second, changing the racial culture of health professions such as psychiatry did not have any substantial impact on the structural inequalities facing the African Americans they served. Third, and perhaps most significantly, the color-blind turn was just not radical enough to generate a thorough deracialization of either the psychiatric profession or the public places that delivered mental health care.

If Americans are serious about creating a postracial culture, they must accept that race is not a biological entity whose significance will diminish once we ignore it. Neither is it a marker of cultural differences that must be tolerated. Instead, we have to be willing to accept that race is a system of power that works most effectively when the people it benefits most deny that it even matters.

Notes

Introduction

Epigraph. Dick Gregory, *From the Back of the Bus* (New York: Avon, 1962), 92.

1. Jonathan Gill, *Harlem: The Four Hundred Year History from Dutch Village to Capital of Black America* (New York: Grove, 2011), 334–84; Allon Schoener, ed., *Harlem on My Mind: Cultural Capital of Black America, 1900–1968* (New York: New Press, 2007), 205–15.

2. William Robert Miller, "The Broadening Horizon: Montgomery, America, and the World," in *Martin Luther King Jr.: A Profile*, ed. C. Eric Lincoln (New York: Hill and Wang, 1970), 56; Gill, *Harlem*, 373–75; Aubre de L. Maynard, *Surgeons to the Poor: The Harlem Hospital Story* (New York: Appleton-Century-Crofts, 1979), 184–92; Hugh Pearson, *When Harlem Nearly Killed King: The 1958 Stabbing of Dr. Martin Luther King Jr.* (New York: Seven Stories Press, 2004).

3. "Mrs. Curry Committed to State Hospital," *New York Amsterdam News*, November 2, 1958, 1; George Barner, "Izola Tries Jailbreak!," *New York Amsterdam News*, October 18, 1958, 1, 11; "Report on Mrs. Curry Next Week," *New York Amsterdam News*, October 18, 1958, 1.

4. George Barner, *New York Amsterdam News*, September 27, 1958, 1; Pearson, *When Harlem Nearly Killed King*, 47–50.

5. Recent literature on African Americans and the history of medicine that have shaped this book include: Gabriel N. Mendes, *Under the Strain of Color: Harlem's Lafargue Clinic and the Promise of an Antiracist Psychiatry* (Ithaca, NY: Cornell University Press, 2015); Mical Raz, *What's Wrong with the Poor: Psychiatry, Race, and the War on Poverty* (Chapel Hill: University of North Carolina Press, 2013); Alondra Nelson, *Body and Soul: The Black Panther Party and the Fight against Medical Discrimination* (Minneapolis: University of Minnesota Press, 2011); Keith Wailoo, *How Cancer Crossed the Color Line* (New York: Oxford University Press, 2011); Karen Kruse Thomas, *Deluxe Jim Crow: Civil Rights and American Health Policy, 1935–1954* (Athens: University of Georgia Press, 2011); Samuel Kelton Roberts, Jr., *Infectious Fear: Politics, Disease, and the Health Effects of Segregation* (Chapel Hill: University of North Carolina Press, 2009); Susan Reverby, *Examining Tuskegee: The Infamous Syphilis Study and Its Legacy* (Chapel Hill: University of North Carolina Press, 2009).

6. Dennis Doyle, "'A Fine New Child': The Lafargue Mental Hygiene Clinic and Harlem's African American Communities, 1946–1958," *Journal of the History of Medicine and Allied Sciences* 64 (April 2009): 173–212; Dennis Doyle, "'Where the Need Is Greatest': Social Psychiatry and Race-Blind Universalism in Harlem's Lafargue Clinic, 1946–1958," *Bulletin of the History of Medicine* 83 (Winter 2009): 746–74.

7. Toni Morrison, *Tar Baby* (New York: Plume, 1982), 231.

8. Elsewhere I have referred to this "cadre of . . . psychiatrists and their liberal allies in New York . . . struggling to increase mental health services for black children" as the "psychiatric network." Doyle, "Where the Need Is Greatest, " 748.

9. Throughout I use the terms "universalism" and "race neutrality" interchangeably.

10. Jacquelyn Dowd Hall, "The Long Civil Rights Movement and the Political Uses of the Past," *Journal of American History* 91 (March 2005): 1233–53; Robert O. Self, *American Babylon: Race and the Struggle for Postwar Oakland* (Princeton, NJ: Princeton University Press, 2003). See also Lauren Rebecca Sklaroff, *Black Culture and the New Deal: The Quest for Civil Rights in the Roosevelt Era* (Chapel Hill: University of North Carolina Press, 2009); Glenda Gilmore, *Defying Dixie: The Radical Roots of Civil Rights* (New York: W. W. Norton, 2009); Thomas Sugrue, *Sweet Land of Liberty: The Forgotten Struggle for Civil Rights in the North* (New York: Random House, 2008); Nikhil Pal Singh, *Black Is a Country: Race and the Unfinished Struggle for Democracy* (Cambridge, MA: Harvard University Press, 2004).

11. Martha Biondi, *To Stand and to Fight: The Struggle for Civil Rights in New York City* (Cambridge, MA: Harvard University Press, 2003); Clarence Taylor, ed., *Civil Rights in New York City: From World War II to the Giuliani Era* (New York: Fordham University Press, 2011).

12. Other scholars, including Susan Reverby, define racialism as "the use of racial categories without emphasis on hierarchy." Reverby, *Examining Tuskegee*, 7. My understanding is that racialism, like race and racism, has a history. In the first half of the twentieth century, racialism could also refer to a kind of biological essentialism, namely, the assumption that significant differences in personal capacities and abilities existed between the races. That is essentially how I use the term in this book. Nevertheless, I do not conflate the terms "racialism" and "racism"—the latter defined here as a system or culture of racial domination.

13. Howard Winant, *Racial Conditions: Politics, Theory, Comparisons* (Minneapolis: University of Minnesota Press, 1994).

14. Ira Katznelson, *When Affirmative Action Was White: An Untold History of Racial Inequality in Twentieth-Century America* (New York: Norton, 2005); David R. Roediger, *Colored White: Transcending the Racial Past* (Berkeley: University of California Press, 2003); Mae M. Ngai, "American Immigration Law: A Reexamination of the Immigration Act of 1924," *Journal of American History* 86 (June 1999): 67–92; Michael K. Brown, *Race, Money, and the American Welfare State* (Ithaca, NY: Cornell University Press, 1999); Matthew Frye Jacobson, *Whiteness of a Different Color: European Immigrants and the Alchemy of Race* (Cambridge, MA: Harvard University Press, 1999); Glenda Gilmore, *Gender and Jim Crow: Women and the Politics of White Supremacy in North Carolina, 1896–1920* (Chapel Hill: University of North Carolina Press, 1996).

15. Thaddeus Russell, "The Color of Discipline: Civil Rights and Black Sexuality," *American Quarterly* 60 (March 2008), 113, 120–21.

16. Peniel E. Joseph, "Introduction: Toward a Historiography of the Black Power Movement," in *The Black Power Movement: Rethinking the Civil Rights-Black Power Era*, ed. Peniel E. Joseph (New York: Routledge, 2006): 1–26; Timothy Tyson, *Radio Free Dixie: Robert F. Williams and the Roots of Black Power* (Chapel Hill: University of North Carolina Press, 1999).

17. Self, *American Babylon*, 14. For more on racial liberalism, see also Mark Brilliant, *The Color of America Has Changed: How Racial Diversity Shaped Civil Rights Reform in California, 1941–1978* (New York: Oxford University Press, 2010); Lorrin Thomas, *Puerto Rican Citizen: History and Political Identity in Twentieth-Century New York City* (Chicago: University of Chicago Press, 2010); Cheryl Lynn Greenberg, *Troubling the Waters: Black-Jewish Relations in the American Century* (Princeton, NJ: Princeton University Press, 2006); Lani Guinier, "From Racial Liberalism to Racial Literacy: *Brown v. Board of Education* and the Interest-Divergence Dilemma," *Journal of American History* 91 (June 2004): 92–118; Ruth Feldstein, *Motherhood in Black and White: Race and Sex in American Liberalism, 1930–1965* (Ithaca, NY: Cornell University Press, 2000); Daryl Michael Scott, *Contempt and Pity: Social Policy and the Image of the Damaged Black Psyche, 1880–1996* (Chapel Hill: University of North Carolina Press, 1997).

18. George Lipsitz, *How Racism Takes Place* (Philadelphia, PA: Temple University Press, 2011), 60.

19. Daniel Martinez HoSang, *Racial Propositions: Ballot Initiatives and the Making of Postwar California* (Berkeley: University of California Press, 2010); Gary Gerstle, "The Crucial Decade: the 1940s and Beyond," *Journal of American History* 92 (March 2006): 1292–99; Gary Gerstle, "The Protean Character of American Liberalism," *American Historical Review* 99 (October 1994): 1043–73.

20. Roger Waldinger, *Still the Promised City? African Americans and New Immigrants in Postindustrial New York* (Cambridge, MA: Harvard University Press, 1999).

21. James Patterson, *Grand Expectations: The United States, 1945–1975* (New York: Oxford University Press, 1997); Robert O. Self, *All in the Family: The Realignment of American Democracy since the 1960s* (New York: Hill and Wang, 2012).

22. On the cultural history of sensibilities and the influence of affect studies on that literature, see Ann Laura Stoler, *Along the Archival Grain: Epistemic Anxieties and Colonial Common Sense* (Princeton, NJ: Princeton University Press, 2009); Lauren Berlant, *The Female Complaint: The Unfinished Business of Sentimentality in American Culture* (Durham, NC: Duke University Press, 2008); Daniel Wickberg, "What Is the History of Sensibilities? On Cultural Histories, Old and New," *American Historical Review* 112 (June 2007): 661–84; Peter N. Stearns, *Anxious Parents: A History of Modern Childrearing in America* (New York: New York University Press, 2004); Amit Rai, *The Rule of Sympathy: Sentiment, Race, and Power, 1750–1850* (New York: Palgrave, 2002).

23. Jason Morgan Ward, *Defending White Democracy: The Making of a Segregationist Movement and the Remaking of Racial Politics, 1936–1965* (Chapel Hill: University of North Carolina Press, 2011); Arnold Hirsch, "Massive Resistance in the Urban North: Trumbull Park, Chicago, 1953–1966," *Journal of American History* 82 (September 1995): 522–50; Thomas J. Sugrue, *The Origins of the Urban Crisis: Race and Inequality in Postwar Detroit* (Princeton, NJ: Princeton University Press, 1996); Thomas J. Sugrue, "Crabgrass-Roots Politics: Race, Rights, and the Reaction against Liberalism in the Urban North," *Journal of American History* 82 (September 1995): 551–77; Gary Gerstle, "Race and the Myth of the Liberal Consensus," *Journal of American History* 82 (September 1995): 579–86; Kenneth Kusmer, "African Americans in the City since World War II: From Industrial to the Post-Industrial Era," *Journal of Urban History* 21 (May 1995): 458–503.

24. Cynthia Young, *Soul Power: Culture, Radicalism, and the Making of a U.S. Third World Left* (Durham, NC: Duke University Press, 2006); Barbara Ransby, *Ella Baker*

and the Black Freedom Movement: A Radical Democratic Vision (Chapel Hill: University of North Carolina Press, 2005); Mary Dudziak, *Cold War Civil Rights: Race and the Image of American Democracy* (Princeton, NJ: Princeton University Press, 2002); John Dittmer, *Local People: The Struggle for Civil Rights in Mississippi* (Urbana: University of Illinois Press, 1995).

25. HoSang, *Racial Propositions*, 268.

26. Homi K. Bhabha, "Culture's In Between," *Art Forum* 32 (December 1993): 167–68, 211–12, 214. For more on the relationship between culture and personal dispositions, see Michael Taussig, *What Color Is the Sacred?* (Chicago: University of Chicago Press, 2009), 12; Gail Bederman, *Manliness and Civilization: A Cultural History of Gender and Race in the United States, 1880–1917* (Chicago: University of Chicago Press, 1995); Pierre Bourdieu, *The Logic of Practice*, trans. Richard Nice (Stanford, CA: Stanford University Press, 1990).

27. For works that address how one historical sensibility can take root within an institution or subculture, see Chandra Mukerji, "Space and the Political Pedagogy at the Gardens of Versailles," *Public Culture* 24 (Fall 2012): 509–34; Christopher Sellers, "Body, Place, and the State: The Making of an 'Environmental' Imaginary in the Post–World War II U.S.," *Radical History Review* 74 (Spring 1999): 31–64.

28. On the public-policy interest in the promotion of psychological health and law-abiding habits in the twentieth century, see Ellen Herman, *Kinship by Design: A History of Adoption in the Modern United States* (Chicago: University of Chicago Press, 2008); Ann Laura Stoler, "Intimations of Empire: Predicaments of the Tactile and Unseen," in *Haunted by Empire: Geographies of Intimacy in North American History*, ed. Ann Laura Stoler (Durham, NC: Duke University Press, 2006); Jackson Lears, *Something for Nothing: Luck in America* (New York: Viking, 2003); Nayan Shah, *Contagious Divides: Epidemics and Race in San Francisco's Chinatown* (Berkeley: University of California Press, 2001); Nikolas Rose, *Inventing Our Selves: Psychology, Power, and Personhood* (New York: Cambridge University Press, 1998).

29. Shah, *Contagious Divides*, 15–16; Rosalind C. Morris, "The Miner's Ear," *Transition* 98 (2008): 110; Michel Foucault, *Discipline and Punish: The Birth of the Prison*, trans. Alan Sheridan (New York: Pantheon, 1977).

30. Ann Laura Stoler, "Interview," by E. Valentine Daniel, *Public Culture* 24 (Fall 2012): 487–508.

31. Warren I. Susman, "'Personality' and the Making of Twentieth-Century Culture," in *Culture as History: The Transformation of American Society in the Twentieth Century* (New York: Pantheon, 1984), 274–81; Jackson Lears, "The Ad Man and the Grand Inquisitor: Intimacy, Publicity, and the Managed Self in America, 1880–1940," in *Constructions of the Self*, ed. George Levine (New Brunswick, NJ: Rutgers University Press, 1992), 107–41; Ellen Herman, *Romance of American Psychology: Political Culture in the Age of Experts* (Berkeley: University of California Press, 1995); Nancy Schnog, "On Inventing the Psychological," in *Inventing the Psychological: Toward a Cultural History of Emotional Life in America*, eds. Joel Pfister and Nancy Schnog (New Haven, CT: Yale University Press, 1997), 5.

32. Elizabeth Lunbeck, *The Psychiatric Persuasion: Knowledge, Gender, and Power in Modern America* (Princeton, NJ: Princeton University Press, 1994); Kathleen W. Jones, *Taming the Troublesome Child: American Families, Child Guidance, and the Limits of Psychiatric Authority* (Cambridge, MA: Harvard University Press, 1999); Margo

Horn, *Before It's Too Late: The Child Guidance Movement in the United States, 1922–1945* (Philadelphia, PA: Temple University Press, 1989).

33. Nathan G. Hale, Jr., *Freud and the Americans: The Beginnings of Psychoanalysis in the United States, 1876–1917* (New York: Oxford University Press, 1971); Nathan G. Hale, Jr., *The Rise and Crisis of Psychoanalysis in the United States: Freud and the Americans, 1917–1985* (New York: Oxford University Press, 1995); Celia Brickman, *Aboriginal Populations in the Mind: Race and Primitivity in Psychoanalysis* (New York: Columbia University Press, 2003); Jonathan Michel Metzl, *Prozac on the Couch: Prescribing Gender in the Era of Wonder Drugs* (Durham, NC: Duke University Press, 2003); F. C. Gosling, *Before Freud: Neurasthenia and the American Medical Community, 1870–1910* (Urbana: University of Illinois Press, 1987).

34. Shah, *Contagious Divides*; Wailoo, *How Cancer Crossed the Color Line*.

35. Wailoo, *How Cancer Crossed the Color Line*, 3.

36. Ibid; Roberts, *Infectious Fear*; Bederman, *Manliness and Civilization*; Anne C. Rose, *Psychology and Selfhood in the Segregated South* (Chapel Hill: University of North Carolina Press, 2009); Brickman, *Aboriginal Populations in the Mind*; Emily Martin, *Bipolar Expeditions: Mania and Depression in American Culture* (Princeton, NJ: Princeton University Press, 2007); Matthew Gambino, "'These Strangers within Our Gates': Race, Psychiatry and Mental Illness among Black Americans at St. Elisabeths Hospital in Washington, DC, 1900–1940," *History of Psychiatry* 19 (2008): 387–408; Jackson Lears, *No Place of Grace: Antimodernism and the Transformation of American Culture* (Chicago: University of Chicago Press, 1994); Marianna Torgovnick, *Gone Primitive: Savage Intellects, Modern Lives* (Chicago: University of Chicago Press, 1990); Sander L. Gilman, *Difference and Pathology: Stereotypes of Sexuality, Race, and Madness* (Ithaca, NY: Cornell University Press, 1985).

37. For more on how racial exceptionalism works, see Michael Taussig, *Mimesis and Alterity: A Particular History of the Senses* (New York: Routledge, 1993), 151; Matt Wray, *Not Quite White: White Trash and the Boundaries of Whiteness* (Durham, NC: Duke University Press, 2006), 9.

38. Wherever possible, this book indicates that informal assumptions and formal political ideologies are two different things. This distinction takes on a critical importance in the last three chapters. New York's antiracist psychiatrists all assumed that blacks and whites were psychological equals. But in their political ideology, not all of those antiracist clinicians were racial liberals.

39. "Interview with Dr. Winsor, Resident Psychiatrist," March 30, April 1, 1937, 5, folder 39, box 4, Justine Wise Polier Papers, Schlesinger Library, Radcliffe Institute for Advanced Study, Cambridge, MA (hereafter JWP). See also Gerald Markowitz and David Rosner, *Children, Race, and Power: Kenneth and Mamie Clark's Northside Center* (Charlottesville: University of Virginia Press, 1996); Gerald Markowitz and David Rosner, "Race, Foster Care and the Politics of Abandonment in New York City," *American Journal of Public Health* 87 (November 1997): 1844–49.

40. The racial liberals in this book accepted the universality of psychodynamic theory as a self-evident truth. For more on the cultural construction of universality as a concept, see Judith Butler, "Restaging the Universal: Hegemony and the Limits of Formalism," in *Contingency, Hegemony, Universality: Contemporary Dialogues on the Left*, ed. Judith Butler, Ernesto Laclau, and Slavoj Zizek (New York: Verso, 2000), 38.

41. On the cultural construction of imagination, see Dilip Paramesshawar Gaonkar, "Toward New Imaginaries: An Introduction," *Public Culture* 14 (Winter 2002): 10; Charles Taylor, "Cultures of Democracy and Citizen Efficacy," *Public Culture* 19 (Winter 2007): 119; Charles Taylor, *Modern Social Imaginaries* (Durham, NC: Duke University Press, 2004); Charles Taylor, "Modernity and Difference," in *Without Guarantees: In Honor of Stuart Hall*, ed. Paul Gilroy, Lawrence Grossberg, and Angela McRobbie (London: Verso, 2000), 365, 371; Cornelius Castoriadis, *The Imaginary Institution of Society*, trans. Kathleen Blarney (Cambridge: Massachusetts Institute of Technology Press, 1998), 364, 369.

42. Keith Wailoo's *How Cancer Crossed the Color Line* and Nayan Shah's *Contagious Divides* are among the exceptions to that trend.

43. Raz, *What's Wrong with the Poor*.

44. Jonathan M. Metzl, *The Protest Psychosis: How Schizophrenia Became a Black Disease* (Boston, MA: Beacon Press, 2009); John Dittmer, *The Good Doctors: The Medical Committee for Human Rights and the Struggle for Social Justice in Health Care* (New York: Bloomsbury Press, 2009); Keith Wailoo, *Dying in the City of the Blues: Sickle Cell Anemia and the Politics of Race and Health* (Chapel Hill: University of North Carolina, 2001). See also Nancy Tomes, "Merchants of Health: Medicine and Consumer Culture in the United States, 1900–1940," *Journal of American History* 88 (2001): 519–47.

Chapter One

1. Pearce Bailey, "A Contribution to the Mental Pathology of the United States," *Archives of Neurology and Psychiatry* 7 (February 1922): 183. See also William M. Bevis, "Psychological Traits of the Southern Negro with Observations as to Some of His Psychoses," *American Journal of Psychiatry* 78 (July 1921): 74–78.

2. Benjamin Malzberg, "Migration and Mental Disease among Negroes in New York State," *American Journal of Physical Anthropology* 21 (January–March 1936): 112; Benjamin Malzberg, "Mental Disease among Negroes in New York State," *Human Biology* 7 (December 1935): 471–513; Gerald N. Grob, "Psychiatry's Holy Grail: The Search for the Mechanisms of Mental Diseases," *Bulletin of the History of Medicine* 72 (1998): 197; Gerald N. Grob, *The Mad among Us: A History of the Care of the America's Mentally Ill* (New York: Free Press, 1994), 185.

3. E. Y. Williams, "The Incidence of Mental Disease in the Negro," *Journal of Negro Education Quarterly* 6 (1937): 377–92. See Jeanne Spurlock, "Early and Contemporary Pioneers," in *Black Psychiatrists and American Psychiatry*, ed. Jeanne Spurlock (Washington, DC: American Psychiatric Association, 1999), 6–7.

4. Claude McKay, *Harlem: Negro Metropolis* (New York: E. P. Dutton, 1940), 15; Sharifa Rhodes-Pitts, *Harlem Is Nowhere: A Journey to the Mecca of Black America* (New York: Little Brown, 2011), 17–20, 258; Claudia Marie Calhoon, "Tuberculosis, Race, and the Delivery of Health Care in Harlem, 1932–1939," *Radical History Review* 73 (Spring 2001): 101–19.

5. Gill, *Harlem*, 174–85; Gilbert Osofsky, *Harlem: The Making of a Ghetto* (New York: Harper, 1966); Cheryl L. Greenberg, *"Or Does It Explode?": Black Harlem in the Great Depression* (New York: Oxford University Press, 1991), 14–16; Jervis Anderson, *This Was Harlem: A Cultural Portrait, 1900–1950* (New York: Farrar, Straus Giroux, 1982),

49–56; Irma Watkins-Owens, *Blood Relations: Caribbean Immigrants and the Harlem Community, 1900–1930* (Bloomington: University of Indiana Press, 1994), 39–44; McKay, *Harlem*, 24–26.

6. Dr. Kenneth B. Clark, report, "Proposed Study of Public Schools in the Harlem Community, 1953," 1, 2, 3, folder 10, box 93, Kenneth B. Clark Papers, Manuscript Division, Library of the United States Congress, Washington, DC (hereafter LOC-CLARK).

7. Jacqueline Leavitt and Susan Seagert, *From Abandonment to Hope: Community-Household in Harlem* (New York: Columbia University Press, 1990), 15.

8. Ibid., 15; McKay, *Harlem*, 21–28; Gill, *Harlem*, 284–85; Watkins-Owens, *Blood Relations*, 52; David L. Lewis, *When Harlem Was in Vogue* (New York: Knopf, 1981), 165; Roi Ottley and William J. Weatherby, *The Negro in New York: An Informal Social History, 1626–1940* (New York: Praeger, 1967), 182–87.

9. Clare Corbould, "Streets, Sounds and Identity in Interwar Harlem," *Journal of Social History* 40 (Summer 2007): 859–82. See also Clare Corbould, *Becoming African Americans: Black Public Life in Harlem, 1919–1939* (Cambridge, MA: Harvard University Press, 2009), 88–106, 162–95; Watkins-Owens, *Blood Relations*; Ottley and Weatherby, *Negro in New York*, 190–94, 214–15; Gill, *Harlem*, 240–41; McKay, *Harlem*, 24, 30–31; 150–51.

10. McKay, *Harlem*, 32–85; Lewis, *When Harlem Was in Vogue*, 221–24, 299–301; Ottley and Weatherby, *Negro in New York*, 251–54; Gill, *Harlem*, 308; Cheryl L. Greenberg, "God and Man in Harlem," *Journal of Urban History* 21 (May 1995): 519–20; Jill Watts, *God, Harlem, U.S.A.: The Father Divine Story* (Berkeley: University of California Press, 1992); Robert Weisbrot, *Father Divine and the Struggle for Racial Equality* (Urbana: University of Illinois Press, 1983).

11. Anderson, *This Was Harlem*, 273–75, 280–84; Gill, *Harlem*, 276–85, 310–24; Corbould, *Becoming African Americans*, 7, 15, 188–95; George Chauncey, Jr., *Gay New York: Gender, Urban Culture and the Making of the Gay World, 1890–1940* (New York: Basic Books, 1994), 246–53, 310; Eric Garber, "A Spectacle in Color: The Lesbian and Gay Subculture of Jazz Age Harlem," in *Hidden from History: Reclaiming the Gay and Lesbian Past*, ed. Martin Duberman, Martha Vicinus, and George Chauncey, Jr. (New York: Meridian, 1989), 318–31.

12. Sklaroff, *Black Culture and the New Deal*, 5.

13. Lewis, *When Harlem Was in Vogue*, 110; Greenberg, *"Or Does It Explode?"* 178–79, 214–21; Sugrue, *Sweet Land of Liberty*, 12–19.

14. Sugrue, *Sweet Land of Liberty*, 19–29; Gill, *Harlem*, 309; Brown, *Race, Money*, 25–28, 63–96; Jacqueline Jones, *Labor of Love, Labor of Sorrow: Black Women, Work and the Family, from Slavery to the Present* (New York: Vintage, 1995), 205–31.

15. Greenberg, *"Or Does It Explode?"*; Calhoon, "Tuberculosis, Race," 106–7; Gill, *Harlem*, 282–94. See also Virginia W. Wolcott, "The Culture of the Informal Economy: Numbers Runners in Inter-War Detroit," *Radical History Review* 69 (Fall 1997): 46–75.

16. Janet Abu-Lughod, *Race, Space, and Riots in Chicago, New York, and Los Angeles* (New York: Oxford University Press, 2007), 139–41.

17. Cheryl L. Greenberg, "The Politics of Disorder: Reexamining Harlem's Riots of 1935 and 1943," *Journal of Urban History* 18 (August 1992): 395–441.

18. Greenberg, *"Or Does It Explode?"* 214–21; Thomas Kessner, *Fiorello H. LaGuardia and the Making of Modern New York* (New York: McGraw-Hill, 1989), 373–77; Gill, *Harlem*, 329–34; Abu-Lughod, *Race, Space, and Riots*, 149.

19. Williams, "Incidence of Mental Disease in the Negro," 378–79; Philip Sigmund Wagner, "A Comparative Study of Negro and White Admissions to the Psychiatric Pavilion of the Cincinnati General Hospital," *American Journal of Psychiatry* 95 (July 1938): 176.

20. Greenberg, *"Or Does It Explode?"* 16; James N. Gregory, *The Southern Diaspora: How the Great Migrations of Black and White Southerners Changed America* (Chapel Hill: University of North Carolina Press, 2005).

21. Walter Bromberg, *Psychiatry between the Wars, 1918–1945: A Recollection* (Westport, CT: Greenwood Press, 1982), 131.

22. Rose, *Psychology and Selfhood*, 23.

23. Sara Lightfoot Lawrence, *Balm in Gilead: Journey of a Healer* (New York: Merloyd-Lawrence, 1988), 27.

24. Simon Fuller, "A Study of Neurofibrils in Dementia Paralytics, Dementia Senilis, Chronic Alcoholism, Cerebral Uses, and Microcephalic Idiocy," *American Journal of Insanity* 63 (1907): 415–68. This was the first article published in the United States by a psychiatrist of African descent.

25. Ralph Martin, "Doctor's Dream in Harlem," *New Republic*, June 3, 1946, 798.

26. Badia Sahar Ahad, *Freud Upside Down: African American Literature and Psychoanalytic Culture* (Urbana: University of Illinois Press, 2010), 13–38.

27. John S. Hughes, "Labeling and Treating Black Mental Illness in Alabama, 1861–1910," *Journal of Social History* 58 (August 1992): 435–60; Metzl, *Protest Psychosis*, 30–34.

28. Martin, *Bipolar Expeditions*, 127; Metzl, *Protest Psychosis*, xi.

29. Homi Bhabha, "Of Mimicry and Man: The Ambivalence of Colonial Discourse," in *October: The First Decade*, ed. Annette Michelson (Cambridge: Massachusetts Institute of Technology Press, 1987), 318.

30. Rose, *Psychology and Selfhood*, 19–20, 27, 62–110; Ann Laura Stoler, *Race and the Education of Desire: Foucault's History of Sexuality and the Colonial Order of Things* (Durham, NC: Duke University Press, 1995), 91, 205–7; Carl N. Degler, *In Search of Human Nature* (New York: Oxford University Press, 1991).

31. Stoler, *Along the Archival Grain*, 21.

32. Robin D. G. Kelley, *Thelonious Monk: The Life and Times of an American Original* (New York: Free Press, 2009), 83.

33. Lunbeck, *Psychiatric Persuasion*, 121–26, 150, 205.

34. Stoler, *Along the Archival Grain*, 254.

35. Martin, *Bipolar Expeditions*, 213. See also Grace Elizabeth Hale, *Making Whiteness: The Culture of Segregation in the South, 1890–1940* (New York: Vintage, 1998), 10, 73, 79, 81, 298.

36. E. M. Green, "Manic-Depressive Psychosis in the Negro," *American Journal of Insanity* 73 (April 1917): 620. See also Bevis, "Psychological Traits of the Southern Negro," 74. Bevis noted: "Much of their usual behavior seems only a step from the simpler types of [dementia praecox]." See also Metzl, *Protest Psychosis*, 29, 34.

37. Paul Schilder and Sam Parker, "Pupillary Disturbances in Schizophrenic Negroes," *Archives of Neurology and Psychiatry* 25 (March 1931): 840; John E. Lind, "Phylogenetic Elements in the Psychoses of the Negro," *Psychoanalytic Review* 4 (January 1917): 330–31; Arrah B. Evarts, "Dementia Precox in the Colored Race," *Psychoanalytic Review* 1 (October 1914): 396; Nolan D. C. Lewis and Lewis D.

Hubbard, "Epileptic Reactions in the Negro," *American Journal of Psychiatry* 88 (January 1932): 648, 673, 676; Nolan D. C. Lewis and Lewis D. Hubbard, "Manic Depressive Reactions in Negroes," *Proceedings of the Association of Research in Nervous and Mental Disease* 11 (1931): 777–79; Mary O'Malley, "Psychosis in the Colored Race: A Study in Comparative Psychiatry," *American Journal of Insanity* 71 (October 1914): 309, 311, 323–26, 330, 336; Bevis, "Psychological Traits of the Southern Negro," 74, 77, 78; Green, "Manic-Depressive Psychosis in the Negro," 621, 625, 626; Simon P. Rosenthal, "Racial Differences in the Mental Diseases," *Journal of Abnormal and Social Psychology* 28 (October–December 1933): 312–13. See also Martin V. Summers, "'Suitable Care of the African When Afflicted with Insanity': Race, Madness, and Social Order in Historical Perspective," *Bulletin of the History of Medicine* 84 (Spring 2010): 75–77, 84–87; Metzl, *Protest Psychosis,* 29–31.

38. O'Malley, "Psychosis in the Colored Race," 336.

39. Stoler, *Along the Archival Grain,* 40.

40. Bevis, "Psychological Traits of the Southern Negro," 78; Lewis and Hubbard, "Epileptic Reactions in the Negro," 654; Scott, *Contempt and Pity,* 14.

41. Jacques M. Quen, "Asylum Psychiatry, Neurology, Social Work, and Mental Hygiene: An Explanatory Study in Interprofessional History," *Journal of the History of the Behavioral Sciences* 13 (January 1977): 9–11; Jack D. Pressman, "Psychiatry and Its Origins," *Bulletin of the History of Medicine* 71 (1997): 131; Norman Dain, *Clifford W. Beers: Advocate for the Insane* (Pittsburgh, PA: University of Pittsburgh Press, 1980), 111, 151, 239, 249, 331; Gerald N. Grob, *Mental Illness and American Society, 1875–1940* (Princeton, NJ: Princeton University Press, 1987), 144–66; Stephen Robertson, *Crimes against Children: Sexual Violence and Legal Culture in New York City, 1880–1960* (Chapel Hill: University of North Carolina Press, 2005), 149; Horn, *Before It's Too Late,* 16–19.

42. Ruth M. Alexander, *The "Girl Problem": Female Sexual Delinquency in New York, 1900–1930* (Ithaca, NY: Cornell University Press, 1995), 63.

43. Robert Bendiner, "Psychiatry for the Needy," *Tomorrow,* April 1942, 22.

44. Ottley and Weatherby, *Negro in New York,* 272–73; McKay, *Harlem,* 122–25; Gill, *Harlem,* 285.

45. A. Peter Bailey, *The Harlem Hospital Story: 110 Years of Struggle against Illness, Struggle, and Genocide* (Richmond, VA: Native Sun, 1991), 41.

46. McKay, *Harlem,* 122–24; Greenberg, *"Or Does It Explode?"* 15.

47. Horn, *Before It's Too Late,* 2–3, 42–43.

48. Jones, *Taming the Troublesome Child,* 92–119, particularly 149; Horn, *Before It's Too Late,* 32–34; Robert M. Mennel, *Thorns and Thistles: Juvenile Delinquency in the United States, 1825–1940* (Hanover, NH: University Press of New England, 1973), 161–70; Karen W. Tice, *Tales of Wayward Girls and Immoral Women: Case Records and the Professionalization of Social Work* (Urbana: University of Illinois Press, 1998), 51, 84; Markowitz and Rosner, *Children, Race, and Power,* 13–17, 61–62.

49. Jones, *Taming the Troublesome Child,* 52–53, 62–90, 190, 212; Horn, *Before It's Too Late,* 39–42, 145–53, 175–78.

50. New York Bureau of Child Guidance, *Five-Year Report, 1932–1937* (New York: Board of Education, 1938), 10.

51. Ibid., 10, 18–21. See also Markowitz and Rosner, *Children, Race, and Power,* 13.

52. Khalil Gibran Muhammad, *The Condemnation of Blackness: Race, Crime, and the Making of Modern Urban America* (Cambridge, MA: Harvard University Press, 2010), 224–25. See also 9–13, 231.

53. Ibid., 3–9, 152–54.

54. A BCG Harlem unit was created only after Board of Education Commissioner Judge John Marshall and his Committee on Delinquency concluded in 1936 that Harlem's rising delinquency rates might indicate a need there for child guidance services. On June 24, 1936, the Board of Education authorized a child-guidance team for P.S. 24 on East 128th Street in Harlem. Although it was technically in operation by 1937, the Harlem BCG unit did not have a full-time psychiatrist or a full child-guidance team before 1938. New York Bureau of Child Guidance, *Five-Year Report, 1932–1937*, 10, 18–21.

55. Muhammad, *Condemnation of Blackness*, 230 (see also 231, 273).

56. Ibid., 231; Alexander, *"Girl Problem,"* 57–58; Greenberg, *"Or Does It Explode?"* 34–37.

57. Justine Wise Polier, *A View from the Bench: The Juvenile Court* (New York: National Council on Crime and Delinquency, 1964), 83. See also Markowitz and Rosner, "Race, Foster Care," 1845.

58. Markowitz and Rosner, "Race, Foster Care," 1845.

59. On the Hudson State Training School for Girls, see Cheryl D. Hicks, "'Bright and Good Looking Colored Girl': Black Women's Sexuality and 'Harmful Intimacy' in Early Twentieth-Century New York," *Journal of the History of Sexuality* 18 (September 2009): 418–56; Cheryl D. Hicks, *Talk with You Like a Woman: African American Women, Justice, and Reform in New York, 1890–1935* (Chapel Hill: University of North Carolina Press, 2010).

60. "Interview with Dr. Winsor, Resident Psychiatrist," 1, March 30, April 1, 1937, folder 39, box 4, JWP; "Interview with Miss Ruth Topping, Associate Administrator and Case Worker in the Clinic Unit," March 8, March 31, 1937, 1–2, folder 39, box 4, JWP; Williams to John Warren Hill, July 1, 1940, folder 63, box 6, JWP.

61. Summers, "Suitable Care of the African," 58–91. See also Degler, *In Search of Human Nature*, 181–87.

62. Greenberg, *"Or Does It Explode?"* 192; Alexander, *"Girl Problem,"* 58; Williams, "Incidence of Mental Disease in the Negro," 387.

63. Walter Bromberg, "Marihuana Intoxication: A Clinical Study of Cannabis Sativa Intoxication," *American Journal of Psychiatry* 91 (September 1934): 303–40; Bromberg, *Psychiatry between the Wars*, 110; Regina Kunzel, *Criminal Intimacy: Prison and the Uneven History of Modern American Sexuality* (Chicago: University of Chicago Press, 2008); Metzl, *Protest Psychosis*, 100–103.

64. Walter Bromberg, "Psychotherapy in a Court Clinic," *American Journal of Orthopsychiatry* 11 (October 1941): 772–73.

65. Lauretta Bender, *A Visual Motor Gestalt Test and Its Clinical Use* (New York: American Orthopsychiatric Association, 1938), 153.

66. Lauretta Bender, "Behavior Problems in Negro Children," *Psychiatry* 2 (May 1939): 213; Markowitz and Rosner, "Race, Foster Care," 1845.

67. Martin, "Doctor's Dream in Harlem," 798.

68. These first two hires were nurses. Greenberg, *"Or Does It Explode?"* 88–89. The chief psychologist David Wechsler and the psychiatrist Frank Curran, head of the adolescent ward, were two of the more racially prejudiced staff members.

69. Lauretta Bender and Zuleika Yarrell, "Psychoses among Followers of Father Divine," *Journal of Nervous and Mental Disease* 87 (1938): 435; Lauretta Bender and Martin A. Spalding, "Behavior Problems in Children from the Homes of Followers of Father Divine," *Journal of Nervous and Mental Disease* 91 (April 1940): 464; Bromberg, "Marihuana Intoxication," 319.

70. Martin, "Doctor's Dream in Harlem," 798.

71. Bender and Yarrell, "Psychoses among Followers of Father Divine," 427–28, 442.

72. Bender, *A Visual Motor Gestalt Test*, 155–56.

73. Gill, *Harlem*, 293; Mezz Mezzrow and Bernard Wolfe, *Really the Blues* (New York: Random House, 1946); Larry Sloman, *Reefer Madness: The History of Marijuana in America* (Indianapolis, IN: Bobbs-Merrill, 1979); Lester Grinspoon, *Marihuana Reconsidered* (Cambridge, MA: Harvard University Press, 1971).

74. Gilman, *Difference and Pathology*, 129–44; Summers, "Suitable Care of the African," 72–74.

75. Bromberg, "Marihuana Intoxication," 313–23. See also Martin, *Bipolar Expeditions*, 127. For more on the logic of racial exceptionalism, see Stoler, *Along the Archival Grain*, 40.

76. Lauretta Bender, *Aggression, Hostility, and Anxiety in Children* (Springfield, IL: Charles C. Thomas, 1953), 24, 77.

77. Lauretta Bender, *Child Psychiatric Techniques* (Springfield, IL: Charles C. Thomas, 1952), 85.

78. Bender, *Aggression, Hostility, and Anxiety in Children*, 101, 109, 110, 128; Bender, *Child Psychiatric Techniques*, 211.

79. Bender, *Aggression, Hostility, and Anxiety in Children*, 24, 109–10.

80. On the Victorian asylum model, see Nancy Tomes, *The Art of Asylum-Keeping: Thomas Story Kirkbride and the Origins of American Psychiatry* (New York: Cambridge University Press, 1984; repr., Philadelphia: University of Pennsylvania Press, 1994); Ellen Dwyer, *Homes for the Mad: Life Inside Two Nineteenth-Century Asylums* (New Brunswick, NJ: Rutgers University Press, 1987); Gerald N. Grob, *Mental Institutions in America: Social Policy to 1875* (New York: Free Press, 1975).

81. Metzl, *Protest Psychosis*, xi.

82. Lunbeck, *Psychiatric Persuasion*, 149–50, 194, 204–8.

83. Grob, "Psychiatry's Holy Grail," 197.

84. Christopher Crenner, "Race and Medical Practice in the Kansas City Free Dispensary," *Bulletin of the History of Medicine* 82 (Winter 2008): 820–47.

85. Green, "Manic-Depressive Psychoses in the Negro," 621, 625; Lewis and Hubbard, "Manic Depressive Reactions in Negroes," 779–90; O'Malley, "Psychoses in the Colored Race," 336; Kirby N. Randolph, "Psychiatry versus the Negro," paper presented at the New York Academy of Medicine, New York, February 27, 2001. See also Brickman, *Aboriginal Populations in the Mind*, 88.

86. Laura Tabili, "Race Is a Relationship, and Not a Thing," *Journal of Social History* (Fall 2003): 125–30.

87. John Hartigan Jr., "Culture against Race: Reworking the Basis for Racial Analysis," *South Atlantic Quarterly* 104 (Summer 2005): 543–60; Stoler, *Along the Archival Grain*, 40–41; Paul Gilroy, "Cosmopolitanism, Blackness, and Utopia," *Transition* 98 (2008): 116–35; Paul Gilroy, *Postcolonial Melancholia* (New York:

Columbia University Press, 2005), 39–42; Paul Gilroy, *Against Race: Imagining Political Culture beyond the Color Line* (Cambridge, MA: Belknap Press, 2000), 42–53; Frantz Fanon, *Black Skin, White Masks*, trans. Charles Lam Markmann (New York: Grove Press, 1967), 111, 112.

88. Shah, *Contagious Divides*, 7.

89. Metzl, *Protest Psychosis*, 207.

90. For this same racial dynamic at work in early twentieth-century nonmedical writing, see Pablo Mitchell, *Coyote Nation: Sexuality, Race, and Conquest in New Mexico, 1880–1920* (Chicago: University of Chicago Press, 2006), 22.

91. Randolph, "Psychiatry versus the Negro." According to Randolph, postbellum psychiatrists generally deferred to Southern asylum superintendents on the "Negro problem," their alleged familiarity with African Americans earning them expert status.

92. Lewis and Hubbard, "Epileptic Reactions in the Negro," 676.

93. Rosenthal, "Racial Differences in the Mental Diseases," 303. See also Otto Klineberg, *Race Differences* (New York: Harper, 1935), 241–51; Daniel J. Kevles, *In the Name of Eugenics: Genetics and the Uses of Human Heredity* (Cambridge, MA: Harvard University Press, 1997), 135–58; Summers, "Suitable Care of the African"; Degler, *In Search of Human Nature*, 181–87.

94. Stoler, *Along the Archival Grain*, 253; Taussig, *What Color Is the Sacred?*, 188.

95. Bevis, "Psychological Traits of the Southern Negro," 71.

96. Gambino, "These Strangers within Our Gates."

97. Stoler, *Along the Archival Grain*, 186.

98. Ibid., 24, 39. See also Degler, *In Search of Human Nature*.

99. Jack P. Pressman, *Last Resort: Psychosurgery and the Limits of Medicine* (New York: Cambridge University Press, 1998), 19–21; Jones, *Taming the Troublesome Child*, 52–53.

100. For more on whiteness as the norm in US psychiatry, see Wailoo, How *Cancer Crossed the Color Line;* Johannes Fabian, *Time and the Other: How Anthropology Makes Its Object* (New York: Columbia University Press, 1983), x, 1–21; Corbould, *Becoming African Americans*, 166–83; Rose, *Psychology and Selfhood*, 9, 13, 53–55, 90–93, 109–10, 184; Roberts, *Infectious Fear*, 42–55; Brickman, *Aboriginal Populations in the Mind*, 4–5, 54–58, 66–67, 72; Gambino, "These Strangers within Our Gates," 389–90; Bederman, *Manliness and Civilization*, 79–120, 148; Lears, *No Place of Grace*, 144–49; Lears, *Something for Nothing*, 202–3, 213.

101. Evarts, "Dementia Precox in the Colored Race," 388. See also Bender, *Child Psychiatric Techniques*, 124–26, 129, 130–31.

102. Brickman, *Aboriginal Populations in the Mind*, 12–14, 65–83, 88–89; Stephen Jay Gould, *I Have Landed* (New York: Norton, 2002), 147–58; Lears, *Something for Nothing*, 213; Torgovnick, *Gone Primitive*, 8, 204.

103. Brickman, *Aboriginal Populations in the Mind*, 89. Over time, certain ostensibly race-neutral words can become "keywords" loaded or embedded with racialized meaning. Nancy Fraser and Linda Gordon, "A Genealogy of *Dependency*: Tracing a Keyword of the U.S. Welfare State," *Signs* 19 (Winter 1994): 309–36; and Stoler, *Along the Archival Grain*, 35.

104. Green, "Manic-Depressive Psychosis in the Negro," 620. See also Lind, "Phylogenetic Elements," 330–31; John E. Lind, "The Dream as Simple

Wish-Fulfillment in the Negro," *Psychoanalytic Review* 1 (October 1914): 295, 296, 300; and Metzl, *Protest Psychosis*, 103.

105. Bender, "Behavior Problems in Negro Children," 215.

106. Lind, "Dream as a Simple Wish-Fulfillment," 296–300; O'Malley, "Psychosis in the Colored Race," 311, 314; Evarts, "Dementia Precox in the Colored Race," 388.

107. Wray, *Not Quite White*, 2–9, 14–16. See also Lunbeck, *Psychiatric Persuasion*; and Laura Hirshbein, "Sex and Gender in Psychiatry: A View from History," *Journal of Medical Humanities* 31 (2010): 155–70.

108. Summers, "Suitable Care of the African," 86; Rose, *Psychology and Selfhood*, 19, 62–64, 89–90, 109–10.

109. Brickman, *Aboriginal Populations in the Mind*, 89.

110. Summers, "Suitable Care of the African," 87.

111. Schilder and Parker, "Pupillary Disturbances in Schizophrenic Negroes"; Bender, "Behavior Problems in Negro Children," 213–28; Green, "Manic-Depressive Psychosis in the Negro," 620; Evarts, "Dementia in the Colored Race," 396, 397, 404; Bevis, "Psychological Traits of the Southern Negro," 69–78; O'Malley, "Psychosis in the Colored Race," 316, 323, 330; Lind, "Phylogenetic Elements," 304, 323.

112. Sigmund Freud, *Introductory Lectures on Psychoanalysis*, trans. and ed. James Strachey (New York: Liveright, 1977), 297–310, 368; Freud, *Three Essays on the Theory of Sexuality*, trans. and ed. James Strachey (New York: Basic Books, 1975), 14–24, 33–34.

113. Corbould, *Becoming African Americans*, 168.

114. Mitchell, *Coyote Nation*, 144; Stoler, *Race and the Education of Desire*, 150–51, 156–58, 177–78, 183.

115. Lewis and Hubbard, "Epileptic Reactions in the Negro," 647, 657, 676; Rosenthal, "Racial Differences in the Mental Diseases," 312–33. See also Brickman, *Aboriginal Populations in the Mind*, 105; Elizabeth Lunbeck, "American Psychiatrists and the Modern Man, 1900 to 1920," *Men and Masculinities* 1 (July 1998): 58–86; Lunbeck, *Psychiatric Persuasion*, 205; Stoler, *Race and the Education of Desire*, 93, 173, 177; Hirshbein, "Sex and Gender in Psychiatry," 156–63.

116. Williams, "Incidence of Mental Disease in the Negro," 388, 389; Ernest Y. Williams, "Some Observations on the Psychological Aspects of Suicide," *Journal of Social and Abnormal Psychology* 31 (October–November 1936): 260–65; Ernest Y. Williams, "Thieves and Punishment," *Journal of Criminal Law and Criminology* 26 (May 1935): 52–60. Alan P. Smith, "Mental Hygiene in the American Negro," *Journal of the National Medical Association* 23 (January–March 1931): 1–10; Alan P. Smith, "The Availability of Facilities for Negroes Suffering from Mental and Nervous Disease," *Journal of Negro Education* 6 (1937): 450–54; Charles Prudhomme, "The Problem of Suicide in the American Negro," *Psychoanalytic Review* 25 (1938): 378; Walker M. Allen, "Paul Laurence Dunbar, a Study in Genius," *Psychoanalytic Review* 25 (1938): 53–82; R. A. Billings, "The Negro and His Church," *Psychoanalytic Review* 21 (1934): 425–41; Ellen Dwyer, "Psychiatry and Race during World War II," *Journal of the History of Medicine and Allied Sciences* 61 (April 2006): 117–43; Ahad, *Freud Upside Down*, 7–10, 13–34, 39–43, 74–77, 82–109; Scott, *Contempt and Pity*, 6–7, 28–32; 64–69; Rose, *Psychology and Selfhood*, 42, 79–81, 99–106, 111; Charles Prudhomme and David F. Musto, "Historical Perspectives on Mental Health and Racism in the United States,"

in *Racism and Mental Health*, ed. Charles V. Willie, Bernard S. Kramer, and Bertram S. Brown (Pittsburgh, PA: University of Pittsburgh Press, 1973), 42–43.

117. Dwyer, "Psychiatry and Race during World War II," 122. For examples of this literature, see Wagner, "A Comparative Study of Negro and White Admissions," 169, 179, 182; and Bender, "Behavior Problems in Negro Children."

118. Michelle Brattain, "Race, Racism, and Antiracism: UNESCO and the Politics of Presenting Science to the Postwar Public," *American Historical Review* 112 (December 2007): 1397. See also Elazar Barkan, *The Retreat of Scientific Racism: Changing Concepts of Race in Britain and the United States between the World Wars.* New York: Cambridge University Press, 1993.

119. Dennis Doyle, "'Racial Differences Have to Be Considered': Lauretta Bender, Bellevue Hospital, and the African American Psyche, 1936–1952," *History of Psychiatry* 21 (June 2010): 206–23; Alexandra Adler, "The Work of Paul Schilder," in *Paul Schilder: Mind Explorer*, ed. Donald A. Shaskan and William L. Roller (New York: Human Sciences Press, 1985), 69–81; Lauretta Bender, "Childhood Schizophrenia," *American Journal of Orthopsychiatry* 17 (1947): 40–56; Lauretta Bender, "Schizophrenia in Childhood—Its Recognition, Description, and Treatment," *American Journal of Orthopsychiatry* 26 (1956): 499–506.

120. Greenberg, "God and Man in Harlem," 519–20; Watts, *God, Harlem, U.S.A.*, 11–12, 87, 110–12; 135–37; McKay, *Harlem*, 32–72.

121. Watts, *God, Harlem, U.S.A.*, 97; McKay, *Harlem*, 32–49, 61–72; John Hoshor, *God in a Rolls Royce: The Rise of Father Divine, Madman, Menace, or Messiah* (New York: Hillman-Curl, 1936); Robert A. Parker, *The Incredible Messiah: The Deification of Father Divine* (Boston, MA: Little, Brown, 1937); Hadley Cantril and Muzafer Sherif, "The Kingdom of Father Divine," *Journal of Abnormal and Social Psychology* 33 (1938): 147–67.

122. Hoshor, *God in a Rolls Royce.* See also Watts, *God, Harlem, U.S.A.*, 138.

123. Bender and Yarrell, "Psychoses among Followers of Father Divine," 418–49; Bender, "Behavior Problems in Negro Children," 213–28; Bender and Spalding, "Behavior Problems in Children," 460–72.

124. "18 Followers of Divine Are Called Insane," *New York Amsterdam News*, May 18, 1935, 1; "16 of Divine Cult Show Mental Ills," *New York Times*, May 17, 1935, 3. See also K. F. Duncan to Drs. Lauretta Bender and Zuleika Yarrell, May 29, 1935, file 1, box 11, Lauretta Bender Papers, Special Collections, Brooklyn College Library, Brooklyn, New York (hereafter LBP).

125. "18 Followers of Divine," 1.

126. Laypersons wrote to Dr. Bender after reading about her APA paper in a mainstream news source. K. F. Duncan to Drs. Lauretta Bender and Zuleika Yarrell, May 29, 1935; J. Raymond Henderson to Drs. Buleika [*sic*] Yarrell and Lauretta Bender, December 5, 1935; Albert Ludlow Kramer, letter addressed to "Drs.," May 25, 1935, letter forwarded to Lauretta Bender, file 1, box 11, series 4, LBP; Cantril and Sharif, "Kingdom of Father Divine"; Parker, *Incredible Messiah;* Hoshor, *God in a Rolls Royce*, xii.

127. Bender's 1940 article drew fire from some of Father Divine's "angels" in Harlem for insinuating that the Peace Mission movement could damage the mental health of children. McKay, *Harlem*, 38; Watts, *God, Harlem, U.S.A.*, xii. See John Lamb to Dr. Joseph Broadman, April 23, 1940, 1; Sweet Love to Drs. Bender and Spalding, May 10, 1940; Miss Sweet Inspiration to Drs. Lauretta Bender and M. A.

Spaulding [sic], May 28, 1940; Miss Beautiful Smile to [Lauretta Bender], May 5, 1940, file 1, box 11, series 4, LBP. See "Ignorance of the Bellevue Hospital Doctors Who Misrepresented Father's Influence Expose," *The New Day*, May 16, 1940, 65–66; "Letter to Drs. Bender and Paulding [sic] of Bellevue Hospital Describes the Care Given to Children in the Promised Land," *The New Day*, June 6, 1940, 63–65, file 2, box 11, series 4, LBP.

128. Bender and Yarrell, "Psychoses among Followers of Father Divine," 425, 443. See also 424, 444, 447–49.

129. Bender, "Behavior Problems in Negro Children," 225.

130. Stoler, *Along the Archival Grain*, 278; Stoler, "Interview," 500–504.

131. Doyle, "Racial Differences Have to Be Considered," 209. See also Johannes Fabian, *Out of Our Minds: Reason and Madness in the Exploration of Central Africa* (Berkeley: University of California Press, 2000), 227; and Stoler, *Along the Archival Grain*, 38, 62.

132. Bender, "Behavior Problems in Negro Children." Bender and her fellow racial agnostics were people who, in the anthropologist Ann Laura Stoler's words, "*suddenly find themselves having difficulty thinking* in certain ways." In this instance, she no longer could uncritically accept racialism. Stoler, *Along the Archival Grain*, 36, 278 (see also 30, 40, 42, 51, 58); Stoler, "Interview," 500; Judith Butler, *Bodies That Matter: On the Discursive Limits of Sex* (New York: Routledge, 1993), 10; and Christopher Sellers, "Thoreau's Body: Towards an Embodied Environmental History," paper presented at 2nd Plenary Session, Annual Meeting of the American Society for Environmental History, Baltimore, MD, March 1997, copy in author's possession.

133. See Doyle, "Racial Differences Have to Be Considered," 206–23.

134. Bender, "Behavior Problems in Negro Children," 227.

135. Ibid., 213.

136. Degler, *In Search of Human Nature*, 186–87.

137. Megan Vaughan, *Curing Their Ills: Colonial Power and African Illness* (Stanford, CA: Stanford University Press, 1992), 12, 109, 115–25, 202; Abram Kardiner, *The Psychological Frontiers of Society* (New York: Columbia University Press, 1945).

138. Bender, "Behavior Problems in Negro Children," 224, 225. On cultural anthropology's influence on Bender's work, see Jules Henry to Lauretta Bender, November 24, 1948, folder 2, box 8, series 3, LBP; Jules Henry, "Environment and Symptom Formation," *American Journal of Orthopsychiatry* 17 (October 1947): 628–51; Lauretta Bender to Dr. S. Bernard Wortis, September 23, 1943, file 1, box 6, LBP; Lauretta Bender to Dr. B. Liber, August 4, 1949, file 1, box 6, LBP; Lauretta Bender and Franziska Boas, "Creative Dance in Therapy," *American Journal of Orthopsychiatry* 11 (1941): 235–45; Lauretta Bender to Mr. Moe, May 8, 1950, file 1, box 5, LBP; Georgene H. Seward to Lauretta Bender, July 25, 1957, file 17, box 11, series 4, LBP; Georgene Seward, photocopy of table of contents from *Clinical Studies of Culture Conflict*, [May 16, 1957], file 17, box 11, series 4, LBP.

139. Lauretta Bender, "Group Activities on the Children's Ward as Method of Psychotherapy," paper presented at the annual meeting of the American Psychiatric Association, St. Louis, Missouri, May 1936, 5, file 9, box 17, series 7, LBP.

140. Summers, "Suitable Care of the African," 78; Bender, "Behavior Problems in Negro Children," 214, 218–21, 227–28; Bender, "Group Activities on the Children's Ward," 5, LBP.

141. Doyle, "Racial Differences Have to Be Considered," 209–18.

142. Ibid., 214. See Bender, "Behavior Problems in Negro Children," 218, 228; Bender, *A Visual Motor Gestalt Test,* vii–viii, ix, 3–6, 14, 17–18, 108.

143. Doyle, "Racial Differences Have to Be Considered."

144. Schilder and Parker, "Pupillary Disturbances in Schizophrenic Negroes"; Bender, *Aggression, Hostility and Anxiety in Children,* 91–115; Lauretta Bender and Frank J. Curran, "Children and Adolescents Who Kill," *Journal of Clinical Psychopathology* 1 (1940): 297–322.

145. Robin D. G. Kelley, *Yo Mama's Disfunktional! Fighting the Culture Wars in Urban America* (Boston, MA: Beacon Press, 1997), 3.

146. Stoler, *Along the Archival Grain,* 39.

Chapter Two

1. Justine Wise Polier, *Everyone's Children, Nobody's Child* (New York: Charles Scribner's Sons, 1941), 191 (see also 190, 192–94).

2. Ibid., 191, 193 (see also 5, 85, 91, 144–46).

3. Rose, *Inventing Our Selves,* 9–20, 29–34, 59–60, 62–78; Jones, *Taming the Troublesome Child,* 199; Robertson, *Crimes against Children,* 4–7, 141, 148–49, 206–8.

4. Alan Brinkley, *The End of Reform: New Deal Liberalism in Recession and War* (New York: Vintage, 1995), 6–11; Jennifer Mittelstadt, "Philanthropy, Feminism, and Left Liberalism," *Journal of Women's History* 20 (Winter 2008): 105, 108–10; Walter A. Jackson, *Gunnar Myrdal and America's Conscience: Social Engineering and Racial Liberalism, 1938–1987* (Chapel Hill: University of North Carolina Press, 1990), xix, 3; Gerstle, "Protean Character of American Liberalism," 1044–45, 1067–73.

5. According to Walter Jackson, racial liberals believed in the "effectiveness of state action in improving the status of blacks" (*Gunnar Myrdal,* 126). See also Brinkley, *End of Reform,* 164–67; and Self, *American Babylon.* For the range of political and intellectual influences that made racial liberalism possible, see Gerstle, "Protean Character of American Liberalism," 1045; Degler, *In Search of Human Nature,* 201–4; Sugrue, *Sweet Land of Liberty,* 190; Greenberg, *Troubling the Waters,* 8, 9, 30–37; Markowitz and Rosner, *Children, Race, and Power,* 28, 36–37, 54–55.

6. Mason B. Williams, *City of Ambition: FDR, La Guardia, and the Making of Modern New York* (New York: Norton, 2013), xi.

7. Herman, *Kinship By Design,* 208–9.

8. According to the historian Todd Shepard, some public policies and practices have been able to promote the "institutionalization of 'confidence'" in new ideas and assumptions. Todd Shepard, *The Invention of Decolonization: The Algerian War and the Remaking of France* (Ithaca, NY: Cornell University Press, 2008), 167.

9. The terms "psychiatric point of view" and "mental hygiene point of view" were commonly used by the New York-based medical and legal professionals mentioned in this chapter.

10. Feldstein, *Motherhood in Black and White,* 38.

11. Justine Wise Polier, "How I Became Interested in Racial Justice," *Opportunity* 26 (Spring 1948): 63.

12. Herman, *Kinship by Design*, 40–45, 205–6; Melvin I. Urofsky, *A Voice That Spoke for Justice: The Life and Time of Stephen S. Wise* (Albany: State University of New York Press, 1982), 71, 100; Nina Bernstein, *The Lost Children of Wilder: The Epic Struggle to Change Foster Care* (New York: Vintage, 2001), 52–54; Greenberg, *Troubling the Waters*, 24, 36.

13. Joyce Antler, *The Journey Home: Jewish Women and the American Century* (New York: Free Press, 1997), 186–88. See also Justine Wise Polier, *Juvenile Justice in Double Jeopardy: The Distanced Community and Vengeful Retribution* (Hillsdale, NJ: Lawrence Erlbaum Associates, 1989), 108.

14. "Mrs. Tulin Named Justice by Mayor," *New York Times* (hereafter *NYT*), July 8, 1935, 4; "Shake-up in Police to Aid Racket War," *NYT*, July 9, 1935, 2; "Mrs. Tulin Studies New Role on Bench," *NYT*, July 10, 1935, 8.

15. Jackson, *Gunnar Myrdal*, xv. On Polier's liberal credentials, see Joyce Antler, "Justine Wise Polier and the Prophetic Tradition," in *Women and American Judaism: Historical Perspectives*, ed. Pamela S. Nadell and Jonathan D. Sarna (Boston, MA: Brandeis University Press, 2001), 268–90.

16. "Mrs. Tulin to Advise Knauth on the Law," *NYT*, April 10, 1935, 10.

17. Jackson, *Gunnar Myrdal*, xv, 5.

18. Greenberg, *"Or Does It Explode?"* 147, 148, 153–55, 183–84; Ronald H. Bayor, *Fiorello La Guardia: Ethnicity and Reform* (Arlington Heights, IL: Harlan Davidson, 1993), 130–34.

19. "Mrs. Tulin Studies New Role on Bench," 8; "Shake-up in Police to Aid Racket War," 2.

20. Charles Garrett, *The La Guardia Years: Machine and Reform Politics in New York City* (New Brunswick, NJ: Rutgers University Press, 1961), 81–113, 132–35, 252–55, 266–67; Edward J. Flynn, *You're the Boss* (New York: Viking Press, 1947), 138–41.

21. Urofsky, *A Voice That Spoke for Justice*, 250–52; Antler, *Journey Home*, 190; Bayor, *Fiorello La Guardia*, 101–4, 106, 144; Williams, *City of Ambition*, 235.

22. Mary P. Ryan, *Mysteries of Sex: Tracing Women and Men through American History* (Chapel Hill: University of North Carolina Press, 2006), 176.

23. On maternalist reform, see Herman, *Kinship by Design*, 86; Ryan, *Mysteries of Sex*, 176–84; Estelle Freedman, *Maternal Justice: Miriam Van Waters and the Female Reform Tradition* (Chicago: University of Chicago Press, 1996), xii–xiii, 57, 58, 86; Linda Gordon, *Pitied but Not Entitled: Single Mothers and the History of Welfare* (Cambridge, MA: Harvard University Press, 1994), 55–57, 103; Robin L. Muncy, *Creating a Female Dominion in American Reform, 1890–1935* (New York: Oxford University Press, 1991), 98, 101, 109, 140, 141, 154–56, 161.

24. Herman, *Kinship by Design*, 206.

25. Bernstein, *Lost Children of Wilder*, 50.

26. Ibid., 56–67; Herman, *Kinship by Design*, 40.

27. Polier, *Juvenile Justice*, 129; Bernstein, *Lost Children of Wilder*, 50–58; Markowitz and Rosner, "Race, Foster Care," 1845; Markowitz and Rosner, *Children, Race, and Power*, 8–9; Herman, *Kinship by Design*, 207–8.

28. Justine Wise Polier, "Memorandum to the Mayor," July 19, 1938, Appendix B, folder 256, box 22, JWP. Two Catholic institutions did take in some delinquent African American teens. See also Bernstein, *The Lost Children of Wilder*, 50, 52, 54, 57; and Markowitz and Rosner, "Race, Foster Care," 1845.

29. Polier, *Everyone's Children*, 238; Polier, "How I Became Interested in Racial Justice," 69; Herman, *Kinship by Design*, 208; Markowitz and Rosner, *Children, Race, and Power*, 10.

30. Regina G. Kunzel, *Fallen Women, Problem Girls: Unmarried Mothers and the Professionalization of Social Work, 1890–1945* (New Haven, CT: Yale University Press, 1993), 41–44, 128, 147–48; Mennel, *Thorns and Thistles*, 161–68; Jones, *Taming the Troublesome Child*, 78, 79, 82, 83, 169, 190, 202; Herman, *Kinship by Design*, 51–52, 87–88; Horn, *Before It's Too Late*, 100–101.

31. Polier, *Juvenile Justice*, 107–8. The court's diagnostic clinic opened in 1917.

32. "Interview with Dr. Winsor, Resident Psychiatrist," 7, JWP; Jones, *Taming the Troublesome Child*, 190.

33. Jones, *Taming the Troublesome Child*, 33–34; Freedman, *Maternal Justice*, 58; Mennel, *Thorns and Thistles*, 129–32, 140–42, 144.

34. Rose, *Inventing Our Selves*, 64; Robertson, *Crimes against Children*, 206–8; Lunbeck, *Psychiatric Persuasion*, 4–7.

35. Rose, *Inventing Our Selves*, 31, 63, 78; Nikolas Rose, *The Politics of Life Itself: Biomedicine, Power, and Subjectivity in the Twenty-First Century* (Princeton, NJ: Princeton University Press, 2008), 52–54; Morris, "Miner's Ear," 110.

36. Regina Kunzel, "White Neurosis, Black Pathology: Constructing Out-of-Wedlock Pregnancy in the Wartime and Postwar United States," in *Not June Cleaver: Women and Gender in Postwar America, 1945–1960*, ed. Joanne Meyerowitz (Philadelphia, PA: Temple University Press, 1994), 321–22; Rickie Solinger, *Wake Up Little Susie: Single Pregnancy and Race before Roe v. Wade* (New York: Routledge, 1992), 9, 21, 24, 25, 43, 86, 87.

37. Paul Livernois, C. S. Desmond, and Lawrence Greenbaum, "Conclusions and Recommendations," September 29, 1936, 1–7, folder 37, box 3, JWP.

38. Committee on Institutions, Board of Visitors, New York City Domestic Relations Court, "Visit to the N.Y. State Training School for Girls," December 3, 1936, 2, 4, folder 37, box 3, JWP. Of the 460 young women institutionalized at Hudson during 1936, the 88 listed as "colored" had all been committed via the New York City court system. In fact, as the committee noted, "most of the Negro girls come from Harlem."

39. New York City, Domestic Relations Court, Committee on Institutions, Report, May 4, 1936, 1, folder 37, box 3, JWP.

40. Committee on Institutions, "Visit to the N.Y. State Training School for Girls," 2, 5, JWP.

41. Mrs. Waite, Mrs. Tinkelpaugh, and Mrs. Rosen, "Memo of Interview with Mr. Harry W. Collins at the Office of the N.Y. State Training School for Boys, in the State Dept. Building, at 80 Center Street," December 9, 1936, 3, folder 39, box 4, JWP.

42. Committee on Institutions, "Visit to the N.Y. State Training School for Girls," 1, JWP.

43. Committee on Institutions, New York City Domestic Relations Court, Board of Justices, "New York Training School Facilities Available for Care and Treatment: Visits to Institution May and June," [1937], 44, folder 41, box 4, JWP.

44. "Interview with Dr. Herbert D. Williams, Superintendent," March 4, March 30, April 1, 1937, 1, folder 39, box 4, JWP; Ms. Waite, Mrs. Tinkelpaugh, and Mrs. Rosen, "Memo of Interview with Mr. Harry W. Collins," 3, JWP; "Interview with Mr.

Schroedel, Executive Assistant Superintendent," March 8 and March 31, 1937, 2, folder 39, box 4, JWP. Schroedel, the head disciplinarian, told the visitors that "corporal punishment is taboo."

45. Committee on Institutions, Board of Justices, New York City Domestic Relations Court, "The New York Training School for Boys: A Summary," 1937, 6, folder 37, box 3, JWP.

46. Ibid., 3, 4.

47. Committee on Institutions, "New York Training School Facilities Available for Care and Treatment," 44, JWP; Rose, *Inventing Our Selves*, 78.

48. Mrs. Waite, Mrs. Tinklepaugh, Mrs. Rosen, "First Visit to State Training School for Boys, Warwick, NY," December 22, 1936, 4, folder 39, box 4, JWP. In its final 1937 report, the committee wished that the clinic could function more as a real child-guidance clinic, handling "more of the everyday problems of the average boy in the Institution than present facilities permit." Committee on Institutions, "New York State Training School for Boys," 3, JWP.

49. The report averred: "If he is successful in permeating the institution with the principles and methods of mental hygiene it would seem that he had achieved more than would be possible through psycho-analysis." "Interview with Dr. Winsor, Resident Psychiatrist," 7, JWP. On the role of the psychological sciences in shaping modern legal expectations of childcare, see Rose, *Inventing Our Selves*, 10–12, 15–16, 19, 21, 33.

50. Polier, *Everyone's Children*, 207.

51. Rose, *Inventing Our Selves*, 92.

52. Advisory Committee on Treatment, Psychiatric Clinic of the Children's Court, Minutes, May 27, 1943, 3, folder 63, box 6, JWP; [Viola W. Bernard], "Obituary for Max Winsor, MD, 1897–1945," *American Journal of Orthopsychiatry* 15 (July 1945): 535–56; [No author], "Dr. Max Winsor, 17 Bank Street," [1945], 1–2; [Evelyn] Seeley, "Winsor: Seeley-schools," 1945, 1–3, folder "Max Winsor Obituary (1897–1945)," box 5, series "Correspondence, Individuals—Alphabetical," Viola W. Bernard Papers, Archives & Special Collections, Health Sciences Library, Columbia University, New York (hereafter VWB); Dr. Viola Bernard, interview by Dr. Spafford Ackerly, May 30, 1973, transcript, 11, folder "VWB's Career in Child Psychiatry," box 1, series "Oral History Transcripts," VWB.

53. "Interview with Dr. Winsor, Resident Psychiatrist," 5, JWP (see also 4, 6); Max Winsor, "Children in Need," *Atlantic Monthly*, July 1943, 59–60.

54. Interview with Dr. Winsor, Resident Psychiatrist," 6, JWP.

55. Kunzel, *Fallen Women, Problem Girls*, 165–66; Jones, *Taming the Troublesome Child*, 190; Herman, *Kinship by Design*, 88, 110, 206, 322; Dain, *Clifford W. Beers*, 194; Viola Bernard, "Interview re: Getting to Know Justine Polier," July 10, 1992, folder "Justine Wise Polier, Biographical Material," box 2 "Justine Wise Polier," series "People," VWB.

56. Polier, *Juvenile Justice*, 111; Jones, *Taming the Troublesome Child*, 58–60; Bernard, "Interview re," VWB; Herman, *Kinship by Design*, 96; Bernstein, *Lost Children of Wilder*, 136. For the source of the quote on Kenworthy, see Polier's dedication to Kenworthy in *Everyone's Children*.

57. Polier, *Everyone's Children*, 111, 207, 224.

58. Freedman, *Maternal Justice*, 58, 60; Kunzel, *Fallen Women, Problem Girls*, 128, 129; Steven Mintz, *Huck's Raft: A History of American Childhood* (Cambridge, MA: Belknap

Press, 2006), 176–78; Lawrence M. Friedman, *American Law in the 20th Century* (New Haven, CT: Yale University Press, 2002), 90–92; Mennel, *Thorns and Thistles*, 131–33, 137–40, 144–47, 149–57.

59. Antler, *Journey Home*, 193. See also Polier, *Everyone's Children*, 111, 207, 224.

60. Rose, *Inventing Our Selves*, 92, 93 (see also 63).

61. Polier, *Everyone's Children*, 73, 77, 78.

62. Board of Justices, Domestic Relations Court, City of New York, Minutes, October 8, 1937, 1, folder 63, box 6, JWP.

63. Ibid. See also Polier, *Juvenile Justice*, 111.

64. Advisory Committee of the Treatment Clinic, untitled recommendations and report, [1943], 24, folder 63, box 6, JWP.

65. Austin H. MacCormick to Hon. W. Bruce Cobb, April 23, 1945, 1, folder 64, box 6, JWP.

66. Advisory Committee of the Treatment Clinic, untitled recommendations and report, [1943], 7, JWP. See also MacCormick to Cobb, April 23, 1945, 2, JWP.

67. Mittelstadt, "Philanthropy, Feminism, and Left Liberalism," 109.

68. Viola W. Bernard, Interview by Milton J. E. Senn, March 16, 1977, transcript, 11, folder "American Child Guidance Clinic Movement, Pediatric-Psychiatric Moments, and the Child Psychiatry Movement," March 16, 1977, box 1, series "Oral History Transcripts," VWB; Axel Madison, *The Marshall Fields: The Evolution of an American Business Dynasty* (Hoboken, NJ: John Wiley & Sons, 2002), 231.

69. Antler, "Justine Wise Polier and the Prophetic Tradition."

70. Board of Justices, Minutes, October 8, 1937, 1, JWP. See also Freedman, *Maternal Justice*, 252.

71. Polier, *Everyone's Children*, 245.

72. Ibid., 73; *Juvenile Justice*, 108; Muncy, *Creating a Female Dominion*, 140.

73. Polier, *Everyone's Children*, 65 (see also 73).

74. Ibid., 73. Polier's explanations of her approach borrowed a great deal from the writings of Kenworthy and three of her associates: Kenworthy's student and the psychiatric social worker Sophia Robison, the Detroit psychiatric social worker and director of the Children's Fund of Michigan's child-guidance clinic Maud E. Watson, and the New York of School of Social Work's professor of education Henry W. Thurston.

75. Ibid., 73.

76. Ibid., 65.

77. Sophia M. Robison, *Juvenile Delinquency: Its Nature and Control* (New York: Holt, 1960), 9, 10. The New York City psychiatric social worker Robison's definition of what she called the "mental hygiene point of view" bears the strongest resemblance to Polier's "individualized approach" to juvenile delinquents.

78. Polier, *Everyone's Children*, 5, 91, 129. For the direct influences on Polier's understanding of this concept, see Maud E. Watson, *Children and Their Parents* (New York: F. S. Crofts, 1932), 82–83; William Healy, *Mental Conflicts and Misconduct* (Boston, MA: Little, Brown, 1930), 321–22; William Healy, Augusta F. Bronner, Edith M. H. Baylor, and J. Prentice Murray, *Reconstructing Behavior in Youth: A Study of Problem Children in Foster Families* (New York: Alfred A. Knopf, 1936), 24. In explaining her approach to juvenile delinquency in *Everyone's Children, Nobody's Child* (1941), Polier relied heavily on the physician Dr. William Healy and the psychologist Augusta

Bronner, directors of Boston's Judge Baker Child Guidance Clinic, referring to them twice by name within the body of the text (84, 91). See also Jones, *Taming the Troublesome Child*, 67–77.

79. Polier, *Everyone's Children*, 85, 91.

80. Ibid., 83. Polier's thinking was indebted to James S. Plant's *Personality and the Cultural Pattern* (New York: Commonwealth Fund, 1937), 25. Plant was a cultural anthropologist and director of the Essex County Juvenile Court Clinic.

81. Polier, *Everyone's Children*, 65. Healy and Bronner, *Reconstructing Behavior*, 19–25; Plant, *Personality and the Cultural Pattern*, 8, 13, 17; Henry W. Thurston, *The Dependent Child: A Story of Changing Aims and Methods in the Care of Dependent Children* (New York: Columbia University Press, 1930), 199–200; Watson, *Children and Their Parents*, 6–7.

82. Polier, *Everyone's Children*, 67.

83. Polier, *Juvenile Justice*, 97, 108–12.

84. W. Bruce Cobb to Justice, Domestic Relations Court, City of New York, June 16, 1943, 5, folder 63, box 6, JWP. Dr. Frank Curran was the head of Bellevue Psychiatric Ward PQ-5.

85. Dr. Frank J. Curran, untitled medical report for the Domestic Relations Court, September 23, 1942, 1, folder 258, box 22, JWP.

86. Ibid., 1–2.

87. Ibid. Polier emphatically marked the passages that contained Curran's most racialist remarks, most likely as an expression of outrage or dismay.

88. Polier, *Everyone's Children*, 207.

89. Ibid., 245.

90. Jonathan Sadowsky, *Imperial Bedlam: Institutions of Madness in Colonial Southwest Nigeria* (Berkeley: University of California Press, 1999), 102–4, 106, 109–10; Summers, "Suitable Care of the African," 58–66, 86–91.

91. Healy, *Mental Conflicts and Misconduct*, 316.

92. Jeffrey L. Gould, *To Die in This Way: Nicaraguan Indians and the Myth of Mestizaje, 1880–1965* (Durham, NC: Duke University Press, 1998). According to Gould, what historical actors considered to be "common sense" was "that part of a worldview that is 'naturalized,' that no longer appears to represent the ideology of particular group" (12).

93. Carl Degler referred to this psychological model of sameness as little more than an "unproven assumption," meaning that no one had bothered to rigorously test it. Degler, *In Search of Human Nature*, 187. On the difference between formal ideology and taken-for-granted assumptions, see Bourdieu, *Logic of Practice*, 52–79; Martin, *Bipolar Expeditions*, 77.

94. Butler, "Restaging the Universal," 38.

95. "Summary of [name withheld]'s Case for Justice Polier," 1938, folder 256, box 22, JWP; Polier, *Everyone's Children*, 147.

96. Watson, *Children and Their Parents*, 95. See also Lunbeck, *Psychiatric Persuasion*.

97. Lunbeck, *Psychiatric Persuasion*, 214, 226; Bederman, *Manliness and Civilization*, 23–36; Brickman, *Aboriginal Populations in the Mind*, 66–67, 69, 71, 72, 75–83; Torgovnick, *Gone Primitive*, 228; Lynn Sacco, *Unspeakable: Father-Daughter Incest in American History* (Baltimore, MD: Johns Hopkins University Press, 2009), 107–9; Summers, "Suitable Care of the African," 66–74, 75–76, 84, 86–89; Martin, *Bipolar*

Expeditions, 213; Vaughan, *Curing Their Ills*, 46, 110–11, 113–14, 115–17, 118, 202; Mitchell, *Coyote Nation*, 144; Metzl, *Protest Psychosis*, 29–31; Gilman, *Difference and Pathology*, 113–20; Gilroy, *Postcolonial Melancholia*, 32; Taussig, *Mimesis and Alterity*, 66–68, 75, 159; Lynette A. Jackson, *Surfacing Up: Psychiatry and Social Order in Colonial Zimbabwe, 1908–1968* (Ithaca, NY: Cornell University Press, 2005), 106–9.

98. Bender, "Behavior Problems of Negro Children," 215. See also Doyle, "Racial Differences Have to Be Considered," 218.

99. Robertson, *Crimes against Children*, 214, 226; Crista DeLuzio, *Female Adolescence in American Scientific Thought, 1830–1930* (Baltimore, MD: Johns Hopkins University Press, 2007), 94–104; Bederman, *Manliness and Civilization*, 35–36; Ann McClintock, *Imperial Leather: Race, Gender, and Sexuality in the Colonial Conquest* (New York: Routledge, 1991), 50–51.

100. Robertson, *Crimes against Children*, 214.

101. Scott, *Contempt and Pity*; Berlant, *Female Complaint*.

102. Kunzel, *Fallen Women, Problem Girls*, 156; Alexander, *"Girl Problem,"* 15, 65, 66, 149, 151; Mary Odem, *Delinquent Daughters: Protecting and Policing Adolescent Female Sexuality in the United States, 1885–1920* (Chapel Hill: University of North Carolina Press, 1995), 43–81, 138–48, 155–56; Hicks, "Bright and Good Looking Colored Girls," 419, 420, 441–43; Robertson, *Crimes against Children*, 13–22, 73–92; Sacco, *Unspeakable*, 186–89, 195.

103. Robertson, *Crimes against Children*, 155, 153.

104. Elizabeth Pleck, *Domestic Tyranny: The Making of Social Policy against Family Violence from Colonial Times to the Present* (New York: Oxford University Press, 1987), 156–57; Sacco, *Unspeakable*, 213–15; Robertson, *Crimes against Children*, 152–55.

105. Polier, *Everyone's Children*, 14; Robertson, *Crimes against Children*, 3–4, 141–49.

106. Polier, *Everyone's Children*, 153.

107. Ibid., 151.

108. Robertson, *Crimes against Children*, 151.

109. Bender, "Behavior Problems in Negro Children," 215.

110. Robertson, *Crimes against Children*, 151 (see also 183).

111. In *Juvenile Justice*, 97, Polier refers to this young African American woman as Joetta, and in *Everyone's Children*, 194–98, as Anita Meeker. She will be hereafter identified by only one of these pseudonyms, Joetta.

112. Dr. Lauretta Bender, untitled medical report to the Domestic Relations Court, September 25, 1939, 1, folder 63, box 6, JWP. See Polier, *Everyone's Children*, 149–58; Polier, *Juvenile Justice*, 100–101. On the House of Good Shepherd and the judicial separation of sexual abuse victims from age peers, see Odem, *Delinquent Daughters*, 148; Anna Meis Knupfer, *Reform and Resistance: Gender, Delinquency, and America's First Juvenile Court* (New York: Routledge, 2001), 157–76; Sacco, *Unspeakable*, 198–295; Freedman, *Maternal Justice*, 87.

113. Polier, *Everyone's Children*, 223.

114. Ibid., 222. See Robertson, *Crimes against Children*, 18–19, 47–49, 62–66.

115. Polier, *Everyone's Children*, 197.

116. Ibid., 196; Robertson, *Crimes against Children*, 153–54; Lauretta Bender, lecture, "Emotional and Social Problems as Factors in Behavior Disorders of School," [n.d.], 1, folder 5, box 13, LBP.

117. Robertson, *Crimes against Children*, 284n52.

118. Bender, untitled medical report to the Domestic Relations Court, September 25, 1939, 2, JWP. Polier was swayed by Bender's opinion that "[Joetta's] attitude to her experience leads the psychiatrist to believe that she is telling the truth on every point." Dr. Bender's understanding of rape as a real and traumatic rather than an imagined event challenges the psychiatrist Dr. Judith Herman's influential argument in *Trauma and Recovery* (New York: Basic Books, 1997) that the idea of rape as a traumatic event disappeared within psychiatry after Freud rejected the thesis, reappearing only when the third wave of feminism politicized rape and revived the concept of rape as trauma.

119. Sacco, *Unspeakable*, 187 (see also 195).

120. Polier, *Everyone's Children*, 197–98.

121. Ibid., 197 (see also 149–58).

122. Rose, *Inventing Our Selves*, 73.

123. James Gilbert, *A Cycle of Outrage: America's Reaction to the Juvenile Delinquent in the 1950s* (New York: Oxford University Press, 1986).

124. Polier, *Juvenile Justice*, 22–23. See also Polier, *Everyone's Children*, 190.

125. Polier, "Memorandum to the Mayor," 1–3, JWP; Polier, *Juvenile Justice*, 21–24; Polier, *Everyone's Children*, 223–24.

126. Polier, "Memorandum to the Mayor," Appendix B, 2, JWP; Polier, *Juvenile Justice*, 20–21; Markowitz and Rosner, "Race, Foster Care," 1845.

127. Polier, "Negro Children," July 12, 1938, 1, folder 256, box 22, JWP; Polier, "Memorandum to the Mayor," 1–2, JWP; Polier, *Juvenile Justice*, 149; Agnes King Inglis to Justine Wise Polier, memo, [1940], 3, folder 257, box 22, JWP; Markowitz and Rosner, *Children, Race, and Power*, 9–11; Markowitz and Rosner, "Race, Foster Care," 1845.

128. Polier, "Memorandum to the Mayor," 3, JWP; Polier, *Everyone's Children*, 238.

129. Domestic Relations Court of the City of New York, Children's Court Division, County of New York, Transcript of delinquency petition before Hon. Justine Wise Polier, July 12, 1938, 3–4, 6–7, 8–9, folder 256, box 22, JWP. See also Polier, "Memorandum to the Mayor," Appendix A, 3, JWP.

130. Polier, *Everyone's Children*, 139.

131. Domestic Relations Court, Transcript of delinquency petition, July 12, 1938, 7, JWP.

132. Ibid., 5–6; Polier, "Memorandum to the Mayor," 2, 3–4, Appendix A, 3, JWP; Markowitz and Rosner, "Race, Foster Care," 1845; Polier, *Juvenile Justice*, 138–39. See also Herman, *Kinship by Design*, 207.

133. Polier, "Memorandum to the Mayor," 4, JWP; Agnes King Linglis to Hon. Justine Wise Polier, memo, [1940], 2–3, folder 257, box 22, JWP.

134. Domestic Relations Court, Transcript of delinquency petition, 8, July 12, 1938, JWP; Polier, "Negro Children," 1, JWP.

135. Domestic Relations Court, Transcript of delinquency petition, July 12, 1938, 6, JWP; Inglis to Polier, memo, [1940], 2, JWP; Polier, *Everyone's Children*, 240–45.

136. Polier, *Everyone's Children*, 240.

137. Ibid., 186–88; 190–98; 220–21; 234–35.

138. Biondi, *To Stand and to Fight*, 40.

139. "Dudley F. Sicher, Ex-Justice Dies," *NYT*, November 16, 1957, 19; Polier, *Juvenile Justice*, xvii; Transcript of Viola W. Bernard tape recording, September 22,

1987, 15–18, folder "Sept. 18, 1987—Bureau of Child Guidance," series "Oral History Transcripts," box 1, VWB; Markowitz and Rosner, *Children, Race, and Power*, 59.

140. Greenberg, *Troubling the Waters*, 92–113; Sugrue, *Sweet Land of Liberty*, 114.

141. "Dudley F. Sicher, Ex-Justice Dies," 19.

142. Hon. Dudley Sicher to Justine Wise Polier, December 7, 1940, folder 257, box 22, JWP.

Chapter Three

1. Claude Brown, *Manchild in the Promised Land* (New York: MacMillan, 1965), 58; Jacqueline A. McLeod, "Persona Non-Grata: Judge Jane Matilda Bolin and the NAACP, 1930–1950," *Afro-Americans in New York Life and History* 29 (January 2005): 7–29; Biondi, *To Stand and to Fight*, 167, 169, 179, 201; Dominic J. Capeci, Jr., *The Harlem Riot of 1943* (Philadelphia, PA: Temple University Press, 1977), 8; Markowitz and Rosner, *Children, Race, and Power*, 7, 9, 59; Marian Wright Edelman, "Judge Jane Bolin," January 26, 2007, http://www.childrensdefense.org/child-research-data-publications/data/marian-wright-edelman-child-watch-column/judge-jane-bolin.html (accessed May 24, 2010).

2. Brown, *Manchild in the Promised Land*, 59, 66, 58.

3. Benjamin Reiss, *Theaters of Madness: Insane Asylums and Nineteenth-Century American Culture* (Chicago: University of Chicago Press, 2008), 11. See also Summers, "Suitable Care of the African."

4. Morris, "Miner's Ear," 110.

5. Muhammad, *Condemnation of Blackness*, 3–9, 152–54.

6. The historian Ellen Herman referred to modern public policies designed to help citizens regulate their own behavior and inner life as "therapeutic government," in *Kinship by Design*, 11, 12–13, 206, 285–86. For more on the historical development of such policies, see Michel Foucault, *Abnormal: Lectures at the College de France, 1974–1975*, trans. Graham Burchell (New York: Picador, 2003), 21, 48–52; Foucault, *Discipline and Punish*, 20–24, 25–30, 296, 298–303, 305; Butler, *Bodies That Matter*, 22; Jacques Donzelot, *The Policing of Families* (New York: Random House, 1979), 94–95; Colin Gordon, "Governmental Rationality: An Introduction," in *The Foucault Effect: Studies in Governmentality*, ed. Graham Burchell, Colin Gordon, and Peter Miller (Chicago: University of Chicago Press, 1991), 1–51; Reiss, *Theaters of Madness*, 10–12; Stoler, *Race and the Education of Desire*, 3, 80, 64–65, 80–84, 96; Rose, *Politics of Life Itself*, 52–54; Rose, *Inventing Our Selves*, 60–66; Loic Waquant, *Punishing the Poor: The Neoliberal Government of Social Insecurity* (Durham, NC: Duke University Press, 2009), xviii, 29–32, 304–5, 324.

7. Viola W. Bernard, "Dr. Max Winsor," 1945, 1, folder "Max Winsor: Obituary (1897–1945)," box 5, series "Professional Correspondence, Individuals—Alphabetical," VWB; New York City Bureau of Child Guidance, *Five-Year Report, 1932–1937*, 20–21. These other two regions were the Lower East Side and the infamous Red Hook section of Brooklyn. The Board of Education authorized the units on June 24, 1936.

8. [Bernard], "Obituary for Max Winsor," 535; Charlotte Winsor, "Introduction," in *Experimental Schools Revisited: Bulletins of the Bureau of Educational Experiments*, ed. Charlotte Winsor (New York: Agathon Press, 1973): 7–8; Mintz, *Huck's Raft*, 175–76.

9. The child study movement, begun by the psychologist G. Stanley Hall in 1897, was the first systematic effort to scientifically study child development. It was an interdisciplinary movement composed of psychologists and laypersons, many of them stay-at-home mothers. Mintz, *Huck's Raft*, 188–90; Freedman, *Maternal Justice*, 36–44; Jones, *Taming the Troublesome Child*, 50–56; Ellen Condliffe Lagemann, *An Elusive Science: The Troubling History of Education Research* (Chicago: University of Chicago Press, 2000), 24–32; 39–50; Mennel, *Thorns and Thistles*, 80–85.

10. Bythe Hinitz, "Margaret Naumburg and the Walden School," and Mary E. Hauser, "Caroline Pratt and the City and Country School," in *Founding Mothers and Others: Women Educational Leaders during the Progressive Era*, ed. Susan Semel and Alan Sadovnick (New York: Palgrave, 2002), 37–60, and 77–92; Lagemann, *An Elusive Science*, 120–30; Winsor, "Introduction," 7–19. Charlotte Winsor and Barbara Biber were two of John Dewey's former students.

11. Seeley, "Winsor," 1945, 1, VWB.

12. Capeci, *Harlem Riot of 1943*, 39–42; Greenberg, *"Or Does It Explode?"* 189–90; Markowitz and Rosner, *Children, Race, and Power*, 6.

13. Dianne Ravitch, *The Great School Wars: A History of the New York City Public Schools*, rev. ed. (Baltimore, MD: Johns Hopkins University Press, 2000), 237. P.S. 24 had been one of seventy schools that adopted the citywide program.

14. Lauri Johnson, "A Generation of Women Activists: African American Female Educators in Harlem, 1930–1950," *Journal of African American History* 89 (Summer 2004): 223–40; Kenneth B. Clark, "A Conversation with James Baldwin," and Gertrude Elise Ayer, "Notes on My Native Sons," in *Harlem: A Community in Transition*, ed. John Henrik Clarke (New York: The Citadel Press, 1964), 123–30, and 137–45; Herb Boyd, *Baldwin's Harlem: A Biography of James Baldwin* (New York: Atria, 2008). James Baldwin was a P.S. 24 student during Ayers's tenure.

15. Seeley, "Winsor," 1945, 2, VWB; Winsor, "Children in Need," 58–61; Max Winsor, "Report to the Joint Advisory Committee of the Special Child Guidance Service Unit in Harlem," June 18, 1942, 19, folder 439, box 35, JWP; Advisory Committee on Treatment, Psychiatric Clinic of the Children's Court, Minutes, May 27, 1943, 3, folder 63, box 6, JWP.

16. Seeley, "Winsor," 1945, 2, VWB; Johnson, "A Generation of Women Activists," 229.

17. Winsor, "Children in Need," 60.

18. Seeley, "Winsor," 1945, 2, VWB.

19. Grob, *Mad among Us*, 237.

20. Herman, *Kinship by Design;* Herman, *Romance of American Psychology;* Jackson, *Gunnar Myrdal.*

21. Seeley, "Winsor," 3, VWB.

22. [Bernard], "Obituary for Max Winsor," 535.

23. See Seeley, "Winsor," 3, VWB.

24. Justine Wise Polier to Hon. Fiorello La Guardia, July 27, 1940, 1, 2, folder 411, box 33, JWP; Bernard, Interview by Senn, 5, VWB.

25. Greenberg, *"Or Does It Explode?"* 191–92.

26. Winsor, "Report to the Joint Advisory Committee," June 18, 1942, 1–2, JWP; Harlem Project Research Committee, *The Role of the School in Preventing and Correcting Maladjustment and Delinquency: A Study in Three Schools* (New York: New York

Foundation, 1949), 1–2, 12; Justine Wise Polier to Hon. Fiorello La Guardia, July 27, 1940, 1–2, JWP.

27. Max Winsor, "Delinquency in Wartime," *American Journal of Orthopsychiatry* 13 (July 1943): 511.

28. Dr. Viola W. Bernard, Interview by Dr. Spafford Ackerly, May 30, 1973, transcript, 9, folder "VWB's Career in Child Psychiatry," box 1, series "Oral History Transcripts," VWB; Winsor, "Report to the Joint Advisory Committee," June 18, 1942, 1–3, JWP; Harlem Project, *Role of the School*, 1–2; Bernard, Interview by Senn, 5, VWB.

29. Since the Progressive Era, psychiatrists and mental hygienists had articulated "a new role for [psychological] experts—that of identifying, recording, assessing risk factors in order to predict future pathology and take action to prevent it." In Rose, *Inventing Our Selves*, 94. See also Robert Castel, "From Dangerousness to Risk," in Burchell, Gordon, and Miller, *Foucault Effect*, 284–87.

30. Herman, *Kinship by Design*, 11.

31. Ibid., 13.

32. Ian Hacking, *Historical Ontology* (Cambridge, MA: Harvard University Press, 2004), 4, 20–23, 26.

33. Between the 1930s and the 1970s, mental health experts exerted more and more influence over public policy, helping to craft responses to a wide range of social problems. See Herman, *Romance of American Psychology;* Raz, *What's Wrong with the Poor*, Castel, "From Dangerousness to Risk," 294–96.

34. According to Kathleen Jones, the child-guidance movement encompassed treatment, prevention, and the handling of juvenile delinquency and "'everyday' misbehavior." *Taming the Troublesome Child*, 208.

35. Muhammad, *Condemnation of Blackness*.

36. Frank O'Brien to Dr. Marion Kenworthy, March 20, 1940, folder 411, box 33, JWP.

37. Harold G. Campbell to the Board of Education [New York City], September 18, 1940, 3, folder 411, box 33, JWP.

38. Polier, *Juvenile Justice*, 7, 22–24, 28, 40; Jones, *Taming the Troublesome Child*, 208, 224–25; Gilbert, *A Cycle of Outrage*, 14, 28; Dominic J. Capeci, Jr., "Fiorello H. La Guardia and the Harlem 'Crime Wave' of 1941," *The New York Historical Society Quarterly* 64 (January 1980): 7–29; Capeci, *Harlem Riot of 1943*, 9–10.

39. Dr. V. Bernard, Interview by Dr. M. Kilpatrick, November 2, 1991, interview no. 3, transcript, 9–10, folder "Oral History (VWB Life Story)," box 2, series "Oral History Transcripts," VWB.

40. Polier to Hon. James Marshall, August 6, 1940, 1, folder 411, box 33, JWP.

41. Polier to La Guardia, July 27, 1940, 2, JWP.

42. Polier, *Everyone's Children*, 179 (see also 167–68).

43. Polier to La Guardia, July 27, 1940, 2, JWP.

44. Polier, *Everyone's Children*, 73.

45. Peter D. Norton, *Fighting Traffic: The Dawn of the Motor Age in the American City* (Cambridge, MA: MIT Press, 2008), 116–17; Morton J. Horwitz, *The Transformation of American Law, 1870–1960: The Crisis of Orthodoxy* (New York: Oxford University Press, 1992), 27–30.

46. Polier, *Everyone's Children*, 73.

47. Polier to La Guardia, July 27, 1940, 1, JWP. See also Frank O'Brien to Dr. Marion Kenworthy, March 20, 1940, 1, JWP.

48. Markowitz and Rosner, *Children, Race, and Power*, 38–39.

49. Herman, *Kinship by Design*, 86; Jones, *Taming the Troublesome Child*, 180.

50. Agnes Murtha to Justine Wise Polier, September 3, 1940, folder 411, box 33, JWP.

51. Dr. Max Winsor to Justine Wise Polier, August 7, 1940, folder 411, box 33, JWP.

52. Polier considered Fiorello a personal friend, even ending her letters to him with the overly familiar "Love, Justine." Polier to La Guardia, July 27, 1940, JWP.

53. Polier to La Guardia, July 27, 1940; Fiorello La Guardia to Mrs. Justine Wise Polier, August 7, 1940, folder 411, box 33, JWP; James Marshall to Fiorello La Guardia, August 27, 1940, folder 411, box 33, JWP; Justine Wise Polier to Hon. James Marshall, August 6, 1940, folder 411, box 33, JWP; Campbell to the Board of Education, September 18, 1940, 1, JWP. See also Fiorello La Guardia to Mrs. Justine Wise Polier, August 7, 1940, folder 411, box 33, JWP; James Marshall to Fiorello La Guardia, August 27, 1940, folder 411, box 33, JWP; Maurice G. Postley to Hon. Justine Wise Polier, October 10, 1940, folder 411, box 33, JWP.

54. Garrett, *La Guardia Years*, 200, 204.

55. Dominic J. Capeci, Jr., "From Different Liberal Perspectives: Fiorello H. La Guardia, Adam Clayton Powell, Jr., and Civil Rights in New York City, 1941–1943," *Journal of Negro History* 62 (April 1977): 160–73; Ravitch, *Great School Wars*, 236–37.

56. Justine Wise Polier to Hon. James Marshall, August 26, 1940, 2, folder 411, box 33, JWP. The choice to promote Winsor's proposal primarily as an antidelinquency policy targeting Harlem makes sense, given that her fellow Domestic Relations Court justice Stephen S. Jackson had already convinced La Guardia to back another antidelinquency project proposed for West Harlem in May. Capeci, *Harlem Riot of 1943*, 9.

57. As the historian Ellen Herman argues: "Therapeutic governments transcended divisions of right and left, representing a commitment to statist solutions that coexisted with conflicts over the appropriate size of government" (*Kinship by Design*, 11).

58. Campbell to the Board of Education, September 18, 1940, 1, JWP.

59. Jones, *Taming the Troublesome Child*, 180.

60. Campbell to the Board of Education, September 18, 1940, 2–3, JWP; Winsor, "Report to the Joint Advisory," June 18, 1942, 2–3, JWP; Harlem Project, *Role of the School*, 12–13.

61. Foundation to Further Child Education, untitled report in incorporation, May 15, 1941, 4, folder 411, box 33, JWP; Winsor, "Report to the Joint Advisory Committee," June 18, 1942, 2–3, JWP; Harlem Project, *Role of the School*, 12–13.

62. Winsor, "Report to the Joint Advisory," June 18, 1942, 3, JWP. Regarding delinquency, 371 male students from P.S. 184 (15.5 percent of that school's 2,400 students) and 347 male students from P.S. 139 (17.8 percent of that school's 1,950 students) were known to at least one of four child agencies as "having manifested some definitive overt misbehavior or maladjustment" (12).

63. Ibid., 3.

64. Ibid., 3, 8, 9, 10, 11, 14, 15; Harlem Project Research Committee, Harlem Project Interim Report, 18, folder 437, box 35, JWP.

65. Winsor, "Report to the Joint Advisory Committee," June 18, 1942, 3–8.

66. Ibid.

67. Ibid., 5.

68. Winsor, "Children in Need," 59. Winsor also notes this same case on page 16 of "Report to the Joint Advisory Committee, June 18, 1942, JWP.

69. Winsor, "Children in Need," 59.

70. Winsor, "Delinquency in Wartime," 511.

71. Winsor, "Children in Need," 61.

72. Winsor, "Delinquency in Wartime," 511.

73. Seeley, "Winsor," 2, VWB.

74. Ibid.; Winsor, "Delinquency in Wartime," 511–13; Winsor, "Children in Need," 59–61.

75. Winsor, "Report to the Joint Advisory Committee," June 18, 1942, 15, JWP.

76. Horn, *Before It's Too Late*, 126 (see also 119–20, 127, 130); and Regina Markell Morantz-Sanchez, *Sympathy and Science: Women Physicians in American Medicine* (New York: Oxford University Press, 1985), 238, 239.

77. Viola W. Bernard, Interview by Dr. W. M. Kirkpatrick, May 13, 1990, transcript, interview no. 2, 11, folder "Oral History, VWB Life Story," box 2, series "Oral History Transcripts," VWB.

78. Ibid., 25. She spent her first residency with Dr. Thomas Brennan at the Grasslands Hospital in Westchester, New York.

79. Bernard, Interview by Senn, 4, VWB; Bernard, Kilpatrick interview no. 2, 25–26, 29–32, VWB; Bernard, Kirkpatrick interview no. 3, 3, 17, VWB.

80. Bernard, Interview by Senn, 4–5, VWB.

81. Bernard, Interview by Ackerly, 1–3, 6, 13, VWB; Bernard, Interview by Senn, 1, VWB; Bernard, Kirkpatrick interview no. 2, 19, VWB; Bernard, Kirkpatrick interview no. 3, 2–3, VWB; Viola W. Bernard, "Some Applications of Psychoanalysis to Social Issues," *Psychoanalytic Review* 85 (February 1998): 139–70.

82. Bernstein, *Lost Children of Wilder*, 50–53; Herman, *Kinship by Design*, 103, 205–9.

83. Polier and Bernard lived in the same building on 4th street in 1940 when Polier and Winsor were planning the Special Harlem Unit. Viola W. Bernard, Interview by Prof. David Rosner and Prof. Gerry Markowitz, July 10, 1992, 1–2, folder "Justine Wise Polier, Biographical Material," box 2, series "People—Justine Wise Polier," VWB. In a letter dated September 18, 1940, Max Winsor informed Justine Wise Polier that "Dr. Bernard is now part of the staff." Max Winsor to Justine Wise Polier, September 18 1940, 2, folder 411, box 33, JWP.

84. Bernard, Interview by Senn, 3, VWB.

85. Bernard, Kirkpatrick interview no. 2, 17–18, VWB; Bernard, "Some Applications of Psychoanalysis to Social Issues," 143; Bernard, Interview by Senn, 2, 3, VWB.

86. Viola W. Bernard, "Detection and Management of Emotional Disorders in Children," *Mental Hygiene* 26 (July 1942): 368–82.

87. Viola W. Bernard, "Normal Psychosexual Development of a Child," February 3, 1944, 3, folder "Talks and Courses/Spence Chapin Adoption Nursery, 'Normal Psychosexual Development of a Child,'" box 1, series "Talks and Courses," VWB.

88. Viola W. Bernard to Charlotte Biber Winsor, March 18, 1970, folder "Charlotte Biber Winsor—Obituary (1899–1982)," box 5, series "Professional Correspondence—Individuals, Alphabetical," VWB.

89. Bernard, Interview by Senn, 5, VWB.

90. Bernard, Kirkpatrick interview no. 2, 30, VWB.

91. [Bernard], "Obituary for Max Winsor," 535.

92. Bernard, "Some Applications of Psychoanalysis to Social Issues," 151–52.

93. Bernard, "Detection and Management of Emotional Disorders in Children," 370 (see also 371–76).

94. Bernard, Kirkpatrick interview no. 3, 11–12, VWB; Bernard, Interview by Ackerly, 10–11, VWB.

95. Viola Bernard, speech written for Conference "October 8, 1942, P.S. 194 Joint Kindergarten Project," folder "Talks and Courses/P.S. 194 Joint Kindergarten Project-Conference Utility of Project Records, 1942," box 1, series "Talks and Courses," VWB. See also Bernard, Kilpatrick interview no. 3, 11–12, VWB; Bernard, Interview by Ackerly, 10–11, VWB.

96. Bernard, speech written for Conference "October 8, 1942, P.S. 194 Joint Kindergarten Project," VWB.

97. Bernard later recalled in a talk on May 4, 1983: "The clinical setting [in Harlem] gave me an invaluable opportunity to relate to black children and their families and to gain some understanding of the psychosocial contexts of their lives, not only through interviews at the clinic or school, but also by making home visits." Bernard, "Some Applications of Psychiatry and Psychoanalysis to Social Issues," 143.

98. Robison, *Juvenile Delinquency*, 47–54.

99. Bernard, speech written for Conference "October 8, 1942, P.S. 194 Joint Kindergarten Project," VWB.

100. Bernard, Interview by Senn, 9–10, VWB.

101. Viola W. Bernard, "Conference Notes," Conference on Utility of P.S. 194 Joint Kindergarten Project Records, October 8, 1942, typescript, folder "Talks and Courses/P.S. 194 Joint Kindergarten Project-Conference Utility of Project Records, 1942," box 1, series "Talks and Courses," VWB. See also Bernard, Interview by Senn, 9–10, VWB; Kirkpatrick interview no. 3, 11–12, VWB.

102. Reiss, *Theaters of Madness*, 10–11.

103. Bernard, "Conference Notes," 1, 2, VWB.

104. Ibid., 1, 2.

105. Bernard, "Detection and Management of Emotional Disorders in Children," 380–81; Polier, "How I Became Interested in Racial Justice," 63.

106. Rose, *Psychology and Selfhood*; Lawrence W. Levine, *Black Culture and Black Consciousness: Afro-American Folk Thought from Slavery to Freedom* (New York: Oxford University Press, 1977).

107. Mintz, *Huck's Raft*, 351–52; Lisa Levenstein, *A Movement without Marchers: African American Women and the Politics of Poverty in Postwar Philadelphia* (Chapel Hill: University of North Carolina Press, 2008), 144–47; Wilma King, *African American Childhoods: Historical Perspectives from Slavery to Civil Rights* (New York: Palgrave MacMillan, 2005).

108. Al-Tony Gilmore, *Bad Nigger! The National Impact of Jack Johnson* (Port Washington, NY: Kennikat Press, 1975), 12; Robin D. G. Kelley, *Race Rebels: Culture, Politics, and the Black Working Class* (New York: The Free Press, 1994); Cecil Brown, *Stagolee Shot Billy* (Cambridge, MA: Harvard University Press, 2004), 14–15.

109. Yvonne P. Chireau, *Black Magic: Religion and the African American Conjuring Tradition* (Berkeley: University of California Press, 2006); Jeffrey E. Anderson, *Conjure in African American Society* (Baton Rouge: University of Louisiana Press, 2005).

110. Brown, *Manchild in the Promised Land*, 39, 41.

111. Ibid., 40.

112. Viola W. Bernard to Mrs. M. [Margaret] Ives, December 8, 1944, folder "Community Service Society, Consultancies, 1943–48," box 1, series "Community Service Society," VWB.

113. Ibid.

114. Viola W. Bernard to Dr. Virginia Moore, September 4, 1942, folder 468, box 38, JWP.

115. Bernard, Interview by Senn, 10–11, VWB.

116. Justine Wise Polier, unpublished manuscript, "The Anatomy of Three Institutions; History of Wiltwyck School," February 1979, 2, 3, 4, folder 467, box 38, JWP; Wiltwyck School for Boys Inc., Minutes of the Intake Policy Committee Meeting, November 4, 1942, folder 468, box 38, JWP; Wiltwyck School for Boys, Minutes of First Meeting of Board of Directors, June 11, 1942, folder "Minutes, Board of Directors, 1942," box 1, series "Wiltwyck School for Boys, Inc.," VWB; Paul Blanshard and Edwin J. Lukas, *Probation and Psychiatric Care for Adolescent Offenders* (New York: Society for the Prevention of Crime, 1942).

117. Polier, "Anatomy of Three Institutions," 6–7, JWP; Wiltwyck School for Boys Inc., Minutes of the Intake Policy Committee Meeting, November 4, 1942, JWP; Justine Wise Polier to Hon. J. Milton Patterson, April 21, 1944, folder 470, box 38, JWP.

118. Polier, "Anatomy of Three Institutions," 1, JWP.

119. Bernard to Moore, September 4, 1942, JWP.

Chapter Four

1. Max Winsor to Viola Bernard, November 30, 1941, folder "Bureau of Child Guidance, 1941, 1948, 1953," box 1, series "Board of Education," VWB.

2. The liaison teacher experiment placed six special teachers in six problem schools in Harlem, the Bronx, and Brooklyn. Winsor, "Report to the Joint Advisory Committee," June 18, 1942, 3, JWP.

3. Winsor, "Report to the Joint Advisory Committee," June 18, 1942, 3–6, JWP; Harlem Project, *Role of the School*, 12–13. See Polier, *Everybody's Children*, 158–81.

4. Biondi, *To Stand and to Fight*, 6, 33, 37, 38; Penny Von Eschen first employed the phrase "black popular front" in *Race against Empire: Black Americans and Anticolonialism, 1937–1957* (Ithaca, NY: Cornell University Press, 1997), 19. See also Sugrue, *Sweet Land of Liberty*, 30–31; Singh, *Black Is a Country*, 102–19.

5. Self, *American Babylon*, 13.

6. Gregory, *Southern Diaspora*, 247. See also Self, *American Babylon*, 330; Biondi, *To Stand and to Fight*, 15–16; Greenberg, *Troubling the Waters*, 8–13, 123–24; Seth Forman, *Blacks in the Jewish Mind: A Crisis of Liberalism* (New York: New York University Press, 1998), 100–109.

7. Nat Brandt, *Harlem at War: The Black Experience in WW II* (New York: Syracuse University Press, 1996), 165–67; Kelley, *Thelonious Monk*, 65, 85; Scott DeVeaux, *The Birth of Bebop: A Social and Musical History* (Berkeley: University of California Press, 1997), 287. The police imposed this unexpected dragnet of Harlem's small-time criminals in November after an apartment in La Guardia's East Harlem building had been robbed. On the Second Great Black Migration, see Gregory, *Southern Diaspora*, 5, 16–23, 32–38.

8. Muhammad, *Condemnation of Blackness*, 12, 231–32.

9. CWCCH, "The Story of the City-Wide Citizens' Committee on Harlem," May 23, 1943, 3, 4–6, folder "City-Wide Committee on Harlem, 1942–1945," box 1, series "Racism," VWB; CWCCH, "Tentative Report of the Sub-Committee on Crime and Delinquency," June 1942, 1–2, folder "City-Wide Citizens' Committee on Harlem, 1942–1945," box 1, series "Racism," VWB. See Brandt, *Harlem at War*, 165–66.

10. According to Biondi, "in New York, movement leaders called for broad social change, economic empowerment, group advancement, and colonial freedom from the beginning" (*To Stand and to Fight*, 272).

11. CWCCH, "Story of the City-Wide Citizens' Committee on Harlem," May 23, 1943, 3, VWB.

12. Ibid., 5.

13. Freda Kirchwey, "Editorial," *The Nation*, June 6, 1942, 644–46. According to Kirchwey, the CWCCH addressed a crisis of national significance with immediate relevance to concerned citizens in other metropolitan areas. Walter White, the NAACP's executive director since 1931, served as the CWCCH's cochair. Walter White, *A Man Called White: The Autobiography of Walter White* (1948; repr., Athens: University of Georgia Press, 1995), 240. See also Self, *American Babylon*, 13, 17–18, 330–33, on the relationship between national and local black freedom struggles in the urban North during World War II.

14. Sugrue, *Sweet Land of Liberty*, 71–77, 170–81.

15. CWCCH, "Story of the City-Wide Citizens' Committee on Harlem," 7, VWB.

16. Biondi, *To Stand and to Fight*, 16; Self, *American Babylon*, 106–7; Gregory, *Southern Diaspora*, 261–62. According to Martha Biondi, "the Black Popular Front aimed to change mainstream institutions and practices in order to increase opportunities for Blacks" (16).

17. Polier, "How I Became Interested in Racial Justice," 68; [Bernard], "Obituary for Max Winsor," 535; Polier, *Everybody's Children*.

18. Jacqueline A. McLeod, *Daughter of the Empire State: The Life of Judge Jane Bolin* (Urbana: University of Illinois Press, 2011), 71.

19. Gregory, *Southern Diaspora*, 261–62.

20. Markowitz and Rosner, "Race, Foster Care," 1845–46.

21. Biondi, *To Stand and to Fight*, 18.

22. Paul Blanshard to Viola Bernard, January 15, 1942, folder "City-Wide Citizens' Committee on Harlem, Subcommittee on Crime and Delinquency," box 1, series "Racism," VWB.

23. Seeley, "Winsor," 2, VWB; Antler, "Justine Wise Polier and the Prophetic Tradition," 285–86; White, *A Man Called White*, 330–33.

24. CWCCH, "Story of the City-Wide Citizens' Committee on Harlem," 3, VWB.

25. Winsor, "Delinquency in Wartime," 510–11; Justine Wise Polier, "Wartime Needs of Children and Federal Responsibility," *Federal Probation* 8 (April–June 1944): 9–12. See also Gilbert, *A Cycle of Outrage*, 25–29; Brandt, *Harlem at War*, 166–68.

26. CWCCH, "Tentative Report of the Sub-Committee on Crime and Delinquency," June 1942, 1, VWB.

27. Ibid., 7.

28. CWCCH, Report of Subcommittee, "Psychiatric Recommendations as Related to Negro Children," March 26, 1942, 1–2, folder "City-Wide Citizens' Committee on Harlem, Subcommittee on Crime and Delinquency, 1942–1945," box 1, series "Racism," VWB.

29. Ibid., 1.

30. Gilbert, *A Cycle of Outrage*, 26–27.

31. Ibid., 33–40.

32. Polier, *Juvenile Justice*, 40 (see also 28); Bayor, *Fiorello La Guardia*, 158–65; Williams, *City of Ambition*, 319.

33. "Mayor Is Critical of Psychiatrists," *NYT*, April 16, 1943, 23.

34. Ibid., 32–33, 40.

35. Williams, *City of Ambition*, 263–64, 325.

36. Polier, *Juvenile Justice*, 111.

37. Ibid., 112.

38. W. Bruce Cobb to the Justices, Domestic Relations Court, City of New York, June 22, 1943, folder 49, box 5, JWP; Robert Lansdale to Hon. Justine Wise Polier, November 22, 1943, folder 49, box 5, JWP.

39. Doris I. Byrne, Press Release, March 7, 1945, 3, folder 64, box 6, JWP.

40. Viola W. Bernard, MD, to Mr. Walter White, NAACP, April 15, 1942, folder "City-Wide Citizens' Committee on Harlem, Subcommittee on Crime and Delinquency, 1942–1945," box 1, series "Racism," VWB.

41. CWCCH, "Psychiatric Recommendations as Related to Negro Children," VWB.

42. For Winsor and his fellow racial liberals in the Harlem Special Child Guidance Service Unit, the adult black patient had been little more than an abstraction that they thought themselves "capable of apprehending independently of the *concrete existence*" of actual adult black patients. Daniel Bertrand Monk, "Hives and Swarms: On the 'Nature' of Neoliberalism and the Rise of the Ecological Insurgent," in *Evil Paradises: Dreamworlds of Neoliberalism*, ed. Mike Davis and Daniel Bertrand Monk (New York: Free Press, 2007), 271.

43. Lears, *Something for Nothing*, 230–31, 238, 356.

44. According to Sugrue, wartime "black activists found common ground, particularly in their emphasis on black economic opportunity" (Sugrue, *Sweet Land of Liberty*, 30). See also Ronald Takaki, *Double Victory: A Multicultural History of America in World War II* (Boston, MA: Little, Brown, 2000), 38–50; Biondi, *To Stand and to Fight*, 4; Hall, "Long Civil Rights Movement," 1246–48; Feldstein, *Motherhood in Black and White*, 165.

45. Biondi, *To Stand and to Fight*, 16, 17, 18, 21, 22, 32, 66, 218–19, 277–78.

46. Feldstein, *Motherhood in Black and White*, 37, 38, 39.

47. CWCCH, "Psychiatric Recommendations as Related to Negro Children," 1–2, VWB.

48. Ibid., 1, VWB.

49. Ibid., 1–2; CWCCH, "Tentative Report of the Sub-Committee on Crime and Delinquency," June 1942, 5–7, VWB; CWCCH, "Story of the City-Wide Citizens' Committee on Harlem," 8–9, 12, 20–21, VWB; CWCCH, "Findings and Recommendations, Closed Meeting of the City-Wide Citizens' Committee on Harlem," May 29, 1944, 3–4, folder "City-Wide Citizens' Committee on Harlem, Subcommittee on Crime and Delinquency, 1942–1945," 3–4, box 1, series "Racism," VWB.

50. Arnold Beichman, "Mayor's 'Economy' Budget Decried Again in Harlem," *PM*, April 28, 1942, mimeographed newspaper clipping, folder "Racism, City-Wide Citizens' Committee on Harlem, 1942–1945," box 1, series "Racism," VWB.

51. Polier, *Juvenile Justice*, 111.

52. CWCCH, "Psychiatric Recommendations as Related to Negro Children," 2, VWB.

53. CWCCH, "Tentative Report of the Sub-Committee on Crime and Delinquency," June 1942, 6, 7, VWB; CWCCH, "Story of the City-Wide Citizens' Committee on Harlem," 8, VWB.

54. Austin H. MacCormick to Shelby Harrison [name crossed out], June 14, 1943, 2, folder 63, box 6, JWP.

55. Polier, *Juvenile Justice*, 7, 22–24, 28, 40; Brandt, *Harlem at War*, 183–215; Capeci, *Harlem Riot of 1943*, 144–45, 158, 175, 176; Williams, *City of Ambition*, 352–53; White, *A Man Called White*, 233–41; Sugrue, *Sweet Land of Liberty*, 69–70; Gill, *Harlem*, 329–34; Kelley, *Thelonious Monk*, 85–86; Gilmore, *Defying Dixie*, 374.

56. Abu-Lughod, *Race, Space, and Riots*, 149–51, 273; Williams, *City of Ambition*, 319; Capeci, *Harlem Riot of 1943*, 115–33.

57. Advisory Committee of the Treatment Clinic, Minutes, April 5, 1944, 3, folder 63, box 6, JWP; Herbert B. Wilcox, MD, to Honorable John Warren Hill, April 1, 1942, folder 63, box 6, JWP; George B. Stevenson, MD, to Dr. Helen Montague, May 26, 1943, folder 63, box 6, JWP; John Warren Hill to Dr. Helen Montague, May 26, 1943, folder 63, box 6, JWP; W. Bruce Cobb to Dr. Helen Montague, May 26, 1943, folder 63, box 6, JWP; Advisory Committee on Treatment, Psychiatric Clinic of the Children's Court, Minutes, November 11, 1943, folder 63, box 6, JWP.

58. Advisory Committee of the Treatment Clinic, Minutes, December 7, 1944, 2, folder 64, box 6, JWP. Since 1943, Justice W. Bruce Cobb, the new presiding justice of the Children's Court, worried that if he asked La Guardia to provide additional funding for the treatment clinic, the mayor might vengefully retaliate and close down the diagnostic clinic.

59. Advisory Committee of the Treatment Clinic, Minutes, December 7, 1944, 3, JWP.

60. W. Bruce Cobb to Hon. Fiorello H. La Guardia, June 1, 1945, folder 64, box 6, JWP; Austin H. MacCormick to Hon. Bruce W. Cobb, April 23, 1945, folder 64, box 6, JWP.

61. Winsor, "Report to the Joint Advisory Committee," June 18, 1942, 11, 13, JWP; Max Winsor to Marshall Field, November 1, 1941, folder 258, box 22, JWP.

62. CWCCH, "Psychiatric Recommendations as Related to Negro Children," 1–2, VWB; CWCCH, "Tentative Report of the Sub-Committee on Crime and Delinquency," June 1942, 7. VWB.

63. Harlem Project, *Role of the School*, 2–5.

64. Lears, *Something for Nothing*, 226–39.

65. Harlem Project, *Role of the School*, ix, 2–5.

66. Ravitch, *Great School Wars*, 236, 238.

67. Kessner, *Fiorello H. La Guardia*, 476.

68. Frank J. O'Brien, MD, "Report of the Meeting Arranged by Superintendent Wade to Consider the Proposal of the New York Foundation," February 24, 1943, 1–2, folder 438, box 35, JWP; Harlem Project, *Role of the School*, ix.

69. CWCCH, "Findings and Recommendations, Closed Meeting of the City-Wide Citizens' Committee on Harlem," May 29, 1944, 3, VWB.

70. Harlem Project, *Role of the School*, ix, x, 35–41.

71. Ibid., ix.

72. Ibid., 3–4.

73. Ibid., 138 (see also 66 and 108–9).

74. Ibid., 35–39, 61, 70–71, 102, 115, 137, 145.

75. Ibid., 39.

76. Ibid., 136.

77. Ibid., 43, 54, 62, 88–90, 94, 98, 107, 137, 142, 145–46.

78. Polier, *Everyone's Children*, 179; Board of Education of the City of New York, "Extended School Services through the All-Day Neighborhood Schools," *Curriculum Bulletin*, 1947–48, no. 2, folder "Bureau of Reference, Research, and Statistics (Relevant 1947–1948)," box 4, series "New York City Board of Education," VWB.

79. Harlem Project, *Role of the School*, 42–54, 137.

80. Ibid., 42–49, 53–55, 110–11, 116; Gill, *Harlem*, 286; Ann Petry, *The Street* (1946; repr., Boston, MA: Beacon Press, 1985). All-day school programs were also known as the all-day neighborhood schools or community schools.

81. Rudolph M. Wittenberg, "Rethinking the Clinic Function in a Public School Setting," *American Journal of Orthopsychiatry* 14 (October 1944): 725; Harlem Project, *Role of the School*, 20, 24, 29, 106–8, 115, 147–54; CWCCH, "Findings and Recommendations," May 29, 1944, 3, VWB; Gill, *Harlem*, 286.

82. Harlem Project, *Role of the School*, 6, 109.

83. Ibid., 111.

84. Bernard, Interview by Ackerly, 14, VWB; Bernard, Kirkpatrick interview no. 3, 14, VWB.

85. Dr. Viola Bernard, Untitled list of statistics regarding Negro psychiatrists up until 1942, [n.d.], mimeograph, folder "City-Wide Citizens' Committee on Harlem, Subcommittee on Crime and Delinquency, 1942–1945," box 1, series "Racism," VWB. See also Vanessa Northington Gamble, *Making a Place for Ourselves: The Black Hospital Movement, 1920–1945* (New York: Oxford University Press, 1995); Bailey, *Harlem Hospital Story*.

86. Vanessa Northington Gamble, *The Black Community Hospital: Contemporary Dilemmas in Historical Perspective* (New York: Garland, 1989), 24–26; 39–43; Gamble, *Making a Place for Ourselves*, xv–xviii, 143, 153, 181, 196.

87. CWCCH, "Psychiatric Recommendations as Related to Negro Children," 2, VWB; Advisory Committee on Treatment, Psychiatric Clinic of the Children's Court, Minutes, December 9, 1943, 1, folder 63, box 6, JWP. One meeting of Judge Polier's Advisory Committee for the Children's Court treatment clinic addressed the "fact that the Psychiatric Institute does not accept Negroes for treatment."

88. Bernard, "Some Applications of Psychiatry and Psychoanalysis to Social Issues," 151–52; Bernard, Kirkpatrick interview no. 2, May 13, 1990, 25–26, folder "Oral History," VWB; Mendes, *Under the Strain of Color*, 96–98.

89. [Viola Bernard], recommendation for Dr. Charles Brown to the Institute of International Relations, February 27, 1947, folder "Support for Training (including Funding), 1944–1954, (Some Gaps), 1969, 1976, 1983, 1993–1994," box 4, series "Racism," VWB.

90. Viola W. Bernard, "Mental Hygiene and the Negro Community," [1947 or 1948], 4–5, folder "Mental Hygiene and the Negro Community (1947–1948)," box 1, series "VWB Publications," VWB.

91. Ibid., 5.

92. Ibid.

93. Bernard, Kirkpatrick interview no. 2; [Bernard], recommendation for Dr. Charles Brown to the Institute of International Relations, February 27, 1947, VWB.

94. Morantz-Sanchez, *Sympathy and Science*, 317, 330–39; Regina Morantz-Sanchez, "Physicians," In *Women, Health, and Medicine in America: A Handbook*, ed. Rima Apple (New York: Garland, 1990), 477–95.

95. Viola W. Bernard, "Notes on Criticisms and Suggestions for the Report on Negro Psychiatry," June 11, 1947, folder "National Urban League, 1946–1948," box 3, series "Racism," VWB; [Viola W. Bernard], "Negro Psychiatrists in Training," July 1947, folder "Racism—City-Wide Citizens' Committee on Harlem, Subcommittee on Crime and Delinquency, 1942–1945," box 1, series "Racism," VWB.

96. Viola W. Bernard, "Chronology of Professional Background Activities That Bear on Interracial Issues," [ca. 1970], folder "VWB Chronology of Professional Background Activities That Bear on Interracial Issues, 1940–1970," box 1, series "Racism," VWB; Bernard, "Some Applications of Psychiatry and Psychoanalysis to Social Issues,"152.

97. Mrs. Lloyd H. Ziegler to Dr. Charles Wilkinson, December 17, 1946, folder "Support for Training (include Funding), 1944–1954, (Some Gaps), 1969, 1976, 1983, 1993–1994," box 4, series "Racism," VWB. Wilkinson did become a psychiatrist and even served as president of the Group for the Advancement of Psychiatry.

98. Clarence E. Pickett to Viola W. Bernard, December 24, 1946, folder "Correspondences, Articles," box 1, series "Margaret Morgan Lawrence, MD," VWB. See also Lawrence, *Balm in Gilead*.

99. Viola W. Bernard, MD, to Lt. Garnett [*sic*] Ice, AMC, June 28, 1944; Garnet T. Ice, 1st Lt. M.C. to Dr. Viola W. Bernard, October 21, 1944; Viola W. Bernard to Capt. Garnett [*sic*] Ice, M.C., April 10, 1946; Garnet T. Ice, Captain, MC to Viola W. Bernard, MD, April 12, 1946; [Viola W. Bernard] to Capt. Garnett [*sic*] Ice, April 29, 1946, folder "Support for Training (including Funding), 1944–1954, (Some Gaps), 1969, 1976, 1983, 1993–1994," box 4, series "Racism," VWB.

100. Garnet T. Ice to Dr. Viola Bernard, February 15, 1947, VWB. See also her return correspondence to this letter, [Viola W. Bernard] to Garnet Ice, February 20, 1947, VWB.

101. [Viola W. Bernard], "Negro Psychiatrists, New York City," November 1949, folder "Support for Training (including Funding), 1944–1954, (Some Gaps), 1969, 1976, 1983, 1993–1994," box 4, series "Racism," VWB.

102. Bernard, "Some Applications of Psychiatry and Psychoanalysis to Social Issues," 153.

103. Bernard, "Notes on Criticisms and Suggestions for the Report on Negro Psychiatry," June 11, 1947, VWB. These three clinical sites were the Menninger Clinic in Kansas, a clinic in Boston, and Dr. Howard Potter's ward at the Long Island College of Medicine.

104. Bernard, "Chronology of Professional Background," [ca. 1970], VWB.

105. Bernard, "Some Applications of Psychiatry and Psychoanalysis to Social Issues,"153; Garnet T. Ice, 1st Lt. M.C. to Dr. Viola W. Bernard, October 21, 1944; Viola W. Bernard, MD, to Lt. G. T. Ice, A.M.C., November 10, 1944, folder "Support for Training (including Funding), 1944–1954, (Some Gaps), 1969, 1976, 1983, 1993–1994," box 4, series "Racism," VWB.

106. [Bernard], recommendation for Dr. Charles Brown to the Institute of International Relations, February 27, 1947; Viola W. Bernard, MD, to Dr. Charles Brown, February 13, 1947; Viola W. Bernard to Dr. Charles Brown, February 17, 1947; folder "Support for Training (including Funding), 1944–1954, (Some Gaps), 1969, 1976, 1983, 1993–1994," box 4, series "Racism," VWB.

107. Bernard, "Some Applications of Psychiatry and Psychoanalysis to Social Issues," 153.

108. Franklin C. McLean, MD, to Dr. Viola Bernard, December 11, 1951; Viola W. Bernard, MD, to Dr. Franklin C. McLean, December 20, 1951; Franklin C. McLean to Dr. June A. Jackson, January 3, 1952; Viola W. Bernard, MD, to Dr. June A. Jackson, February 4, 1952; June A. Jackson to Dr. Viola W. Bernard, March 22, 1952; [Bernard], "Negro Psychiatrists, New York City," VWB. In a 1985 interview, Dr. June Jackson Christmas recalled that Bernard had offered her psychoanalytic training at Columbia. Although she appreciated the offer, Christmas located psychoanalytic training for herself elsewhere in New York City.

109. Rutherford B. Stevens, "Racial Aspects of Emotional Problems of Negro Soldiers," *American Journal of Psychiatry* 103 (1947): 493–98.

110. Viola W. Bernard to Dr. Sandor Rado, March 14, 1949, folder "Support for Training (including Funding), 1944–1954, (Some Gaps), 1969, 1976, 1983, 1993–1994," box 4, series "Racism," VWB.

111. Grob, *The Mad among Us*, 198–201. The Group for the Advancement of Psychiatry was a national organization that William Menninger had organized in 1946. Bernard, Interview by Senn, 28, VWB.

112. Bernard to Dr. Sandor Rado, VWB.

113. Viola W. Bernard to Dr. Margaret Lawrence, January 23, 1947, folder "Correspondences, Articles," box 1, series "Margaret Morgan Lawrence, MD," VWB. Lawrence had asked Bernard to check on the status of her application at the New York State Psychiatric Institute. The letter reveals that a month before the journalist Albert Deutsch released his exposé, Bernard speculated that racism might have been responsible for the rejection of Lawrence's application. In a February 10, 1947, interview in the liberal newspaper *PM*, Lewis openly admitted to the journalist and CWCCH ally Albert Deutsch that the publicly funded Psychiatric Institute did exclude blacks as a matter of policy. According to an annotated news clipping found in Viola W. Bernard's papers, Dr. Bernard apparently used the "article by Al Deutsch to get Lewis to accept Margaret Lawrence as first black resident at P.I." Viola

W. Bernard to Dr. Margaret M. Lawrence, February 17, 1949; Viola W. Bernard to Dr. Nolan C. Lewis, February 21, 1947; Viola W. Bernard to Dr. Margaret M. Lawrence, May 8, 1947, Viola W. Bernard, MD, to Dr. Nathaniel Ross, January 6, 1948; folder "Correspondences, Articles," box 1, series "Margaret Morgan Lawrence, MD," VWB; Albert Deutsch, "State Psychiatric Institute Here Bars Negro Patients and Doctors," *PM*, February 10, 1947, 24 [annotated news clipping], folder "The Physician's Forum, VWB Discussion, 'Discrimination in Medicine,' 1946–47," box 2, series "Talks and Courses," VWB.

114. Bernard to Dr. Nathaniel Ross, January 6, 1948, VWB.

115. Ibid. Bernard prevailed on Dr. Nathaniel Ross, who had previously expressed an interest in providing "analytic training for a qualified Negro," to accept Dr. Lawrence for training.

116. [Viola W. Bernard] to Mr. Wolf Schwabacher, March 29, 1945, folder "Racism—City-Wide Citizens' Committee on Harlem, 1942–1945," box 1, series "Racism," VWB.

117. Anthony S. Chen, "'The Hitlerian Rule of Quotas': Conservatism and the Politics of Fair Employment Legislation in New York State, 1941–1945," *Journal of American History* 92 (March 2006): 1242; Cornelius L. Bynum, *A. Philip Randolph and the Struggle for Civil Rights* (Urbana: University of Illinois Press, 2010), 163–86; Gilmore, *Defying Dixie*, 358–64; Hall, "Long Civil Rights Movement," 1244–48; Singh, *Black Is a Country*, 98–100; White, *A Man Called White*, 186–94; Sklaroff, *Black Culture and the New Deal*, 151–52; Kelley, *Thelonious Monk*, 83; Brinkley, *End of Reform*, 167; Takaki, *Double Victory*, 40–42.

118. CWCCH, "Tentative Report of the Sub-Committee on Crime and Delinquency," June 1942, 4–5; Markowitz and Rosner, "Race, Foster Care," 1845; Eve P. Smith, "Willingness and Resistance to Change: The Case of the Race Discrimination Amendment of 1942," *Social Service Review* 69 (March 1995): 31–56; Antler, "Justine Wise Polier and the Prophetic Tradition," 280.

119. CWCCH, Sub-Committee on Crime and Delinquency, "Minutes of Meeting," October 13, 1942, folder "City-Wide Citizens' Committee on Harlem, 1942–1945," box 1, series "Racism," VWB.

120. CWCCH, Sub-Committee on Crime and Delinquency, "Minutes of Meeting," October 23, 1943, folder "City-Wide Citizens' Committee on Harlem, 1942–1945," box 1, series "Racism," VWB.

121. [Justine Wise Polier] to Mr. Harold F. Strong, April 6, 1944, folder 258, box 22, JWP; Justine Wise Polier to Hon. W. Bruce Cobb, memorandum, April 6, 1944, folder 258, box 22, JWP; [Justine Wise Polier], "Memorandum re: Children's Village," May 19, 1944, folder 258, box 22, JWP. See also Polier, *Juvenile Justice*, 137–57; and Markowitz and Rosner, "Race, Foster Care," 1846–49.

122. Petry, *Street*, 387, 405, 408–10.

123. W. Bruce Cobb to Fiorello H. La Guardia, March 17, 1943, folder 49, box 5, JWP; W. Bruce Cobb to Justices, Domestic Relations Court, City of New York, June 22, 1943, folder 49, box 5, JWP.

124. Markowitz and Rosner, "Race, Foster Care," 1846; CWCCH, Sub-Committee on Crime and Delinquency, "Minutes of Meeting," October 23, 1943, JWP. On October 23, 1943, Polier brought the SPCC crisis to the CWCCH's attention, urging it to take "immediate action."

125. Committee on Institutions to Hon. W. Bruce Cobb, memorandum, June 23, 1944, folder 49, box 5, JWP.

126. Joseph E. Maguire, Hubert T. Delany, Justine Wise Polier, W. Bruce Cobb, and William B. Herlands, "Shelter Care of Children by the New York Society for the Prevention of Cruelty to Children," January 4, 1944, 20, 53, folder 51, box 5, JWP (see also pages ii and 14).

127. Ibid., 7.

128. Untitled Press Release for Sunday A.M. Papers, January 16, 1944, 1, folder 51, box 5, JWP.

129. Ibid., 6–7; Adrian P. Burke to W. Bruce Cobb, April 10, 1945, folder 33, box 3, JWP; Committee on Institutions to Hon. W. Bruce Cobb, memorandum, June 23, 1944, JWP; Markowitz and Rosner, "Race, Foster Care," 1846.

130. Biondi, *To Stand and to Fight*, 17, 28, 39; McLeod, *Daughter of the Empire State*, 35–36, 61, 71–104; Von Eschen, *Race against Empire*, 18, 66, 116; Brandt, *Harlem at War*, 210; Markowitz and Rosner, *Children, Race, and Power*, 5, 7, 25, 59.

131. Kenneth W. Mack, "Law and Mass Politics in the Making of the Civil Rights Lawyer, 1931–1941," *Journal of American History* 93 (June 2006): 56.

132. Committee on Institutions, Report to the Board of Justices on Visit to the New York State Training School, Saturday, April 28, 1945, [May 1945], 2, 3, 4, 5–6, folder 39, box 4, JWP. In Polier's own 1987 account of this inspection, she misremembered the date of the inspection as 1938 (*Juvenile Justice*, 40).

133. Mary Sherwood to Judge W. Bruce Cobb, June 28, 1943, folder 39, box 4, JWP; [Committee on Institutions], memorandum "Regarding Conference between Judge Delany, Judge Polier, Mr. and Mrs. Grant, Former Cottage Parents New York State Training School," November 1, [1943], folder 40, box 4, JWP; [Committee on Institutions], memorandum "On Conference with Dr. Jolowicz, Psychiatrist at the New York State Training School," August 24, 1945, folder 40, box 4, JWP.

134. [Committee on Institutions], memorandum "On Conference with Dr. Jolowicz, Psychiatrist at the New York State Training School," 1, 2, JWP; [Committee on Institutions], memorandum "Regarding Conference between Judge Delany, Judge Polier" [1943], 1, 2, JWP.

135. W. Bruce Cobb to Raymond W. Houston, Esq., July 19, 1945, folder 39, box 4, JWP; W. Bruce Cobb to Hon. Lawrence C. Greenbaum, September 27, 1945, folder 40, box 4, JWP.

136. Polier, *Juvenile Justice*, 40.

137. The political theorist Nancy Fraser argues that "in cases where misrecognition involves denying the common humanity of some participants" in a society, and where such denials disqualify those participants from equal access to public resources, then "the remedy is universalist recognition" of those participants' full humanity. Nancy Fraser and Axel Honneth, *Redistribution or Recognition? A Political-Philosophical Exchange* (New York: Verso, 2003), 45–46.

Chapter Five

1. Leslie J. Reagan, Nancy Tomes, and Paula Treichler, "Introduction: Medicine, Health, and Bodies in American Film and Television," in *Medicine's Moving Pictures:*

Medicine, Health, and Bodies in American Film and Television (Rochester, NY: University of Rochester Press, 2007), 1–18.

2. Hilde Mosse, "Review of *The Quiet One,*" *American Journal of Psychotherapy* 3 (April 1949): 317, 318.

3. Sugrue, *Sweet Land of Liberty,* xxi, xxv–xxvi, 213–18; Elizabeth Lasch-Quinn, *Race Experts: How Racial Etiquette, Sensitivity Training, and New Age Therapy Hijacked the Civil Rights Revolution* (New York: Norton, 2001), 35, 39, 48, 49; Feldstein, *Motherhood in Black and White,* 44–60; Daryl Michael Scott, "Postwar Pluralism, *Brown v. Board of Education,* and the Origins of Multicultural Education," *Journal of American History* 91 (June 2004): 69–82.

4. Fraser and Honneth, *Redistribution or Recognition?,* 31.

5. Annelise Orleck, *Storming Caesar's Palace: How Black Mothers Fought Their Own War on Poverty* (Boston, MA: Beacon Press, 2005), 81–87; Jill Quadagno, *The Color of Welfare: How Racism Undermined the War on Poverty* (New York: Oxford University Press, 1996), 17–32; Brown, *Race, Money,* 170–77; 186–202; Solinger, *Wake Up Little Susie,* 12–18, 26–28.

6. Wiltwyck School for Boys, Inc., "Statement on the Wiltwyck School for Boys, Inc.," [1948], 3, folder "Administration, 1948, 1954–56," box 1, series "Wilwtwck School for Boys, Inc.," VWB.

7. Bernard to Moore, September 4, 1942, JWP; Wiltwyck Intake Policy Committee, Minutes of Meeting, November 4, 1942, folder 468, box 38, JWP.

8. Lee C. Dowling to Mrs. Louis S. Weiss, May 5, 1948, 2, folder "Administration, 1948, 1954–63," box 1, series "Wiltwyck School for Boys, Inc.," VWB.

9. Ibid., 2, 3.

10. Ibid., 2, 4.

11. Fritz Mayer, "Confidential: C. Conclusions and Recommendations," [Copy #3], 3, folder "Survey of the Program, Correspondence, 1947–1948," box 3, series "Wiltwyck School for Boys, Inc.," VWB.

12. Mrs. William Goodman to Richard Wright, May 7, 194[4], folder 2029, box 139, Richard Wright Papers, Beinecke Rare Book and Manuscript Library, Yale University, New Haven, CT (hereafter RWPYU).

13. Viola W. Bernard to Dr. Charles Brown, October 17, 1945, folder "Administration, 1948, 1954–1963," box 4, series "Wiltwyck School for Boys, Inc.," VWB.

14. Justine Wise Polier to Richard Wright, June 21, 1945, July 10, 1945, folder 1551, box 104, RWPYU; Wiltwyck School for Boys, Inc., "Our Children: Wiltwyck School for Boys, Inc., 1944–1945 Report," June 1945, RWPYU; Wiltwyck School for Boys, Inc., "Wiltwyck School for Boys," printed brochure, 1945, folder 2029, box 139; RWPYU; Arnold Rampersad, "Afterword," in Richard Wright, *Rite of Passage* (New York: Harper Trophy, 1994), 135–42; Jay Garcia, *Psychology Comes to Harlem: Rethinking the Race Question in Twentieth-Century America* (Baltimore, MD: Johns Hopkins University Press, 2012), 1–2, 64–69.

15. Jack Maeder to Robert Cooper, April 25, 1944, folder 470, box 38, JWP; Hans Maeder, untitled manuscript, [May 11, 1944], folder 470, box 38, JWP; Hans Maeder to Mr. Cooper, May 11, 1944, folder 470, box 38, JWP.

16. Memorandum, Robert L. Cooper to Mrs. Pratt, May 16, 1944, folder 470, box 38, JWP.

204   NOTES TO PP. 99–101

17. Dorothy A. Stearns to Dr. Robert L. Cooper, May 25, 1944; Donald Axon to Dr. Robert L. Cooper, May 25, 1944; Mr. and Mrs. Ben Cohen to Dr. Cooper, May 26, 1944, folder 470, box 38, JWP.

18. Sugrue, *Sweet Land of Liberty*, 179.

19. Dorothy K. Whyte to Dr. Lauretta Bender, April 3, 1946, folder 17, box 11, series 4, LBP.

20. James DeJongh, *Vicious Modernism: Black Harlem and the Literary Imagination* (New York: Cambridge University Press, 1994), 89, 133; David Serlin, *Replaceable You: Engineering the Body in Postwar America* (Chicago: University of Chicago Press, 2004), 113. For depictions of Harlem as a slum, see Roi Ottley, *"New World A-Coming": Inside Black America* (New York: Houghton Mifflin, 1945); Roi Ottley, "Slum-Shocked and Café Au Lait Society," *New York Amsterdam News*. May 1944, 11-A; Jack Lait and Lee Mortimer, *New York: Confidential!* (New York: Dell, 1951), 91–114.

21. Sugrue, *Sweet Land of Liberty*, xxi.

22. Walter Adams, "The Negro Patient in Psychiatric Treatment," *American Journal of Orthopsychiatry* 20 (April 1950): 305. For evidence that racialism was still acceptable within the literature, see E. J. Wiggins and R. S. Lyman, "Manic Psychosis in a Negro: With Special Reference to the Role of the Psychogenic and Sociogenic Factors," *American Journal of Psychiatry* 100 (May 1944): 781–87; Lt. Colonel Herbert S. Ripley and Major Stewart Wolf, "Mental Illness among Negro Troops Overseas," *American Journal of Psychiatry* 103 (1947): 499–512.

23. Grob, *Mad among Us*, 191–97.

24. Laynard Holloman, "On the Supremacy of the Negro Athlete in White Athletic Competition," *Psychoanalytic Review* 30 (1943): 157–62; Adams, "Negro Patient," 305–10; W. Loyd Warner, Buford H. Junker, and Walter A. Adams, *Color and Human Nature: Negro Personality Development in a Northern City* (Washington DC: American Council of Education, 1941); Stevens, "Racial Aspects of Emotional Problems of Negro Soldiers," 493–98; Helen V. McLean, "Racial Prejudice," *American Journal of Orthopsychiatry* 14 (October 1944): 706–13; McLean, "Psychodynamic Factors in Race Relations," *Annals of the American Academy of Political and Social Science* 244 (March 1946): 159–66; McLean, "The Emotional Health of Negroes," *Journal of Negro Education* 18 (1949): 283–90. McLean was married to Franklin McLean, the physiologist who ran the National Medical Fellowship for minority physicians.

25. Adams, "Negro Patient," 310 (see also 108); McLean, "Emotional Health of Negroes," 283, 285; McLean, "Psychodynamic Factors in Race Relations," 159.

26. Dwyer, "Psychiatry and Race during World War II," 122.

27. McLean, "Emotional Health of Negroes," 284, 290. See also Warner, Junker, and Adams, *Color and Human Nature*.

28. McClintock, *Imperial Leather*, 61.

29. Carolyn Herbst Lewis, *Prescription for Heterosexuality: Sexual Citizenship in the Cold War Era* (Chapel Hill: University of North Carolina Press, 2010), 5; Joanne Meyerowitz, *How Sex Changed: A History of Transsexuality in the United States* (Cambridge, MA: Harvard University Press, 2002), 98–99, 105; Metzl, *Prozac on the Couch*, 77, 79–81.

30. Green, "Manic-Depressive Psychosis in the Negro," 620; Evarts, "Dementia Precox in the Colored Race," 396, 397, 404; Bevis, "Psychological Traits of the Southern Negro," 69–78; O'Malley, "Psychosis in the Colored Race," 316, 323, 330;

Lind, "Phylogenetic Elements," 304, 323; Lewis and Hubbard, "Epileptic Reactions in the Negro," 647, 648, 657, 676; Rosenthal, "Racial Differences in the Mental Diseases," 312–13; Klineberg, *Race Differences*, 250–51.

31. McLean, "Psychodynamic Factors in Race Relations," 164.

32. Metzl, *Prozac on the Couch*, 6–12, 14–15, 17, 20–22, 24.

33. Marilyn E. Hegarty, *Victory Girls, Khaki-Wackies, and Patriotutes: The Regulation of Female Sexuality during World War II* (New York: New York University Press, 2007), 1–2, 4–5, 7–8, 110–27; Elaine Tyler May, *Homeward Bound: American Families in the Cold War Era* (New York: Basic Books, 1988); Metzl, *Prozac on the Couch*, 80; Meyerowitz, *How Sex Changed*, 41, 68.

34. Doris Sommer, *Foundational Fictions: The National Romances of Latin America* (Berkeley: University of California Press, 1991), 12, 18, 23; Anne McClintock, "No Longer in a Future Heaven: Nationalism, Gender and Race," in *Becoming National: A Reader*, ed. Geoff Eley and Ron Grigor Suny (New York: Oxford University Press, 1996), 261–62; Nira Yuval-Davis, *Gender and Nation* (Thousand Oaks, CA: Sage, 1997), 43–46.

35. Feldstein, *Motherhood in Black and White*.

36. Metzl, *Prozac on the Couch*, 77.

37. McLean, "Emotional Health of Negroes," 286. See also Adams, "Negro Patient," 309; Stevens, "Racial Aspects of Emotional Problems of Negro Soldiers," 493, 495, 496.

38. McLean, "Emotional Health of Negroes," 287; Kunzel, "White Neurosis, Black Pathology," 321; Solinger, *Wake Up Little Susie*, 9, 12–18, 21, 24, 86, 321; Paula Giddings, *When and Where I Enter: The Impact of Black Women on Race and Sex in America* (New York: William Morrow, 1984), 251–53.

39. Maeder, untitled manuscript, [May 11, 1944], 1, JWP.

40. For example, see Mary Braggiotti, "Laughter Conquers Evil," *New York Post*, March 28 1945, 30. Profiling Robert L. Cooper and Wiltwyck, Braggiotti states outright: "There is no race problem at Wiltwyck," and quotes Cooper as saying that "race is completely unimportant among both the children and the staff."

41. Harlem Project, *Role of the School*, 3–4.

42. Ibid., 91.

43. Ibid., 71–72, 76, 81–85.

44. Ibid., 90 (see also 91–95, 98–99).

45. Ibid., 88, 91 (see also 88–92).

46. Ibid., 21 (see also 61, 95).

47. Bernard to Moore, September 4, 1942, JWP.

48. Reagan, Tomes, and Treichler, "Introduction," 2, 5, 11.

49. Sandra S. Phillips, "Helen Levitt's New York," in *Helen Levitt*, ed. Sandra S. Phillips and Maria Morris Hambourg (San Francisco: San Francisco Museum of Modern Art; New York: Metropolitan Museum of Art, 1991), 17.

50. Jane Livingston, *The New York School: Photographs, 1936–1963* (New York: Stewart, Tabnori, and Chang, 1992), 4, 303. The New York School was part of a larger movement of neorealist street photographers striving to capture—in documentary fashion—authentic moments in the lives of common people in the 1930s and 1940s.

51. James Thrall Soby to Dr. Lauretta Bender, March 17, 1943, file 4, box 17, LBP. See also Phillips, "Helen Levitt's New York," 30.

52. Janice Loeb, "Proposal for a Film on the Children of Wiltwyck," September 19, 1945, folder "*The Quiet One*—General, 1946–1950," [n.d.], box 1, series "Mental Health Films," VWB.

53. Phillips, "Helen Levitt's New York," 29, 39; Serlin, *Replaceable You*, 22–24.

54. Soby to Bender, March 17, 1943, LBP.

55. Phillips, "Helen Levitt's New York," 29.

56. Reagan, Tomes, and Treichler, "Introduction," 5. Within the medical film genre, it became fairly common for filmmakers to "try to move audiences to adopt a new perspective or take action with regard to a current health controversy."

57. Loeb, "Proposal for a Film on the Children of Wiltwyck."

58. Reagan, Tomes, and Treichler, "Introduction," 6.

59. Loeb, "Proposal for a Film on the Children of Wiltwyck." According to Loeb the two producers and Wiltwyck's board were in "agreement as to the value of Wiltwyck and the values implicit in its activities." See also Philips, "Helen Levitt's New York," 32, 47.

60. Reagan, Tomes, and Treichler, "Introduction," 11.

61. Ibid., 10, 11.

62. Loeb, "Proposal for a Film on the Children of Wiltwyck."

63. Reagan, Tomes, and Treichler, "Introduction," 11.

64. Gertrude Binder to Dr. Viola W. Bernard, September 20, 1946; Gertrude Binder to Judge Polier, December 10, 1946; Viola W. Bernard to Gertrude Binder, December 18, 1946; Gertrude Binder to Mrs. Lash, Judge Polier, Dr. Bernard, December 26, 1946, folder "*The Quiet One*—General, 1946–1950," [n.d.], box 1, series "Mental Health Films," VWB.

65. Reagan, Tomes, and Treichler, "Introduction," 11.

66. Viola W. Bernard to Gertrude Binder, February 17, 1947, folder "*The Quiet One*—General, 1946–1950," [n.d.], box 1, series "Mental Health Films," VWB. Even though Dr. Bernard found it "very time consuming," she allowed Levitt and Loeb to "pick my brains mental-hygiene wise."

67. Viola W. Bernard to Fred G. Wale, February 2, 1950, folder "*Roots of Happiness*, 1949–1984," box 1, series "Mental Health Films," VWB.

68. Viola W. Bernard, "The Production of Films for Mental Health Education: Psychiatrist's Experience," *American Journal of Orthopsychiatry* 20 (October 1950): 779, 780.

69. Viola W. Bernard to Gertrude Binder, December 18, 1946, folder "*The Quiet One*—General, 1946–1950," [n.d.], box 1, series "Mental Health Films," VWB; Viola W. Bernard's annotated copy of Film Documents Inc., "Proposed Treatment for a Film on the Wiltwyck Child," December 26, 1926, folder "*The Quiet One*—General, 1946–1950," [n.d.], box 1, series "Mental Health Films," VWB; Bernard, "Production of Films for Mental Health Education," 780.

70. Bernard to Wale, February 2, 1950, VWB; Livingston, *New York School*, 373. Edna Meyers, a Jewish American, was a remedial tutor at the Northside Center, where Viola Bernard was on the Board of Directors. Edna was also an analysand of Dr. Alexander Thomas, an antiracist psychiatrist and the husband of the Northside Center's psychiatric social worker Stella Chess. Markowitz and Rosner, *Children, Race, and Power*, 49–50.

71. Maria Morris Hambourg, "Helen Levitt: A Life in Part," in Phillips and Hambourg, *Helen Levitt*, 58–59.

72. Loeb, "Proposal for a Film on the Children of Wiltwyck," VWB.

73. Viola W. Bernard's annotated copy of Helen Levitt and Janice Loeb, "Proposed Treatment for a Film on the Wiltwyck Child," December 26, 1946, 13, folder "*The Quiet One*—General, 1946–1950," [n.d.], box 1, series "Mental Health Films," VWB.

74. Ibid.

75. Ibid., 1–7, 13.

76. Ibid., 13; Viola W. Bernard to Dr. Arthur H. Ruggles, April 29, 1950, folder "*The Quiet One*—General, 1946–1950," [n.d.], box 1, series "Mental Health Films," VWB.

77. Levitt and Loeb, "Proposed Treatment for a Film on the Wiltwyck Child," 13; "Script for *The Wanderer: A Film about the Life of a Wiltwyck Child*," May 15, 1947; Transcript, *The Quiet One*, 1948, folder "*The Quiet One*—General, 1946–1950," [n.d.], box 1, series "Mental Health Films," VWB.

78. The part of Clarence was played by a Wiltwyck counselor named Clarence Cooper.

79. *The Quiet One*, dir. Sidney Meyers, Film Documents, 1948.

80. Bernard to Ruggles, April 29, 1950, VWB.

81. Bernard, "Production of Films for Mental Health Education," 780.

82. Bernard to Ruggles, April 29, 1950, VWB.

83. Bernard, "Production of Films for Mental Health Education," 780.

84. *The Quiet One*, dir. Meyers, 1948.

85. Bernard to Ruggles, April 29, 1950, VWB.

86. Bernard, "Production of Films for Mental Health Education," 779; Viola W. Bernard to Bill Levitt, November 16, 1948, folder "*The Quiet One*—General, 1946–1950," [n.d.], box 1, series "Mental Health Films," VWB. Bernard did confide in Helen Levitt's husband and collaborator, Bill, that she did not expect all audiences to be able to get beyond Donald's skin color and recognize his common humanity in the depth of his emotional distress.

87. Ernst Papanek, "Report of the Executive Director to the Board of Directors, September 1949 to June 1951," June 5, 1951, 9, folder "Administration, 1948, 1954–1963," box 1, series "Wiltwyck School for Boys, Inc.," VWB. See also Viola W. Bernard to Dr. Harry Weinstock, October 15, 1948; Viola W. Bernard to Dr. Carl Binger, October 13, 1948, folder "*The Quiet One*—General, 1946–1950," [n.d.], box 1, series "Mental Health Films," VWB; and Reagan, Tomes, and Treichler, "Introduction," 4.

88. Viola W. Bernard to Dr. Devid Levy, July 30, 1948, folder "*The Quiet One*—General, 1946–1950," [n.d.], box 1, series "Mental Health Films," VWB; Bernard, "Production of Films for Mental Health Education," 779.

89. Arthur H. Ruggles to Dr. Viola W. Bernard, May 11, 1950; Viola W. Bernard to Bill Levitt, November 16, 1948; Adele Franklin to Dr. Viola W. Bernard, December 1, 1946; Jane Judge to Viola W. Bernard, November 30, 1948; George S. Goldman, MD, to Dr. Viola W. Bernard, December 10, 1948; Harold Boris to Dr. Bernard, [n.d.]; Edith B. Jackson, MD, to William Levitt, January 20, 1949; Mildred Buchwalder Beck to Dr. Viola W. Bernard, November 30, 1948; Viola W. Bernard to Janice Loeb and Bill Levitt, December 3, 1948; Janice Loeb to Dr. Viola W. Bernard, December 15,

1948, folder "*The Quiet One*—General, 1946–1950," [n.d.], box 1, series "Mental Health Films," VWB.

90. Anthony Bower, "Review of *The Quiet One*," *The Nation*, January 29, 1949, 137–38; Robert Hatch, "Review of *The Quiet One*," *The New Republic*, March 28, 1949, 298–30; Bernard to Ruggles, April 29, 1950, VWB.

91. Bosley Crowther, "Review of *The Quiet One*," *NYT*, February 14, 1949, 15.

92. Doyle, "A Fine New Child," 173–212; Doyle, "Where the Need Is Greatest," 746–74.

93. Bendiner, "Psychiatry for the Needy," 22–25; Mendes, *Under the Strain of Color*, 96–100.

94. Fredric Wertham to Richard Wright, August 1, 1945, folder 1677, box 108, RWPYU; Florence Hesketh to Richard Wright [ca. 1946], 1–2, box 108, folder 1676, RWPYU; Florence Hesketh to Richard and Ellen Wright, [ca. 1946 or 1947], 3, box 108, folder 1676, RWPYU; Fredric Wertham, "Rx Lafargue Clinic," undated note card, white envelope with note cards, folder 10, box 52, Dr. Fredric Wertham Papers, Manuscript Division, Library of the United States Congress, Washington, DC (hereafter FWP); Mendes, *Under the Strain of Color*, 96–100.

95. Florence Hesketh to Richard Wright, July 27, 1947, box 108, folder 1676, RWPYU.

96. Wertham to Wright, August 1, 1945, RWPYU.

97. Hesketh to Wright, [ca. 1946], 2, RWPYU.

98. Fredric Wertham, "Rx Earl—Lafargue," undated note card, white envelope with note cards, folder 10, box 52, FWP.

99. Fredric Wertham to Hilde Mosse, "Rx Lafargue Clinic," undated note card, white envelope with note cards, folder 10, box 52, FWP; Dr. Ann Clark to Fredric Wertham, note card size memorandum, June 14, 1945, 1–5, folder 10, box 52, FWP; Fredric Wertham, "Richard Wright, 10-2-45," memorandum, October 2, 1945, 1–5, white envelope with memo notes, folder 7, box 62, FWP; "Conference Notes," transcript, November 30, 1948, folder 11, box 51, FWP; Hilde Mosse, "Re: Wiltwyck," typed memorandum, June 24, 1956, 1–2, folder 4, box 63, FWP.

100. "The Report of the Harlem Project," handwritten Lafargue Clinic conference notes, 6, folder 10, box 52, FWP.

101. The scholar Gabriel Mendes partially attributes the divide to the New York racial liberals' doubts that a clinic run by white psychiatrists would be the right fit for Harlem's black community (*Under the Strain of Color*, 95–97).

102. Hilde Mosse to Florence Hesketh, August 13, 1957, 3, folder 4, box 63, FWP; Hilde Mosse, "Ideas for a Paper for International Congress of Psychiatry in Vienna, 1961," July 22, 1960, 2, folder "Ms. by Hilde Mosse, 1961," box 4, Lafargue Clinic Records, Manuscripts, Archives and Rare Books Division, Schomburg Center for Research in Black Culture, New York Public Library, Astor, Lennox and Tilden Foundation, New York (hereafter LFC-SCRBC); David James Fisher, PhD to Dennis Doyle, May 4, 2012, letter in author's possession.

103. Therese Pol, "Psychiatry in Harlem," *The Protestant*, June–July 1947, 30.

104. Doyle, "A Fine New Child," 173–212; Doyle, "Where the Need Is Greatest," 746–74. See also Hilde Mosse, MD, "Child Psychiatry and Social Action: An Integral Part of the History of American Child Psychiatry" (unpublished manuscript), 1981, 5, folder "Manuscript by Hilde Mosse, 1981," box 4, LFC-SCRBC; Richard Kluger,

Simple Justice: The History of Brown v. Board of Education and Black America's Struggle for Equality (New York: Alfred A. Knopf, 1976), 439–42; Gilbert, *A Cycle of Outrage*, 91–108; Mendes, *Under the Strain of Color;* Garcia, *Psychology Comes to Harlem*, 49–74; Catherine A. Stewart, "Crazy for This Democracy": Psychoanalysis, African American Blues Narratives, and the Lafargue Clinic," *American Quarterly* 65 (June 2013): 371–95.

105. Florence Hesketh to Richard Wright, [1946], folder 1676, box 108, RWPYU. Florence Hesketh, Fredric Wertham's wife, jokingly referred to both Wright and her husband as the "two 'publicity directors' of the Board."

106. Richard Wright, "Psychiatry Comes to Harlem," *Free World* 12 (September 1946): 45–51; Earl Brown, "Timely Topics," *New York Amsterdam News*, February 15, 1947, 13. See also [Earl Brown], "Clinic for Sick Minds: Basement of a Harlem Church Is Haven for Mentally Ill," *Life*, February 24, 1948, 99–100, 102.

107. In 1946, the Harvard graduate Earl Brown was an editor and columnist with Harlem's *New York Amsterdam News* and a writer for *Life*. In 1949 he was elected city councilman in New York City as a Democrat. See Biondi, *To Stand and to Fight*, 154. On Ellison and Lafargue Cinic, see Kenneth Spencer, "Sans Funds, Lafargue Clinic Lives," *People's Voice*, July 13, 1946, clipping, folder "Clippings Re. Lafargue," box 3, LFC-SCRBC; Martin, "Doctor's Dream in Harlem," 799; Mosse, "Child Psychiatry and Social Action," 5, LFC-SCRBC; Ralph Ellison, "Harlem Is Nowhere," in *Shadow and Act* (New York: Random House, 1964), 292–302.

108. Richard R. Dier, "Harlem Mental Hygiene Clinic Drawing Support," *New Jersey Afro-American*, March 30, 1946, 11; Constance Curtis, "Harlem's Mental Health Clinic Doing OK," *New York Amsterdam News*, April 13, 1946, 1, 23; S. I. Hayakawa, "Second Thoughts," *Chicago Defender*, January 4, 1947, January 11, 1947; Lillian Scott, "Patients Wait in Line for Treatment at Famed Inter-racial Clinic in Harlem," *Chicago Defender*, January 3, 1948, clipping, folder "Clippings Re. Lafargue," box 3, LFC-SCRBC; Sidney M. Katz, "Jim Crow Is Barred from Wertham's Clinic," *Magazine Digest*, September 1946, 1–5, reprint, folder "Reprints," box 3, LFC-SCRBC; Bendiner, "Psychiatry for the Needy," 22–25; James L. Tuck, "Here's Hope for Harlem," *New York-Herald Tribune*, January 26, 1947, reprint, folder "Clippings Re. Lafargue," box 3, LFC-SCRBC; Wright, "Psychiatry Comes to Harlem," 45–51; "Harlem Pioneers with Mental Clinic," *Headlines and Pictures*, July 1946, clipping, folder "Clippings Re. Lafargue," box 3, LFC-SCRBC; Pol, "Psychiatry in Harlem," 28–30; Martin, "Doctor's Dream in Harlem," 798–800; [Brown], "Clinic for Sick Minds," 99–100, 102; Brown, "Timely Topics," 13; Spencer, "Sans Funds"; Dorothy Norman, "Help for the Troubled in Harlem," *New York Post*, March 16, 1946, 30; "Why Segregate Negro Psychiatry," *New York Post*, September 6, 1946, 34; Lawrence Galton, "Communities on the March," *Woman's Home Companion*, January 1947, clipping, folder "Clippings Re. Lafargue," box 3, LFC-SCRBC; Lloyd and Mary Morain, "Do You Know?" *The Humanist* (Spring 1948): 186; "Psychiatry in Harlem," *Time*, December 1, 1947, 50, 52.

109. Testimony of Witnesses, In the Court of Chancery of the State of Delaware in and for New Castle County, *Belton v. Gebhart*, Civil Action 258, and *Beulah v. Gebhart*, Civil Action 265, October 22, 1951, 154, bound transcript of testimony, box B319, NAACP Papers, part 2, Manuscript Division, Library of the United States Congress, Washington, DC.

110. Katz, "Jim Crow Is Barred from Wertham's Clinic," 5, LFC-SCRBC; Margaret Walker, *Richard Wright, Daemonic Genius: A Portrait of the Man, a Critical Look at His Work* (New York: Warner, 1988), 121–58, 158–59; Fredric Wertham, "An Unconscious Determinant in *Native Son*," *Journal of Clinical Psychopathology* 6 (July 1944): 111–15; McLean, "Psychodynamic Factors in Race Relations."

111. Martin, "Doctor's Dream in Harlem," 798.

112. Fredric Wertham, "Who Will Guard the Guardians?" *The New Republic*, October 29, 1945, 578. See also Degler, *In Search of Human Nature*, 204; Brattain, "Race, Racism, and Antiracism."

113. Rose, *Psychology and Selfhood.*

114. Ibid.

115. Mosse, "Review of *The Quiet One*," 317.

116. Ibid., 318, 317.

117. Ibid., 318.

118. Wright, "Psychiatry Comes to Harlem," 49; Tuck, "Here's Hope for Harlem," LFC-SCRBC; "Harlem Pioneers with Mental Clinic," LFC-SCRBC; Spencer, "Sans Funds," LFC-SCRBC; Martin, "Doctor's Dream in Harlem," 798–800; Curtis, "Harlem's Mental Clinic Doing OK"; Hayakawa, "Second Thoughts," January 4, 1947, January 11, 1947; Mona Walter Agnew, "John L. Fortson's Religion in the News," script, March 15, 1947, folder "Clippings Re. Lafargue," box 3, LFC-SCRBC.

119. "Harlem Pioneers with Mental Clinic," LFC-SCRBC; Wright, "Psychiatry Comes to Harlem," 50; Katz, "Jim Crow Is Barred from Wertham's Clinic," LFC-SCRBC; Curtis, "Harlem's Mental Clinic Doing OK," Bendiner, "Psychiatry for the Needy," 24; Martin, "Doctor's Dream in Harlem," 798–99.

120. Mosse, "Review of *The Quiet One*," 317; Martin, "Doctor's Dream in Harlem," 800, Tuck, "Here's Hope for Harlem," LFC-SCRBC; Wright, "Psychiatry Comes to Harlem," 51; Spencer, "Sans Funds," LFC-SRBC; Hayakawa, "Second Thoughts," January 11, 1947; Katz, "Jim Crow Is Barred from Wertham's Clinic," LFC-SCRBC.

121. Wright, "Psychiatry Comes to Harlem," 51.

122. Stella Chess, Kenneth B. Clark, and Alexander Thomas, "The Importance of Cultural Evaluation in Psychiatric Diagnosis and Treatment," *Psychiatric Quarterly* 27 (1953): 112.

123. Ibid., 103, 105–6, 112; Viola W. Bernard, "Psychoanalysis and Members of Minority Groups," *Journal of the American Psychoanalytic Association* 1 (1953): 263; Hilde Mosse, "Is There an Ishmael Complex?" *American Journal of Psychotherapy* 7 (January 1953): 74; Charles W. Collins, "Psychoanalysis of Groups: Critique of a Study of a Small Negro Sample," *Journal of the National Medical Association* 44 (May 1952): 168; Fredric Wertham, "Psychological Effects of School Segregation," *American Journal of Psychotherapy* 6 (January 1952): 97.

124. Chess, Clark, and Thomas, "Importance of Cultural Evaluation," 106.

125. Brattain, "Race, Racism, and Antiracism, 1397 (see also 1404, 1405, 1408).

126. Chess, Clark, and Thomas, "Importance of Cultural Evaluation," 103; Abram Kardiner and Lionel Ovesey, *The Mark of Oppression: Explorations in the Personality of the American Negro*, rev. ed. (New York: Meridian, 1962), xvii, 78–79; Robison, *Juvenile Delinquency*, 186.

127. Kardiner and Ovesey, *Mark of Oppression*, vi, xi, xii, xv, xviii, 8–9.

128. Wertham, "Who Will Guard the Guardians?" 578, 580; Mosse, "Is There an Ishmael Complex?" 73.

129. Prince Barker, "Psychoanalysis of Groups," *Journal of the National Medical Association* 6 (November 1952): 456.

130. Bernard, "Psychoanalysis of Minority Groups," 266; Jatinder Bains, "Race, Culture, and Psychiatry: A History of Transcultural Psychiatry," *History of Psychiatry* 16 (June 2005): 139–54; Joanne Meyerowitz, "'How Common Culture Shapes the Separate Lives': Sexuality, Race, and Mid-Twentieth-Century Social Constructivist Thought," *Journal of American History* 96 (March 2010): 1057–84.

131. Chess, Clark, and Thomas, "Importance of Cultural Evaluation," 103.

132. Bernard, "Psychoanalysis of Minority Groups," 261.

133. Chess, Clark, and Thomas, "Importance of Cultural Evaluation," 110.

134. Bernard, "Psychoanalysis of Minority Groups," 262.

135. Wiggins and Lyman, "Manic Psychosis in a Negro," 781–87; Ripley, Wolf, "Mental Illness among Negro Troops Overseas," 499–512; Bingham Dai, "Some Problems of Personality Development among Negro Children," in *Personality in Nature, Society, and Culture*, ed. Clyde Kluckholn and Henry A. Murray, 2nd ed. (New York: Alfred A. Knopf, 1967), 545–66; Harvey St. Clair, "Psychiatric Interview Experiences with Negroes," *American Journal of Psychiatry* 108 (1951): 113–19; Helen Mayer Hacker, "Ishmael Complex," *American Journal of Psychotherapy* 6 (July 1952): 494–512; Janet Alterman Kennedy, "Problems Posed in the Analysis of Negro Patients," *Psychiatry* 15 (August 1952): 313–27.

136. Kardiner and Ovesey, *Mark of Oppression*, 81; Lasch-Quinn, *Race Experts*, 115.

137. Most recently, Thomas J. Sugrue reinforced the claim that *The Mark of Oppression* generated no backlash, in *Sweet Land of Liberty*, 214.

138. This early outrage against the black damaged psyche thesis is missing from Daryl Michael Scott's history of liberalism's long engagement with the thesis in *Contempt and Pity*. The 1951–53 outcry over *The Mark of Oppression*'s racist overtones is confirmed in Meyerowitz, "How Common Culture Shapes the Separate Lives," 1080. See also Rutherford B. Stevens, "Psychoanalysis of Groups," *Journal of the National Medical Association* 6 (November 1952): 457; Barker, "Psychoanalysis of Groups," 455; Lighfoot, *Balm in Gilead*, 181.

139. Mosse, "Is There an Ishmael Complex?" 73.

140. Kardiner and Ovesey, *Mark of Oppression*, 11, 22, 81, 222–23, 235, 297, 302–4, 309–11, 313–14, 362, 364, 384, 387.

141. Ibid., 81, 317.

142. Feldstein, *Motherhood in Black and White*, 53–60. See also Kardiner and Ovesey, *Mark of Oppression*, vi, xv, 11–12, 20, 22, 81, 302–4.

143. Bernard, "Psychoanalysis of Minority Groups," 263.

144. Bernard, "Psychoanalysis of Minority Groups," 263; Wertham, "Psychological Effects of School Segregation," 97; Mosse, "Is There an Ishmael Complex?" 73; Collins, "Psychoanalysis of Groups," 168; Barker, "Psychoanalysis of Groups," 456; Lawrence, *Balm in Gilead*, 184.

145. Kardiner and Ovesey, *Mark of Oppression*, 302, 387.

146. Mosse, "Is There an Ishmael Complex?" 73; Mosse, "Ideas for a Paper for International Congress of Psychiatry in Vienna, 1961," LFC-SCRBC; Wertham, "Who Will Guard the Guardians?" 578.

147. Kardiner and Ovesey, *Mark Oppression*, 169, 303–4, 359, 363–69.
148. Mosse, "Is There an Ishmael Complex?" 73.
149. Collins, "Psychoanalysis of Groups," 168.
150. Adams, "Negro Patient," 308.
151. Fraser and Honneth, *Redistribution or Recognition?*, 49.

Chapter Six

1. M. R. Kane to Dr. K. B. Clark, September 20, 1955, folder 6, box 42, LOC-CLARK; Biondi, *To Stand and to Fight*, 150, 161, 179–80, 193–94, 196, 231, 246.

2. "Hubert T. Delany, 89, Ex-Judge and Civil Rights Advocate Dies," *NYT*, December 31, 1990, http://www.nytimes.com/1990/12/31/obituaries/hubert-t-delany-89-ex-judge-and-civil-rights-advocate-dies.html (accessed December 6, 2014).

3. Clarence Taylor, "Conservative and Liberal Opposition to the New York City School-Integration Campaign," in Taylor, *Civil Rights in New York City*, 98–99; Biondi, *To Stand and to Fight*, 246–47; Markowitz and Rosner, *Children, Race, and Power*, 25.

4. Markowitz and Rosner, *Children, Race, and Power*, 18–42.

5. Scott, *Contempt and Pity*, 82–83; 133–36.

6. Kenneth B. Clark to Honorable Hubert T. Delany, September 21, 1955, folder 6, box 42, LOC-CLARK.

7. Joshua Freeman, *Working-Class New York: Life and Labor since World War II* (New York: Free Press, 2000), 72.

8. Richard Iton, *In Search of the Black Fantastic: Politics and Popular Culture in the Post-Civil Rights Era* (New York: Oxford University Press, 2008), 34.

9. Sugrue, *Sweet Land of Liberty*; Hall, "The Long Civil Rights Movement"; Biondi, *To Stand and to Fight*.

10. Dudziak, *Cold War Civil Rights*, 47–78; Waldo E. Martin, Jr., *No Coward Soldiers: Black Cultural Politics and Postwar America* (Cambridge, MA: Harvard University Press, 2005), 14–19; Biondi, *To Stand and to Fight*, 156–225; Iton, *In Search of the Black Fantastic*, 27–73.

11. Biondi, *To Stand and to Fight*, 165–67, 169, 201; Iton, *In Search of the Black Fantastic*, 49–61; Greenberg, *Troubling the Waters*, 193–94; Peniel E. Joseph, *Waiting 'Til the Midnight Hour: A Narrative History of Black Power in America* (New York: Henry Holt, 2006), 2–18.

12. Antler, "Justine Wise Polier and the Prophetic Tradition," 285.

13. Ibid., 285.

14. Freeman, *Working-Class New York*, 86–87.

15. On the Domestic Relations Court's role in battling racial segregation in the public schools in 1958, see Adina Black, "Exposing the 'Whole Segregation Myth': The Harlem Nine and New York City's School Desegregation Battles," in *Freedom North: Black Freedom Struggles Outside the South, 1940–1980*, ed. Jeanne Theoharis and Komozi Woodard (New York: Palgrave Macmillan, 2003), 65–91.

16. According to Lani Guinier, the Red scare convinced racial liberals to mostly work with middle-class civil-rights organizations making "status-based legal challenges that focused on formal equality through the elimination of de jure segregation"

("From Racial Liberalism to Racial Literacy," 101). See also Biondi, *To Stand and to Fight*, 171, 182–83; Greenberg, *Troubling the Waters*, 124.

17. Biondi, *To Stand and to Fight*, 194.

18. "Dudley F. Sicher Retires," *Juvenile Court Judges Journal* 5 (January 1954): 19.

19. The alleged inability of those with low intelligence quotients to express abstract ideas with precision was known as "nonconceptual thinking" (Polier, *Juvenile Justice*, 120); Justine Wise Polier, "Attitudes and Contradictions in our Culture," *Child Welfare* 39 (November 1960): 1–5.

20. Karen Kruse Thomas, "The Hill-Burton Act and Civil Rights: Expanding Hospital Care for Black Southerners, 1939–1960," *Journal of Southern History* 72 (November 2006): 824, 847; Thomas, *Deluxe Jim Crow*, 190–94.

21. Helene Risor, "Twenty Hanging Dolls and a Lynching: Defacing Dangerousness and Enacting Citizenship in El Alto, Bolivia," *Public Culture* 22 (Fall 2010): 468.

22. Fredric Wertham, undated note card marked "Rx Lafargue Clinic," white envelope containing note cards, folder 10, box 52, FWP. See also Gabriel N. Mendes, "An Underground Extension of Democracy," *Transition* 115 (2014): 4–22.

23. Doyle, "A Fine New Child"; Doyle, "Where the Need Is Greatest"; and David James Fisher, PhD, to Dennis Doyle, May 4, 2012, letter in author's possession.

24. Gilbert, *A Cycle of Outrage*, 96; Markowitz and Rosner, *Children, Race, and Power*, 40.

25. Biondi, *To Stand and to Fight*, 278.

26. Markowitz and Rosner, *Children, Race, and Power*, 18–36.

27. Ibid., 38–39.

28. Ibid., 54–64, 65, 69–71.

29. Ibid., 69–79, 82, 84–86. See also Greenberg, *Troubling the Waters*, 47, 159.

30. Polier, *Juvenile Justice*, 143, 145–53; Polier, "Anatomy of Three Institutions," 24, JWP.

31. Wiltwyck School For Boys, Inc., "Service Plan and Supportive Data," October 1963, folder "Committee on the Treatment Program, 1961–1969," box 2, series "Wiltwyck School for Boys, Inc.," VWB.

32. Polier, "Anatomy of Three Institutions," 17–18.

33. Mildred D. Saffell, press release, September 14, 1949, folder "Administration, 1948, 1954–1963," box 1, series "Wiltwyck School for Boys, Inc.," VWB; Papanek, "Report of the Executive Director to the Board of Directors: September 1949 to June 1951," June 5, 1951, VWB; Wiltwyck School for Boys, Inc., "Minutes of the Meeting of the Board of Directors," January 27, 1958, 5, folder "Board of Directors, Minutes, 1942, 1956–1960," box 1, series "Wiltwyck School for Boys, Inc.," VWB.

34. Brown, *Manchild in the Promised Land*, 78–79, 82–84.

35. Ibid., 82, 85, 120.

36. Papanek, "Report of the Executive Director to the Board of Directors: September 1949 to June 1951," VWB; Bernard, Interview by Senn, 13, VWB.

37. Child Welfare League of America, Inc., "Report . . . to the Field Foundation re: Wiltwyck School for Boys, Esopus, New York," October 15, 1952, 2, folder "Administration, 1948, 1954–1963," box 1, series "Wiltwyck School for Boys, Inc.," VWB.

38. Polier, "Anatomy of Three Institutions," 23–25; Polier, *Juvenile Justice*, 120; Robison, *Juvenile Delinquency*, 454–55.

39. Robison, *Juvenile Delinquency*, 454, 461.

40. Child Welfare League of America, Inc., "Report . . . to the Field Foundation," 2, VWB; Robison, *Juvenile Delinquency*, 454.

41. Wiltwyck School for Boys, "Minutes of the Meeting of the Board of Directors," November 25, 1957, 3–4; February 5, 1959, 7–9, folder "Board of Directors, Minutes, 1942, 1956–1960," box 1, series "Wiltwyck School for Boys, Inc.," VWB; Justine Wise Polier to Viola Bernard, July 13, 1959, folder "Professional Advisory Committee, 1941–1960," box 1, series "Wiltwyck School for Boys, Inc.," VWB.

42. Viola W. Bernard to Dr. David S. Thoresen, June 4, 1959, folder "Administration, 1948, 1954–1963," box 1, series "Wiltwyck School for Boys, Inc.," VWB.

43. In part, this drive to place the school under greater psychiatric authority dovetailed with plans to meet the New York City Department of Welfare's stricter requirements for residential treatment centers. In 1959 the school had failed to meet those standards and the Department of Welfare refused to fully reimburse its treatment costs. To meet those standards the school needed additional counselors, caseworkers, and psychiatrists on staff. Wiltwyck School for Boys, "Minutes of the Meeting of the Board of Directors," January 27, 1958, 3; February 5, 1959, 2; March 19, 1959, 3; May 26, 1959, 2–3, 5, 6, folder "Board of Directors, Minutes, 1942, 1956–1960," box 1, series "Wiltwyck School for Boys, Inc.," VWB; Sylvia Liese to Members of Board of Directors, Internal Memorandum, August 10, 1959, 1–2, folder "Administration, 1948, 1954–1963," box 1, series "Wiltwyck School for Boys, Inc.," VWB.

44. Wilwyck School for Boys, "Appendix A: Summary of Staff Research Suggestions," December 31, 1956, folder "Administration, 1948, 1954–1963," box 1, series "Wiltwyck School for Boys, Inc.," VWB; [Lou Gilbert?] to [unnamed], typed notes, December 26, 1958; Thomas L. Brayboy to Judge Sylvia Liese, August 10, 1959; Judge Sylvia Jaffin Liese to Dr. Thomas Brayboy, August 13, 1959, folder "Administration, 1948, 1954–1963," box 1, series "Wiltwyck School for Boys, Inc.," VWB; Wiltwyck School, "Minutes of the Board," January 27, 1958, 5, VWB; Wiltwyck School for Boys, "Minutes of the Meeting of the Board of Directors," April 5, 1960, folder "Board of Directors, Minutes 1942, 1956–1960," box 1, series "Wiltwyck School for Boys, Inc.," VWB.

45. Sylvia Liese to Members of Board of Directors, Internal Memorandum, August 10, 1959, 1–2, folder "Administration, 1948, 1954–1963," box 1, series "Wiltwyck School for Boys, Inc.," VWB. See also Brayboy to Liese, August 10, 1959, VWB.

46. Wiltwyck School for Boys, "Minutes of the Meeting of the Board of Directors," April 5, 1960, 5; September 24, 1959, 4–5, folder "Board of Directors, Minutes, 1942, 1956–1960," box 1, series "Wiltwyck School for Boys, Inc.," VWB.

47. [Edgar Auerswald], proposal, "Study of Families of Children in Residential Treatment," November 1960, 1, folder "Research Proposals and Papers, 'Children in Residential Treatment,' 1960–1963," box 5, series "Wiltwyck School for Boys, Inc.," VWB.

48. Ibid., 1–4, 5; Nathan Levine, "Report to Taconic Foundation," August 15, 1960, 1–3, folder "Administration, 1948, 1956–1963," box 1, series "Wiltwyck School for Boys, Inc.," VWB; Sylvia Liese to Members of Board of Directors, August 10, 1959, VWB.

49. Deborah Weinstein, *The Pathological Family: Postwar America and the Rise of Family Therapy* (Ithaca, NY: Cornell University Press, 2013); Nathan Ackerman, *Treating the Troubled Family* (New York: Basic Books, 1966); [Auerswald], "Study of Families of Children in Residential Treatment," 26–31, VWB; Levine, "Report to Taconic Foundation," 3, VWB.

50. Levine, "Report to Taconic Foundation," 1–6, VWB; [Auerswald], "Study of Families of Children in Residential Treatment," 4–9, VWB; Edgar H. Auerswald, untitled paper, [1962], folder 467, box 38, JWP.

51. [Auerswald], "Study of Families of Children in Residential Treatment," 22–25, VWB.

52. Auerswald, untitled paper, [1962], JWP.

53. Wiltwyck School for Boys, "Minutes of the Meeting of the Board of Directors," May 24, 1962, folder "Board of Directors, Minutes, 1961–63," box 1, series "Wiltwyck School for Boys, Inc.," VWB; Wiltwyck School for Boys, Inc., program, "A Benefit for Wiltwyck School for Boys," April 11, 1965, 4–9, folder "Fundraising Programs, Souvenir 1965–1970," 1975, box 4, series "Wiltwyck School for Boys, Inc.," VWB; Salvador Minuchin, Edgar Auerswald, Charles H. King, and Clara Rabinowitz, "The Study and Treatment of Families Who Produce Multiple Acting-Out Boys," paper presented at the American Orthopsychiatric Association, March 1963, 1–7, folder "Administration, 1948, 1954–1963," box 1, series "Wiltwyck School for Boys, Inc.," VWB; Wiltwyck School For Boys, Inc., "Service Plan and Supportive Data," October 1963, 1–12, file "Committee on the Treatment Program, 1961–1969," box 2, Wiltwyck School for Boys, Inc., VWB; [Auerswald], "Study of Families of Children in Residential Treatment," 11–22, VWB; Auerswald, untitled paper, [1962], 2–9, JWP; Levine, "Report to Taconic Foundation," 1–6, VWB.

54. Oliver Zunz, *Philanthropy in America: A History* (Princeton, NJ: Princeton University Press, 2012), 201, 211.

55. Wiltwyck School for Boys, "Minutes of the Meeting of the Board of Directors," April 5, 1960, 1, folder "Board of Directors, Minutes, 1942, 1956–1960," box 1, series "Wiltwyck School for Boys, Inc.," VWB; Mrs. Robert H. Preiskel to Stephen R. Currier, December 7, 1959, folder "Committee on the Treatment Program," 1960, box 2, series "Wiltwyck School for Boys, Inc.," VWB.

56. Auerswald, untitled paper, [1962], 2–9, JWP; [Auerswald], "Study of Families of Children in Residential Treatment," 1–5, 6–7, 13–14, VWB.

57. Meeting state and local standards enabled Wiltwyck to be reimbursed for the cost of treatment. Peter Kasius to Honorable Justine Wise Polier, folder "Administration, 1948, 1954–1963," box 1, series "Wiltwyck School for Boys, Inc.," VWB; Justine Wise Polier to Board Members, August 6, 1962, folder "Administration, 1948, 1954–1963," box 1, series "Wiltwyck School for Boys, Inc.," VWB; Charles H. King to Dr. Viola Bernard, November 24, 1964, folder "Committee on the Treatment Program, 1961–1964," box 2, series "Wiltwyck School for Boys, Inc."; Wiltwyck School for Boys, Inc., program, "A Benefit for Wiltwyck School for Boys," April 11, 1965, 4, VWB; Minuchin, Auerswald, King, and Rabinowitz, "Study and Treatment of Families Who Produce Multiple Acting-Out Boys," 2, VWB; Auerswald, untitled paper, [1962], 5, JWP.

58. Dennis Doyle, "Black Celebrities, Selfhood, and Psychiatry in the Civil Rights Era: The Wiltwyck School for Boys and the Floyd Patterson House," *Social History of Medicine* 28 (May 2015): 330–50.

59. Wiltwyck School for Boys, "Minutes of the Regular Meeting of the Board of Directors," March 22, 1962, copy annotated by Viola W. Bernard, 3, folder "Minutes, 1961–1963," box 1, series "Wiltwyck School for Boys, Inc.," VWB. Dr. Butts was the Floyd Patterson House psychiatrist. Bernard helped promote his career. Auerswald, untitled paper, [1962], 6, 8, JWP.

60. Polier, "Anatomy of Three Institutions," 28–29, JWP; Auerswald, untitled paper, [1962], 6, 8, 7–9, JWP; "A Benefit for Wiltwyck School for Boys," April 11, 1965, 4–7, VWB.

61. Wiltwyck School for Boys, Inc., "Minutes of the Meeting of the Board of Directors," February 5, 1959, 8–9, VWB.

62. Wiltwyck School for Boys, Inc., "Minutes of the Meeting of the Board of Directors," March 19, 1959, 5; May 26, 1959, 4; September 24, 1959, 4, folder "Board of Directors, Minutes, 1942, 1956–1960," box 1, series "Wiltwyck School for Boys, Inc.," VWB. As late as 1962, the Harlem Neighborhoods Association executive director Milton Yale still held out hope that a relationship between Northside and Wiltwyck could be established. Milton Yale to Charles H. King, February 5, 1962, folder 8, box 48, LOC-CLARK.

63. Markowitz and Rosner, *Children, Race, and Power*, 188; Harlem Neighborhoods Association, "Annual Report: One Year of HANA (April 1960)," 1, folder 653, box 111, M. Moran Weston Papers, Rare Books and Manuscripts Library, Columbia University, New York (hereafter MMW).

64. Harlem Neighborhoods Association, "Annual Report, 1960," 4, MMW.

65. Harlem Neighborhoods Association, "Resolution for a Proposal to Mayor Wagner at HANA Community Meeting, June 15, 1960," 1, folder 653, box 111, MMW.

66. Joseph King and Marion D. Clark, "Summary Findings and Recommendations of the Mental Health Committee in Reference to the Psychiatric Services at Harlem Hospital," May 1961, 1, 2, folder 654, box 111, MMW.

67. John C. Walter, *The Harlem Fox: J. Raymond Jones and Tammany, 1920–1970* (Albany: State University of New York Press, 1989), 122–24, 139, 144, 150–61; Clarence Taylor, *Knocking at Our Own Door: Milton A. Galamison and the Struggle to Integrate New York City Schools* (Lanham, MD: Lexington, 2001), 52–55; Taylor, "Conservative and Liberal Opposition," 95, 97–99, 101, 116; Biondi, *To Stand and to Fight*, 246–47.

68. Leigh Roberts, "Introduction," in *Community Psychiatry*, ed. Leigh M. Roberts, Seymour L. Halleck, and Martin B. Loeb (Madison: University of Wisconsin Press, 1966), 6.

69. Grob, *Mad among Us*, 240–61; Pressman, *Last Resort*, 428–32.

70. Grob, *Mad among Us*, 234–35.

71. Bernard, "Some Applications of Psychoanalysis to Social Issues," 155.

72. Ibid.

73. Ibid., 154–59; Viola W. Bernard, "The Division of Community Psychiatry and the Washington Heights Program," in *Urban Challenges to Psychiatry: The Case History of a Response*, ed. Lawrence C. Kolb, Viola W. Bernard, and Bruce Dohrenwend (Boston, MA: Little, Brown, 1969), 119–37; Bernard, Interview by Senn, 21–26, VWB.

74. Bernard, "Some Applications of Psychoanalysis to Social Issues," 154–55; Bernard, Interview by Senn, 22–24, VWB: Bernard, Interview by Ackerly, 22–25, VWB; Bernard, "Division of Community Psychiatry and the Washington Heights Program," 119–24.

75. Maynard, *Surgeons to the Poor*, 209. Once the affiliation between Harlem Hospital and Columbia University became official, Ray Trussell issued a press release in 1964 touting the advantages of the relationship for the community. Dr. Ray E. Trussell and Sue Halpern, newspaper release, City of New York, Department of Hospitals, February 24, 1964, 7, folder 11, box 7, series "College of Physicians and Surgeons, Office of the Assistant Dean's Records, Archives and Special Collections, Health Sciences Library, Columbia University, New York (hereafter Yahr's Records, CU-HSL).

76. Taylor, "Conservative and Liberal Opposition," 95; Julio Vitullo-Martin, ed., *Breaking Away, the Future of Cities: Essays in Honor of Robert F. Wagner, Jr.* (New York: Twentieth Century Fund, 1996).

77. Maynard, *Surgeons to the Poor*, 209–10. This division of hospital care was typical of many large cities across the country during the 1950s. Rosemary Stevens, *In Sickness and in Wealth: American Hospitals in the Twentieth Century* (Baltimore, MD: Johns Hopkins University Press, 1989), 237, 252–53.

78. Maynard, *Surgeons to the Poor*, 209–12; Elizabeth B. Davis, "Development of a Department of Psychiatry in a General Hospital," in Spurlock, *Black Psychiatrists and American Psychiatry*, 25–57; Elizabeth B. Davis, interview, October 19, 1983, VHS tape recording, Moving Images and Recorded Sound Division, Schomburg Center for Research in Black Culture, New York Public Library, Astor, Lennox and Tilden Foundation, New York (hereafter VT-SCRBC).

79. H. Houston Merritt to Dr. Lawrence C. Kolb, April 2, 1961, folder "Harlem Hospital, 1932–1961," box 322, subseries "Dean's Code 112," Office of the Vice President for Health Sciences/Dean of the Faculty of Medicine, Central Records, 1883–2003, Archives and Special Collections, Health Sciences Library, Columbia University, New York (hereafter VP/Dean, CU-HSL); Davis, "Development of a Department of Psychiatry in a General Hospital," 25–57.

80. Elizabeth B. Davis, "Harlem Psychiatric Unit Marks Second Anniversary," *The Bulletin* [of the New York State District Branches, American Psychiatric Association] 7 (October 1964): 1–2, reprint, folder "Davis, E. B. writings," box 1, Elizabeth B. Davis Papers, Manuscripts, Archives and Rare Books Division, Schomburg Center for Research in Black Culture, New York Public Library, Astor, Lennox and Tilden Foundation, New York (hereafter EBD-SCRBC); Lawrence C. Kolb, MD, to H. Houston Merritt, MD, April 12, 1961, folder "Harlem Hospital, 1932–1961," box 322, subseries "Dean's Code 112," VP/Dean, CU-HSL; [Charles H. King?], "Proposed Plan for Association between Wiltwyck School for Boys, Residential Treatment Center and Department of Psychiatry-Harlem Hospital," [1963], folder "Proposals for Liaison Associations-Harlem Hospital, 1962–1963," box 4, series "Wiltwyck School for Boys, Inc.," VWB; Charles H. King, draft of proposal for "Affiliation of Harlem Hospital and Series: Wiltwyck School for Boys, Inc.," March 23, 1963, folder "Proposals for Liaison Associations-Harlem Hospital, 1962–1963," box 4, series "Wiltwyck School for Boys, Inc.," VWB.

81. Stevens, *In Sickness and in Wealth*, 278–79; W. Michael Byrd and Linda A. Clayton, *An American Health Dilemma: Race, Medicine, and Health Care in the United States, 1900–2000* (New York: Routledge, 2001), 205–6, 311, 329–31.

82. Biondi, *To Stand and to Fight*.

83. Davis, "Harlem Psychiatric Unit Marks Second Anniversary," 1, EBD-SCRBC.

84. Davis, "Development of a Department of Psychiatry in a General Hospital," 26.

85. Kolb was aware of HANA's proposal for an expanded psychiatric unit and welcomed its support. Kolb to Merritt, April 12, 1961, VP/Dean, CU-HSL.

86. Dr. Ray E. Trussell and Sue Halpern [City of New York Department of Hospitals], newspaper release, February 21, 1964, 1, 2, folder 11, box 7, Yahr's Records, CU-HSL.

87. Maynard, *Surgeons to the Poor*, 209–29; Ray E. Trussell, MD, to President Grayson Kirk, April 2, 1961, folder "Harlem Hospital, 1932–1961," box 322, subseries "Dean's Code 112," VP/Dean, CU-HSL; Pearson, *When Harlem Nearly Killed King*, 120–21.

88. Maynard, *Surgeons to the Poor*, 212.

89. H. Houston Merritt, MD, [Joint Committee on Harlem Hospital-Columbia University], "File Memorandum. Conference on July 12, 1961 at Harlem Hospital," folder 8, box 7, Yahr's Records, CU-HSL.

90. City of New York Department of Hospitals, Harlem Hospital-Columbia University Agreement of Psychiatric Affiliation, July 11, 1962, 1, folder "Harlem Hospital Psychiatry, Finances, 1961–1975," box 329, subseries "Dean's Code 112," VP/Dean, CU-HSL.

91. On the older Harlem Hospital physicians' resistance to Columbia control over hiring decisions and Trussell's response to the resistance, see H. Houston Merritt, MD, "File Memorandum' [on the Committee to Study Relationships with Harlem Hospital], April 21, 1961, 1, folder "Harlem Hospital, 1932–1961," box 322, subseries "Dean's Code 112," VP/Dean, CU-HSL; Ray E. Trussell, MD, to Dr. A. Charles Posner, September 5, 1962, folder 8, box 7, Yahr's Records, CU-HSL; Maynard, *Surgeons to the Poor*, 213–19. For the fate of the psychiatrist Dr. Harold Ellis, see Ray E. Trussell, MD, to Dr. Vaughan C. Mason, September 19, 1962, folder 2, box 9, Yahr's Records, CU-HSL; Dr. Ray E. Trussell, Memorandum: To All Members of the Medical Board of Harlem Hospital, November 9, 1962, 1–2, folder 8, box 7, Yahr's Records, CU-HSL.

92. Lawrence C. Kolb, MD, to Dr. Houston Merritt, May 31, 1962, folder 17, box 9, Yahr's Records, CU-HSL; Trussell to Mason, September 19, 1962, Yahr's records, CU-HSL; Trussell, Memorandum: To All Members of the Medical Board of Harlem Hospital, November 9, 1962, Yahr's Records, CU-HSL; Lawrence C. Kolb, MD, to Dr. Ray E. Trussell, November 26, 1962, folder "Harlem Hospital, 1962," box 322, subseries "Dean's Code 112," VP/Dean, CU-HSL; Harlem Hospital Center, "Announcement of Internships and Residencies Harlem Hospital," residency training program booklet, [1962?], 2, folder 5, box 7, Yahr's Records, CU-HSL; Harlem Hospital, *Training in Psychiatry* [New York: Harlem Hospital, 1963], folder "Harlem Hospital, 1963–1965," box 322, subseries "Dean's Code 112," VP/Dean, CU-HSL; William V. Thompson, MD, to Rafael R. Gamso, MD, and Elizabeth B. Davis, MD, May 27, 1964, folder "Harlem Hospital, 1963–1965," box 322, subseries "Dean's Code 112," VP/Dean, CU-HSL; Davis, "Development of a Department of Psychiatry in a General Hospital," 26–37; Stevens, *In Sickness and in Wealth*, 276.

93. Elizabeth B. Davis, Hugh F. Butts, and Trevor Lindo, "Implications for Outcome of Time-Limited Hospital Treatment," 1, paper presented at the annual American Psychiatric Association meeting, Bal Harbour, Florida, May 1969, folder "Papers Presented, Not Published, 1964–1969," Elizabeth B. Davis Papers, Archives and Special Collections, Health Sciences Library, Columbia University, New York (hereafter EBD-CU-HSL).

94. "Proposed Plan for Association between Wiltwyck School for Boys, Residential Treatment Center and Department of Psychiatry-Harlem Hospital," 2, VWB; Nate Levine to Dr. Hagop S. Mashikian, April 5, 1960, Viola W. Bernard to Dr. Jack Mashikian, February 26, 1960, Jack Mashikian to Viola W. Bernard, February 17, 1960, Folder "Committee on the Treatment Program 1960," box 2, series "Wiltwyck School for Boys, Inc.," VWB; [News clipping] "Psychiatrist Opposes Isolation of the Mentally Ill," *Medical Tribune* (August 24, 1967), 4–5, folder "Harlem Hospital, September 1967–December 1967," box 322, subseries "Dean's Code 112," VP/Dean, CU-HSL.

95. Kolb to Merritt, May 31, 1962, Yahr's Records, CU-HSL; Davis, interview, October 19, 1983, VT-SCRBC; Davis, "Development of a Department of Psychiatry in a General Hospital," 40–41; Lawrence, *Balm in Gilead*, 188–96, 196–203, 221–25, 288–94, 304.

96. Margaret Lawrence, interview by Elizabeth Auchincloss, Joanna Chapin, Henry McCurtis, and Viola W. Bernard, March 4, 1989, 4, folder "Interviews with Drs. M.L., Elizabeth Auchincloss, Joanna Chapin, Henry Curtis, 1989–1990," box 1, series "Margaret Lawrence, MD," VWB.

97. June Jackson Christmas, Interview by James Briggs Murray, June 27, 1985, VT-SCRBC.

98. Michael C. Dawson, *Behind the Mule: Race and Class in African-American Politics* (Princeton, NJ: Princeton University Press, 1995).

99. Christmas, Interview by Murray, June 27, 1985, VT-SCRBC.

100. King, draft of proposal for "Affiliation of Harlem Hospital and Series," 3, VWB; "Proposed Plan for Association between Wiltwyck School for Boys, Residential Treatment Center and Department of Psychiatry-Harlem Hospital," 2, VWB.

101. Wiltwyck School for Boys, "Minutes of the Meeting of the Board of Directors," April 25, 1963, 3–4, folder "Board of Directors, Minutes, 1961–1963," box 1, series "Wiltwyck School for Boys, Inc.," VWB.

102. [Eliza]beth Davis to Viola W. Bernard, November 14, 1962, Viola W. Bernard to Dr. Elizabeth Davis, November 21, 1962, folder "Proposals for Liaison Associations-Harlem Hospital, 1962–1963," box 4, series "Wiltwyck School for Boys, Inc.," VWB.

103. "Proposed Plan for Association between Wiltwyck School for Boys, Residential Treatment Center and Department of Psychiatry-Harlem Hospital," 2, VWB; Viola W. Bernard, memorandum, to Justine W. Polier and Charlotte Winsor, March 22, 1963, folder "Proposals for Liaison Associations-Harlem Hospital, 1962–1963," box 4, series "Wiltwyck School for Boys, Inc.," VWB; Edgar H. Auerswald to Viola Bernard, March 29, 1963, Viola W. Bernard to Edgar Auerswald, May 10, 1963, Edgar H. Auerswald to Viola Bernard, May 15, 1963, folder "Administration, 1948, 1954–1963," box 4, series "Wiltwyck School for Boys, Inc.," VWB; Elizabeth B. Davis to Charles H. King, May 20, 1963, Charles H. King to Elisabeth [*sic*] B. Davis, May 23, 1963, folder "Proposals for Liaison Associations-Harlem Hospital, 1962–1963," box 4, series "Wiltwyck School for Boys, Inc.," VWB.

104. "Proposed Plan for Association between Wiltwyck School for Boys, Residential Treatment Center and Department of Psychiatry-Harlem Hospital," 1–2, VWB. The committee's report was named for the cochairwoman Gloria Abbate.

105. Elizabeth B. Davis to Charles H. King, May 20, 1963, Elizabeth B. Davis to Viola W. Bernard, October 16, 1963, folder "Proposals for Liaison Associations-Harlem Hospital, 1962–1963," box 4, series "Wiltwyck School for Boys, Inc.," VWB.

106. Wright, "Psychiatry Comes to Harlem," 45.

Chapter Seven

1. Davis, interview, October 19, 1983, VT-SCRBC.

2. Benjamin Pasamanick, "Some Misconceptions concerning Differences in the Racial Prevalence of Mental Disease," *American Journal of Orthopsychiatry* 33 (January 1963): 75; Ralph Mason Dreger and Kent S. Miller, "Comparative Psychological Studies of Negroes and Whites in the United States: 1959–1965," monograph supplement, *Psychological Bulletin* 70, no. 3, pt. 2 (1968): 39, 47–48; Rose, *Psychology and Selfhood*, 174.

3. Lynn Hunt, *Inventing Human Rights: A History* (New York: Norton, 2007), 200–208; Thomas Jackson, *From Civil Rights to Human Rights: Martin Luther King, Jr. and the Struggle for Economic Justice* (Philadelphia: University of Pennsylvania Press, 2009), 215, 216, 224–27, 359–65.

4. Rose, *Psychology and Selfhood*, 176.

5. Elizabeth B. Davis, "From Family Membership to Personal and Social Identity," paper for "The Negro Family" symposium, University of California at Berkeley, November 6–8, 1964, 1, folder "Papers Presented, Not Published, 1964–1969," EBD-CU-HSL.

6. Thomas, *Puerto Rican Citizen*; Brilliant, *Color of America Has Changed.*

7. Scott, *Contempt and Pity*; Sugrue, *Sweet Land of Liberty.*

8. Alexander Thomas and Samuel Sillen, *Racism and Psychiatry* (New York: Brunner/Mazel, 1972), 65. Lasch-Quinn, *Race Experts*, 115.

9. Thomas and Sillen, *Racism and Psychiatry*, 58.

10. Ibid., 59.

11. William H. Grier and Price M. Cobbs, *Black Rage*, rev. ed. (New York: Basic Books, 1992), 177, 178–79.

12. Thomas and Sillen, *Racism and Psychiatry*, 66.

13. Scott, *Contempt and Pity*, 163–83.

14. Thomas and Sillen, *Racism and Psychiatry*, 58.

15. Metzl, *Protest Psychosis*, 104, 126–28; Rychetta Watkins, *Black Power, Yellow Power, and the Making of Revolutionary Identities* (Jackson: University of Mississippi Press, 2014), 4–7, 15, 24, 33, 36, 45–46, 49.

16. Lasch-Quinn, *Race Experts*, 120. See also Scott, *Contempt and Pity*, 161–85.

17. Grier and Cobbs, *Black Rage*, 210. See also Lasch-Quinn, *Race Experts*, 76–85; Scott, *Contempt and Pity*, 102–3; Thomas and Sillen, *Racism and Psychiatry*, 54–55.

18. Grier and Cobbs, *Black Rage*, 161, 178.

19. Ibid., 154–55.

20. Rose, *Psychology and Selfhood*, 176. For liberal criticism of *Black Rage*, see Hugh F. Butts, "Review of William H. Grier and Price M. Cobbs, *Black Rage*," *Journal of Negro Education* 38 (Spring 1969): 166–68.

21. Berlant, *Female Complaint*, 56.

22. Joseph, "Introduction," 8.

23. Berlant, *Female Complaint*, 6, 57. According to Peniel Joseph, by 1963, the Harlem native "Baldwin became the freedom movement's most revered public intellectual" (Joseph, *Waiting 'Til the Midnight Hour*, 69).

24. Joseph, "Introduction," 3.

25. Dittmer, *Good Doctors*, 100.

26. Alvin F. Poussaint, "The Black Child's Image of the Future," in *Learning for Tomorrow: The Role of the Future in Education*, ed. Alfred Toffler (New York: Vintage, 1972), 60. See also Alvin F. Poussaint, "A Negro Psychiatrist Explains the Negro Psyche," *New York Times Magazine*, August 20, 1967, 52–58, 73–80; Alvin F. Poussaint, "Education and Black Self-Image, No. 4, 1968," in *Freedomways Reader: Prophets in Their Own Country*, ed. Esther Cooper Jackson (Boulder, CO: Westview Press, 2000), 222–28.

27. Robert Coles, *Children in Crisis: A Study of Courage and Fear* (Boston, MA: Little, Brown, 1967), 348. The community psychiatrist June Jackson Christmas, one of Davis's first hires in 1962, made a similar claim. June Jackson Christmas, "Community Psychiatry and Work in the Public Sector, 1962–1980," in Spurlock, *Black Psychiatrists and American Psychiatry*, 52.

28. Dreger and Miller, "Comparative Psychological Studies," 44.

29. Viola W. Bernard, "Some Principles of Dynamic Psychiatry in Relation to Poverty," *American Journal of Psychiatry* 122 (September 1965): 265.

30. Thomas and Sillen, *Racism and Psychiatry*, 59; Berlant, *Female Complaint*, 111, 307n30.

31. Hugh F. Butts, "Skin Color Perception and Self-Esteem," *Journal of Negro Education* 32 (Spring 1963): 122–28; Davis, "From Family Membership to Personal and Social Identity," 5–7, EBD-CU-HSL; Elizabeth B. Davis, "Position Paper," August 21, 1967, 1–5, folder "Papers Presented, Not Published, 1964–1969," EBD-CU-HSL.

32. August de Belmont Hollingshead and Frederick C. Redlich, "Social Stratification and Psychiatric Disorders," *American Sociological Review* 18 (1953): 163–69; August de Belmont Hollingshead and Frederick C. Redlich, *Social Class and Mental Illness* (New York: John Wright and Sons, 1958); John Spiegel, "Some Cultural Aspects of Transference and Countertransference," in *Individual and Family Dynamics*, ed. J. H. Masserman (New York: Grune and Stratton, 1959), 160–82; Normal W. Nell and John Spiegel, "Social Psychiatry," *Archives in General Psychiatry* 14 (1966): 337–45; Alexander H. Leighton, "Poverty and Social Change," *Scientific American* 212 (May 1965): 21–27; Leo Srole, *Mental Health in the Metropolis: The Midtown Manhattan Study* (New York: McGraw-Hill, 1962).

33. Bernard, "Some Principles of Dynamic Psychiatry," 254–55, 261; Viola W. Bernard and DeWitt Crandall, "Evidence for Various Hypotheses of Social Psychiatry," in *Social Psychiatry*, ed. Joseph Zubin and Fritz A. Freyhan (New York: Grune and Stratton, 1968), 201–2; Joe Yamamoto and Marcia Kraft Coin, "On the Treatment of the Poor," *American Journal of Psychiatry* 122 (September 1965): 267; Elizabeth Davis, "Mental Health Services for the Inner City," 2, EBD-CU-HSL; [Auerswald], "Study of Families of Children in Residential Treatment," 4, 7, VWB.

34. Bernard, "Some Principles of Dynamic Psychiatry," 255.

35. Elizabeth B. Davis, "The American Negro: From Family Membership to Personal and Social Identity," paper presented at the 72nd Annual Convention of the National Medical Association, St. Louis, Missouri, August 9, 1967, 8, 13, folder "Davis, E. B., Writings-Papers," EBD-SCRBC; Davis, "From Family Membership to Personal and Social Identity," 6, EBD-CU-HSL. See also Davis, "Position Paper," August 21, 1967, 2, EBD-CU-HSL.

36. Salvador Minuchin, *Families of the Slums: An Exploration of Their Structure and Treatment* (New York: Basic Books, 1967), 21–40.

37. I am indebted to the historian Mical Raz for helping me place the culture of poverty and cultural deprivation models in their proper chronology.

38. Scott, *Contempt and Pity*, 137–55; Raz, *What's Wrong with the Poor;* Herman, *Romance of American Psychology;* Laura Briggs, *Reproducing Empire: Race, Sex, Science, and U.S. Imperialism in Puerto Rico* (Berkeley: University of California Press, 2002), 3–4, 162–88.

39. Minuchin, Auerswald, King, and Rabinowitz, "Study and Treatment of Families Who Produce Multiple Acting-Out Boys," 1–14, VWB. For more on Minuchin, see Weinstein, *The Pathological Family;* and Joan Jacobs Brumberg, *Fasting Girls: The History of Anorexia Nervosa* (New York: Plume, 1989), 29.

40. Minuchin, *Families of the Slums*, 5.

41. Ibid., 349–52.

42. Ibid., 371.

43. Minuchin, Auerswald, King, and Rabinowitz, "Study and Treatment of Families Who Produce Multiple Acting-Out Boys," 10, VWB.

44. Minuchin, *Families of the Slums*, 372.

45. Ibid., 22 (see also ix, x, 5–6, 24–25, 352); Minuchin, Auerswald, King, and Rabinowitz, "Study and Treatment of Families Who Produce Multiple Acting-Out Boys," 4–8, VWB.

46. Minuchin, *Families of the Slums*, 10–11, 144–45, 193, 196–98, 202, 206, 211–15, 220.

47. Ibid., 4–5, 36, 196–98, 213–14, 351, 372–76.

48. Ibid., 351.

49. Ibid., 30.

50. Berlant, *Female Complaint*, 268.

51. Bernard, "Dynamic Psychiatry in Relation to Poverty," 257.

52. Minuchin, *Families Of the Slums*, 29, 144–45, 287, 289, 356–57, 366–67, 370–71.

53. Davis, "Position Paper," August 21, 1967, 4, EBD-CU-HSL.

54. Bernard and Crandall, "Evidence for Various Hypotheses," 203.

55. Kenneth B. Clark, *Dark Ghetto: Dilemmas of Social Power* (New York: Harper & Row, 1965); William Ryan, *Blaming the Victim* (New York: Vintage, 1972).

56. Davis, "American Negro," 7, EBD-SCRBC; Minuchin, *Families of the Slums*, 22; Herbert J. Gans, *The Urban Villagers: Group and Class in the Life of Italian Americans* (New York: Free Press, 1965).

57. Bernard, "Dynamic Psychiatry in Relation to Poverty," 257.

58. Dreger and Miller, "Comparative Psychological Studies," 44.

59. Fraser and Gordon, "A Genealogy of *Dependency*," 310; Scott, *Contempt and Pity*, 144; Herman, *Romance of American Psychology*, 205; Briggs, *Reproducing Empire*, 440; Thomas and Sillen, *Racism and Psychiatry*, 67.

60. Thomas and Sillen, *Racism and Psychiatry*, 67.

61. Davis, "Mental Health Services for the Inner City," 15, EBD-CU-HSL.

62. Davis, interview, October 19, 1983, VT-SCRBC.

63. Biondi, *To Stand and to Fight*, 239. The historical literature on the postwar racialization of residential space in the United States is extensive. For New York, see Nicholas Dagan Bloom, *Public Housing That Worked: New York in the Twentieth Century* (Philadelphia: University of Pennsylvania Press, 2009); Joel Schwartz, *The New York Approach: Robert Moses, Urban Liberals, and Redevelopment of the Inner City* (Columbus: The Ohio State University Press, 1993).

64. Douglas Massey and Nancy A Denton, *American Apartheid: Segregation and the Making of the Underclass* (Cambridge, MA: Harvard University Press, 1993), 49; Michael B. Katz, Mark J. Stern, and Jamie J. Fader, "The New African American Inequality," *Journal of American History* 92 (June 2005): 75–108; Clark, "Proposed Study of Public Schools in the Harlem Community, 1953," 1–3, LOC-CLARK.

65. Biondi, *To Stand and to Fight*, 235–41, 248; Lipsitz, *How Racism Takes Place*, 110–16; Massey and Denton, *American Apartheid*, 60–185.

66. Felicia Kornbluh, *The Battle for Welfare Rights: Politics and Poverty in Modern America* (Philadelphia: University of Pennsylvania Press, 2007), 23; Abu-Lughod, *Race, Space, and Riots*, 171–76, 179; Joseph, *Waiting 'Til the Midnight Hour*, 111–17; Stefan M. Bradley, *Harlem vs. Columbia University: Black Student Power in the Late 1960s* (Urbana: University of Illinois Press, 2009), 18; Sugrue, *Sweet Land of Liberty*, 406; Gill, *Harlem*, 400–402.

67. Jacob Levenson, *The Secret Epidemic: The Story of AIDS and Black America* (New York: Anchor, 2004), 81.

68. Robert Lipsyte, *The Contender* (New York: Bantam, 1980), 1.

69. B. F. Skinner, *Beyond Freedom and Dignity* (New York: Bantam, 1972), 189.

70. Lipsitz, *How Racism Takes Place*, 13, 15, 60, 112 123, 245.

71. Some residents did view central Harlem's problems as intractable. See Claude Brown, "Nobody Wants to Hear That Nonsense in Harlem," *New Republic* 153 (October 16, 1965): 20; Sugrue, *Sweet Land of Liberty*, 410–14.

72. Markowitz and Rosner, *Children, Race, and Power*, 184, 194–99; Joseph, *Wait 'Til the Midnight Hour*, 99.

73. Markowitz and Rosner, *Children, Race, and Power*, 89, 120–25; Taylor, "Conservative and Liberal Opposition," and Martha Biondi, "Brooklyn College Belongs to Us: Black Studies and the Transformation of Public Higher Education in New York City," in Taylor, *Civil Rights in New York City: From World War II to the Giuliani Era*, 95–117, 161–81.

74. Joseph, "Introduction," 3.

75. Klytus Smith, et al., *The Harlem Cultural/Political Movements, 1960–1970: From Malcolm X to Black Is Beautiful* (New York: Gumbs & Thomas, 1995), 1–4, 17–18, 40–41, 46–47, 63, 83, 95–99; Young, *Soul Power*, 55–99; Joseph, *Waiting 'Til the Midnight Hour*, 44, 45, 55, 68, 73, 97–102, 119, 121, 125–26, 147; Bradley, *Harlem vs. Columbia University*, 2, 11, 48, 53–57, 74–75, 88–89.

76. Devin Fergus, *Liberalism, Black Power, and the Making of American Politics, 1965–1980* (Athens: University of Georgia Press, 2009), 233. According to Fergus, racial liberals drew ideas from black leftists in the late 1960s. The historian Lorrin Thomas reasons that this was possible because postwar liberalism was "flexible and able to incorporate many new ideas, especially racial justice in certain forms" (*Puerto Rican Citizen*, 20).

77. Markowitz and Rosner, *Children, Race, and Power*, 197.

78. Herman, *Kinship by Design*.

79. Davis, interview, October 19, 1983, VT-SCRBC.

80. Elizabeth B. Davis, "Implementation of Principles of Community Psychiatry, Its Opportunities and Problems," 3–4, paper presented at meeting of the New Haven Area Mental Health Association, January 29, 1969, folder "Papers Presented, Not Published, 1964–1969," EBD-CU-HSL.

81. Ibid., 4.

82. Parent's Action Committee for Equality, "Memorandum," March 11, 1965, 4, folder 8, box 6, Harlem Neighborhoods Association Papers, Manuscripts, Archives and Rare Books Division, Schomburg Center for Research in Black Culture (hereafter HANA, SCRBC); Davis, "Implementation of Principles of Community Psychiatry," 4, EBD-CU-HSL; Davis, "Mental Health Services for the Inner City," 10, EBD-CU-HSL.

83. Milton Yale, "Report of the Conference of the Mental Health Committee of the Harlem Neighborhoods Association [entitled "Mental Health Needs of Harlem Youth]," June 17, 1963, 1–16, folder 4, box 6, HANA, SCRBC.

84. Joseph King and James Soler, form letter, June 30, 1965, folder 6, box 6, HANA, SCRBC; HANA, flyer for "Community Conference on School Suspensions," January 10, 1968, folder 6, box 6, HANA, SCRBC. See also "Disruptive Child Issue Protested," *School Parent* 24 (October 1967): 3, folder 6, box 6, HANA, SCRBC; Mrs. Thomas B. Hess, memo, April 5, 1967, folder 6, box 5, HANA, SCRBC; Citizens' Committee for Children, "Preserving the Right to an Education for all Children," 1–7, folder 6, box 5, HANA, SCRBC; Citizens' Committee for Children of New York, Inc., "Notes regarding School Suspension Conferences Attended," April 20, 1967, 1–5, folder 6, box 5, HANA, SCRBC; Marvin E. Perkins to Dr. Bernard E. Donovan, November 3, 1966, folder 5, Box 9, Bernard E. Donovan files, Special Collections, Milbank Memorial Library, Teachers College, Columbia University, New York.

85. Davis, "Implementation of the Principles of Community Psychiatry," 3, EBD-CU-HSL. See also James Soler, form letter, November 3, 1965, folder 6, box 6, HANA, SCRBC.

86. James Soler to Dr. Cesarina Paoli, June 18, 1965, folder 6, box 6, HANA, SCRBC.

87. Harlem Neighborhoods Association, Inc., Ad Hoc Committee on School Suspensions, "Summary Minutes," July 14, 1965, 1–2, October 27, [1965], 1–2, folder 7, box 6, HANA, SCRBC.

88. Harlem Neighborhoods Association, Inc., Ad Hoc Committee on School Suspensions, "A Summary Review," [November 1965], 6, folder 7, box 6, HANA, SCRBC. Soler encouraged other activists join the effort by telling them that Harlem Hospital had already gotten involved. James Soler to Dr. Mamie Clark, October 21, 1965, James Soler to Schools Suspension Study Committee [New York City Board of Education], June 18, 1965, folder 6, box 6, HANA, SCRBC; Soler, form letter, November 3, 1965, HANA, SCRBC.

89. See also Lipsitz, *How Racism Takes Place*, 58.

90. Davis, "Implementation of the Principles of Community Psychiatry," 4–5, EBD-CU-HSL.

91. The psychiatrist Virginia Wilking headed the special nursery school.

92. Division of Child Psychiatry, Department of Psychiatry, Harlem Hospital Center, "Protocol for the Further Development of a Psychiatric Pre-school Program," [January 1968], 2, folder "Harlem Hospital Center," box 48, SP-SCRBC; Elizabeth Baillet to Father Weston, January 2, 1968, Virginia Wilking to Father Weston, February 20, 1968, folder "Harlem Hospital Center," box 48, SP-SCRBC; Davis, "Implementation of the Principles of Community Psychiatry," 3, EBD-CU-HSL.

93. Davis, interview, October 19, 1983, VT-SCRBC.

94. Christmas, Interview by Murray, June 12, 1985, VT-SCRBC; Markowitz and Rosner, *Children, Race, and Power,* 122; Dittmer, *Good Doctors,* x, 54; Biondi, "Brooklyn College Belongs to Us," 162–63; Gill, *Harlem,* 387–88.

95. Grob, *Mad among Us,* 257–58, 279, 282; Metzl, *Protest Psychosis,* 134.

96. Christmas, Interview by Murray, June 27, 1985, VT-SCRBC.

97. Grob, *Mad among Us,* 267–68.

98. Bonnie Lefkowitz, *Community Health Centers: A Movement and the People Who Made It Happen* (New Brunswick, NJ: Rutgers University Press, 2007), 6–13; Byrd and Clayton, *An American Health Dilemma,* 219; Dittmer, *Good Doctors,* 62, 63, 65, 82.

99. Christmas, "Community Psychiatry and Work in the Public Sector, 1962–1980," 52.

100. "Psychiatrist Opposes Isolation of the Mentally Ill," 1, VP/Dean, CU-HSL; Christmas, Interview by Murray, June 27, 1985, VT-SCRBC.

101. Sugrue, *Sweet Land of Liberty,* 364–74.

102. "Psychiatrist Opposes Isolation of the Mentally Ill," 1, VP/Dean, CU-HSL.

103. Public Relations, Columbia-Presbyterian Medical Center, newspaper release, May 2, 1967, 1, folder "Harlem Hospital, March, 1967–August 1967," box 322, subseries "Dean's Code 112," VP/Dean, CU-HSL.

104. Christmas, "Community Psychiatry and Work in the Public Sector, 1962–1980," 51, 54. See also June Jackson Christmas, "Group Methods in Training and Practice: Nonprofessional Mental Health Personnel in a Deprived Community," *American Journal of Orthopsychiatry* 36 (April 1966): 410–19; Christmas, Interview by Murray, June 27, 1985, VT-SCRBC; "Psychiatrist Opposes Isolation of the Mentally Ill," 1, VP/Dean, CU-HSL.

105. Christmas, Interview by Murray, June 27, 1985, VT-SCRBC.

106. Ibid.; Department of Psychiatry, Harlem Hospital Center, press release, July 17, 1966, 2, folder "Harlem Hospital, January 1966–August 1966," box 322, subseries "Dean's Code 112," VP/Dean, CU-HSL.

107. Public Relations, Columbia-Presbyterian Medical Center, newspaper release, May 2, 1967, 1–4, VP/Dean, CU-HSL.

108. Lipsitz, *How Racism Takes Place,* 56.

109. Christmas, Interview by Murray, June 27, 1985, VT-SCRBC. In addition, they also helped their clients to wade through the mixed messages directed at people—especially young women—receiving public assistance during an era of heavy backlash against AFDC and other social welfare programs. Kornbluh, *Battle for Welfare Rights,* 25.

110. Christmas, "Community Psychiatry and Work in the Public Sector, 1962–1980," 53.

111. Division of Rehabilitation Services, Department of Psychiatry, Harlem Hospital Center, "A Proposal Submitted to the President's Committee on Urban-Minority Problems, Columbia University," January 1968, 1–7, folder 1, box 10, Yahr's Records, CU-HSL; Mrs. Harriett Carter, "Varying Roles of the Mental Health Aide," 1–15, Mrs. Hilda Wallace, "Purpose, Goals, and Achievement of a Work-for-Pay Program," 1–8, Mrs. Viola Washington, "The Orientation and Work of a New Psychiatric Rehabilitation Worker," 1–10, papers presented at the 5th Annual National Meeting of the Psychiatric Out Patient Center of America, March 22, 1967, folder "Writings, Other Authors," EBD-SCRBC; Christmas, Interview by Murray,

June 27, 1985, VT-SCRBC; newsclippings from the *New York Amsterdam News*, [May 27, 1967], folder "Harlem Hospital, March, 1967–August 1967," box 322, subseries "Dean's Code 112," VP/Dean, CU-HSL; Department of Psychiatry, Harlem Hospital Center, press release, July 17, 1966, VP/Dean, CU-HSL.

112. Christmas, Interview by Murray, June 27, 1985, VT-SCRBC. For the lay workers' individual perspectives, see Carter, "Varying Roles of the Mental Health Aide," 1–15; Wallace, "Purpose, Goals, and Achievement of a Work-for-Pay Program," 1–8; and Washington, "The Orientation and Work of a New Psychiatric Rehabilitation Worker," 1–10, EBD-SCRBC.

113. Lipsitz, *How Racism Takes Place*, 60.

114. Christmas, "Group Methods in Training and Practice," 410; Christmas, "Community Psychiatry and Work in the Public Sector, 1962–1980," 56; Christmas, Interview by Murray, June 27, 1985, VT-SCRBC; June Jackson Christmas, MD to Dr. E. B. Davis, May 2, 1968, folder 1, box 10, Yahr's Records, CU-HSL.

115. Metzl, *Protest Psychosis*, xii.

116. Ibid., x–xiii, 15–16, 25–26, 34–40, 41, 56–57, 93–99, 151–59, 187–92.

117. Metzl, *Protest Psychosis*, 94, 108, 154–59, 190, 202, 203.

118. Laura D. Hirshbein, *American Melancholy: Constructions of Depression in the Twentieth Century* (New Brunswick, NJ: Rutgers University Press, 2009), 64, 110, 117; Hirshbein, "Sex and Gender in Psychiatry," 161.

119. Elizabeth B. Davis, discussion of "Multipregnancies in Multiproblem Families: The Chronic Postpartum Reactions," 3, paper presented at meeting of the American Psychoanalytic Association, May 11, 1968, Boston, Massachusetts, folder "Davis, E. B., Writings-Papers," EBD-SCRBC.

120. Davis, "American Negro," 7, EBD-SCRBC.

121. Ibid. For more on the medical profession's support for the sterilization program, see H. D. Kruse, MD, to Dr. Ray E. Trussell, April 7, 1964, folder 8, box 7, Yahr's Records, CU-HSL.

122. Davis, interview, October 19, 1983, VT-SCRBC.

123. Davis, discussion of "Multipregnancies in Multiproblem Families," 5–9, EBD-SCRBC; Davis, "Implementation of Principles of Community Psychiatry," 8–9, EBD-CU-HSL; Burton Lerner, Raymond Raskin, and Elizabeth B. Davis, "On the Need to Be Pregnant," *International Journal of Psychoanalysis* 48 (1967): 288–97.

124. Davis, discussion of "Multipregnancies in Multiproblem Families," 7, EBD-SCRBC. Davis claimed: "It is well-known that unplanned, and particularly unplanned, out-of-wedlock pregnancies are very common in the low socio-economic sector of the urban Negro population." Davis, "Implementation of Principles of Community Psychiatry," 8, 9, EBD-CU-HSL.

125. Davis, discussion of "Multipregnancies in Multiproblem Families," 6, 7, EBD-SCRBC.

126. Davis, "Implementation of Principles of Community Psychiatry," 9–13, EBD-CU-HSL (see also 3, 4, 5).

127. Elaine Tyler May, *America and the Pill: A History of Promise, Peril, and Liberation* (New York: Basic Books, 2010); Grob, *Mad among Us*, 273–78.

128. Rickie Solinger, *Pregnancy and Power: A Short History of Reproductive Politics in America* (New York: New York University Press, 2005), 186–203; Byrd and Clayton, *An American Health Dilemma*, 284–85, 448–59; Simone M. Caron, "Birth Control and the

Black Community in the 1960s: Genocide or Power Politics," *Journal of Social History* 31 (Spring 1998): 545–69; Dorothy Roberts, *Killing the Black Body: Race, Reproduction, and the Meaning of Liberty* (New York: Pantheon, 1997), 89–103; Robert Weisbord, *Genocide? Birth Control and the Black American* (New York: Greenwood Press, 1975).

129. Solinger, *Pregnancy and Power*, 191–94; Roberts, *Killing the Black Body*, 98–103; Weisbord, *Genocide?* 110–21.

130. Donald P. Swartz, MD to Dr. Jean Pakter, December 21, 1967, folder 23, box 8, Yahr's Records, CU-HSL; Donald P. Swartz, MD, to Dr. J. George Moore, September 14, 1967, folder 23, box 8, Yahr's Records, CU-HSL; James Soler and Donald P. Swartz, MD, "Harlem Neighborhood Family Planning Project: A Proposal to Increase the Patient Load for Family Planning Services at the Harlem Hospital Center," August 15, 1967, folder 23, box 8, Yahr's Records, CU-HSL. See Ray E. Trussell to Dean Houston Merritt, folder 11, box 7, Yahr's Records, CU-HSL. Entering 1967, most of the hospital's population was indigent; 94 percent of Harlem Hospital's patients were eligible for Medicaid.

131. Bradley, *Harlem vs. Columbia University*, 17, 21, 48, 53, 57–166.

132. Ibid., 36, 37.

133. Joseph, "Introduction," 20.

134. Cathy Aldridge, "Harlem Hospital Protests," *New York Amsterdam News*, May 4, 1968, 1; Dick Edwards, "Harlem Genocide? Answer Seems Yes!" *New York Amsterdam News*, July 20, 1968, 1; Barbara Yuncker, "A Tale of 2 Hospitals: Race Was Added to Delays in Construction," *New York Post*, July 8, 1967, 8; Michael Rothfeld to Dr. Truman, folder 23, box 8, Yahr's Records, CU-HSL; Michael Meltsner to Hon. Joseph V. Terenzio, June 23, 1967, folder 3, box 8, Yahr's Records, CU-HSL; Harold G. Logan to H. Houston Merritt, MD, internal memorandum [June 1968], folder 11, box 7, Yahr's Records, CU-HSL; Ray E. Trussell to Charles Brown, MD, February 27, 1967, folder "Harlem Hospital, February 1967," box 322, subseries "Dean's Code 112," VP/Dean, CU-HSL; Ray E. Trussell to Dean Houston Merritt, February 8, 1967, folder 11, box 7, Yahr's Records, CUHSL; Cornelius McDougald to Hon. John V. Lindsay, February 20, 1967, and Arnold J. Boyce to Melvin Yahr [*sic*], April 8, 1967, folder 3, box 8, Yahr's Records, CU-HSL; Harriet Pickens to Hon. Joseph V. Terenzio, January 25, 1967, folder "Harlem Hospital, February 1967," box 322, subseries "Dean's Code 112," VP/Dean, CU-HSL.

135. Bradley, *Harlem vs. Columbia University*, 178–79. Columbia University's administration got wind of this conspiracy theory. To assuage local malcontents, Columbia took out an advertisement in Harlem's *New York Amsterdam News* declaring that Harlem Hospital was still a public institution serving the needs of local residents. In 1967, Dr. Donald Swartz, Harlem Hospital's head of obstetrics and gynecology, had even drafted a preemptive press release in the event that Black Power opposition to birth control and family planning at Harlem Hospital became, in his words, a "situation." Donald P. Swartz to Dr. M. Yahr, memorandum, December 27, 1967, and Donald P. Swartz. MD, "Draft," December 12, 1967, folder 1, box 9, Yahr's Records CU-HSL.

136. Davis, interview, October 19, 1983, VT-SCRBC.

Conclusion

Epigraph. Jorge Luis Borges, *Ficciones* (New York: Grove Press, 1962), 115.

1. Metzl, *Protest Psychosis*, ix–xxi.

2. Ibid.

3. Barbara J. Fields, *Racecraft: The Soul of Inequality in American Life* (New York: Verso, 2012); Jacobson, *Whiteness of a Different Color*, 142–45, 170.

4. Brattain, "Race, Racism, and Antiracism," 1386–1413.

5. Uday S. Mehta, "Liberal Strategies of Exclusion," in *Tensions of Empire: Colonial Cultures in a Bourgeois World*, ed. Frederick Cooper and Ann Laura Stoler (Berkeley: University of California Press, 1997), 62.

6. Thomas, *Puerto Rican Citizen*, 18–20, 222–27, 250.

7. Metzl, *Protest Psychosis*, 104, 200–203.

8. Since the 1970s, the literature on the research, handling, and treatment of black patients has become voluminous. The following is a mere sample: Robert T. Carter, ed., *Theory and Research*, vol. 1 of *Handbook of Racial-Cultural Psychology and Counseling* (Hoboken, NJ: John Wiley, 2005); Robert T. Carter, *The Influence of Race and Racial Identity in Psychotherapy: Towards a Racially Inclusive Model* (New York: John Wiley, 1995); Jeffrey Scott Mio and Gayle Y. Iwamesa, eds., *Culturally Diverse Mental Health: The Challenges of Research and Resistance* (New York: Brunner-Routledge, 2003); Suman Fernando, *Mental Health, Race and Culture*, 2nd ed. (New York: Palgrave, 2002); Alvin F. Poussaint and Amy Alexander, *Lay My Burden Down: Unraveling Suicide and the Mental Health Crisis among African-Americans* (Boston, MA: Beacon Press, 2000); Donald R. Atkinson, George Morten, and Derold W. Sue, *Counseling American Minorities*, 5th ed. (Boston, MA: McGraw Hill, 1998); Dorothy S. Ruiz, ed., *Handbook of Mental Health and Mental Disorder among Black Americans* (New York: Greenwood Press, 1990); Joseph L. White, *The Psychology of Blacks: An Afro-American Perspective* (Englewood Cliffs, NJ: Prentice-Hall, 1984); Reginald L. Jones, *Black Psychology*, 2nd ed. (New York: Harper & Row, 1980); Roger Wilcox, ed., *The Psychological Consequences of Being a Black American: A Sourcebook of Research by Black Psychologists* (New York: Wiley & Sons, 1971).

9. Viola W. Bernard, annotated clipping of Alvin F. Poussaint and James P. Comer, "The Question Every Black Parent Asks: What Shall I Tell My Child?" *Redbook*, January 1971, 64, 110, 111, 112, 113, folder "Black Mental Health and Social Work Issues, Relevant Literature, 1946–1984," box 2, series "Racism," VWB. According to Ann Laura Stoler, "marginalia" can be "moments of breach" where a reader's scribbled comment indicates that "something's not as it should be within" what he or she was reading. Stoler, "Interview," 502–3.

10. James P. Comer and Alvin F. Poussaint, *Raising Black Children: Two Leading Psychiatrists Confront the Educational, Social, and Emotional Problems Facing Black Children* (New York: Plume, 1992), 14, 15.

11. Frances Cress Welsing, *The Isis Papers: The Keys to Color* (Chicago: Third World Press, 1991).

12. Bernard, "Mental Hygiene and the Negro Community," 5, VWB.

13. Metzl, *Prozac on the Couch*; Metzl, *Protest Psychosis*.

14. Brickman, *Aboriginal Populations in the Mind*.

15. Winant, *Racial Conditions*, 27, 53, 67, 75; HoSang, *Racial Propositions*, 264–74; Michelle Alexander, *The New Jim Crow: Mass Incarceration in the Age of Colorblindness* (New York: New Press, 2010), 224–36; Eduardo Bonilla-Silva, *Racism without Racists: Color-Blind Racism and the Persistence of Racial Inequality in the United States*, 3rd ed. (New York: Rowman & Littlefield, 2010), 25–73.

16. Robert C. Schwartz and Kevin P. Feisthamel, "Disproportionate Diagnosis of Mental Disorders among African Americans versus European American Clients: Implications for Counseling Theory, Research, and Practice," *Journal of Counseling & Development* 87 (Summer 2009): 295–301; Metzl, *Protest Psychosis*, ix–xi; Michael K. Brown, Martin Camoy, Elliott Currie, and Troy Duster, *Whitewashing Race: The Myth of a Color-Blind Society* (Berkeley: University of California Press, 2005), 141–44; Mio and Iwamesa, *Culturally Diverse Mental Health*, 150; Poussaint and Alexander, *Lay My Burden Down*, 146; Atkinson, Morten, and Sue, *Counseling American Minorities*, 52–53, 60–61, 65; Ruiz, *Handbook of Mental Health*, 232–33.

Bibliography

Archival Sources

Archives and Special Collections, Health Sciences Library, Columbia University, New York

Viola W. Bernard Papers (VWB)

College of Physicians and Surgeons, Office of the Assistant Dean's Records (Yahr's Records, CU-HSL)

Elizabeth B. Davis Papers (EBD-CU-HSL)

Office of the Vice President for Health Sciences / Dean of the Faculty of Medicine, Central Records, 1883–2003 (VP/Dean, CU-HSL)

Beinecke Rare Book and Manuscript Library, Yale University, New Haven, Connecticut

Richard Wright Papers (RWPYU)

Manuscript Division, Library of the United States Congress, Washington, DC

Kenneth B. Clark Papers (LOC-CLARK)

NAACP Papers, part 2

Dr. Fredric Wertham Papers (FWP)

Manuscripts, Archives, and Rare Books Division, Schomburg Center for Research in Black Culture, New York Public Library, Astor, Lennox, and Tilden Foundation, New York

Elizabeth B. Davis Papers (EBD-SCRBC)

Harlem Neighborhoods Association Papers (HANA, SCRBC)

Lafargue Clinic Records (LFC-SCRBC)

St. Philips Episcopal Church Records (SP-SCRBC)

Rare Books and Manuscripts Library, Columbia University, New York

M. Moran Weston Papers (MMW)

Schlesinger Library, Radcliffe Institute for Advanced Study, Cambridge, Massachusetts

Justine Wise Polier Papers (JWP)

Special Collections, Brooklyn College Library, Brooklyn, New York

Lauretta Bender Papers (LBP)

Special Collections, Milbank Memorial Library, Teachers College, Columbia University, New York

Bernard E. Donovan files

Published Sources

Abu-Lughod, Janet. *Race, Space, and Riots in Chicago, New York, and Los Angeles.* New York: Oxford University Press, 2007.

Adams, Walter. "The Negro Patient in Psychiatric Treatment." *American Journal of Orthopsychiatry* 20 (April 1950): 305–10.

Adler, Alexandra. "The Work of Paul Schilder." In *Paul Schilder: Mind Explorer,* edited by Donald A. Shaskan and William L. Roller, 69–81. New York: Human Sciences Press, 1985.

Ahad, Badia Sahar. *Freud Upside Down: African American Literature and Psychoanalytic Culture.* Urbana: University of Illinois Press, 2010.

Alexander, Michelle. *The New Jim Crow: Mass Incarceration in the Age of Colorblindness.* New York: New Press, 2010.

Alexander, Ruth M. *The "Girl Problem": Female Sexual Delinquency in New York, 1900–1930.* Ithaca, NY: Cornell University Press, 1995.

Allen, Walker M. "Paul Laurence Dunbar, a Study in Genius." *Psychoanalytic Review* 25 (1938): 53–82.

Anderson, Jeffrey E. *Conjure in African American Society.* Baton Rouge: University of Louisiana Press, 2005.

Anderson, Jervis. *This Was Harlem: A Cultural Portrait, 1900–1950.* New York: Farrar Straus Giroux, 1982.

Antler, Joyce. *The Journey Home: Jewish Women and the American Century* (New York: Free Press, 1997.

———. "Justine Wise Polier and the Prophetic Tradition." In *Women and American Judaism: Historical Perspectives,* edited by Pamela S. Nadell and Jonathan D. Sarna, 268–90. Boston, MA: Brandeis University Press, 2001.

Atkinson, Donald R., George Morten, and Derold W. Sue. *Counseling American Minorities.* 5th ed. Boston, MA: McGraw Hill, 1998.

Ayer, Gertrude Elise. "Notes on My Native Sons." In Clarke, *Harlem,* 137–45.

Bailey, A. Peter. *The Harlem Hospital Story: 110 Years of Struggle against Illness, Struggle, and Genocide.* Richmond, VA: Native Sun, 1991.

Bailey, Pearce. "A Contribution to the Mental Pathology of the United States." *Archives of Neurology and Psychiatry* 7 (February 1922): 183–201.

Bains, Jatinder. "Race, Culture, and Psychiatry: A History of Transcultural Psychiatry." *History of Psychiatry* 16 (June 2005): 139–54.

Barkan, Elazar. *The Retreat of Scientific Racism: Changing Concepts of Race in Britain and the United States between the World Wars.* New York: Cambridge University Press, 1993.

Barker, Prince. "Psychoanalysis of Groups." *Journal of the National Medical Association* 6 (November 1952): 455–56.

Bayor, Ronald H. *Fiorello La Guardia: Ethnicity and Reform.* Arlington Heights, IL: Harlan Davidson, 1993.

Bederman, Gail. *Manliness and Civilization: A Cultural History of Gender and Race in the United States, 1880–1917.* Chicago: University of Chicago Press, 1995.

Bender, Lauretta. *Aggression, Hostility, and Anxiety in Children.* Springfield, IL: Charles C. Thomas, 1953.

———. "Behavior Problems in Negro Children." *Psychiatry* 2 (May 1939): 213–28.

————. *Child Psychiatric Techniques.* Springfield, IL: Charles C. Thomas, 1952.

————. "Childhood Schizophrenia." *American Journal of Orthopsychiatry* 17 (1947): 40–56.

————. "Schizophrenia in Childhood—Its Recognition, Description, and Treatment." *American Journal of Orthopsychiatry* 26 (1956): 499–506.

————. *A Visual Motor Gestalt Test and Its Clinical Use.* New York: American Orthopsychiatric Association, 1938.

Bender, Lauretta, and Frank J. Curran. "Children and Adolescents Who Kill." *Journal of Clinical Psychopathology* 1 (1940): 297–322.

Bender, Lauretta, and Martin A. Spalding. "Behavior Problems in Children from the Homes of Followers of Father Divine." *Journal of Nervous and Mental Disease* 91 (April 1940): 460–72.

Bender, Lauretta, and Zuleika Yarrell. "Psychoses among Followers of Father Divine." *Journal of Nervous and Mental Disease* 87 (1938): 418–49.

Berlant, Lauren. *The Female Complaint: The Unfinished Business of Sentimentality in American Culture.* Durham, NC: Duke University Press, 2008.

Bernard, Viola W. "Detection and Management of Emotional Disorders in Children." *Mental Hygiene* 26 (July 1942): 368–82.

————. "The Division of Community Psychiatry and the Washington Heights Program." In *Urban Challenges to Psychiatry: The Case History of a Response*, edited by Lawrence C. Kolb, Viola W. Bernard, and Bruce Dohrenwend, 119–37. Boston, MA: Little, Brown, 1969.

————. "The Production of Films for Mental Health Education: Psychiatrist's Experience." *American Journal of Orthopsychiatry* 20 (October 1950): 776–84.

————. "Psychoanalysis and Members of Minority Groups." *Journal of the American Psychoanalytic Association* 1 (1953): 256–67.

————. "Some Applications of Psychoanalysis to Social Issues." *Psychoanalytic Review* 85 (February 1998): 139–70.

————. "Some Principles of Dynamic Psychiatry in Relation to Poverty." *American Journal of Psychiatry* 122 (September 1965): 254–66.

Bernard, Viola W., and DeWitt Crandall. "Evidence for Various Hypotheses of Social Psychiatry." In *Social Psychiatry*, edited by Joseph Zubin and Fritz A. Freyhan, 172–219. New York: Grune and Stratton, 1968.

Bernstein, Nina. *The Lost Children of Wilder: The Epic Struggle to Change Foster Care.* New York: Vintage, 2001.

Bevis, William M. "Psychological Traits of the Southern Negro with Observations as to Some of His Psychoses." *American Journal of Psychiatry* 78 (July 1921): 74–8.

Bhabha, Homi K. "Culture's In Between." *Art Forum* 32 (December 1993): 167–68, 211–12, 214.

————. "Of Mimicry and Man: The Ambivalence of Colonial Discourse." In *October: The First Decade*, edited by Annette Michelson, 317–25. Cambridge: Massachusetts Institute of Technology Press, 1987.

Billings, R. A. "The Negro and His Church." *Psychoanalytic Review* 21 (1934): 425–41.

Biondi, Martha. "Brooklyn College Belongs to Us: Black Studies and the Transformation of Public Higher Education in New York City." In Taylor, *Civil Rights in New York City*, 161–81.

————. *To Stand and to Fight: The Struggle for Civil Rights in New York City.* Cambridge, MA: Harvard University Press, 2003.

Black, Adina. "Exposing the 'Whole Segregation Myth': The Harlem Nine and New York City's School Desegregation Battles." In *Freedom North: Black Freedom Struggles Outside the South, 1940–1980,* edited by Jeanne Theoharis and Komozi Woodard, 65–91. New York: Palgrave Macmillan, 2003.

Bloom, Nicolas Dagan. *Public Housing That Worked: New York in the Twentieth Century.* Philadelphia: University of Pennsylvania Press, 2009.

Bonilla-Silva, Eduardo. *Racism without Racists: Color-Blind Racism and the Persistence of Racial Inequality in the United States.* 3rd ed. New York: Rowman & Littlefield, 2010.

Borges, Jorge Luis. *Ficciones.* New York: Grove Press, 1962.

Bourdieu, Pierre. *The Logic of Practice.* Translated by Richard Nice. Stanford, CA: Stanford University Press, 1990.

Boyd, Herb. *Baldwin's Harlem: A Biography of James Baldwin.* New York: Atria, 2008.

Bradley, Stefan M. *Harlem vs. Columbia University: Black Student Power in the Late 1960s.* Urbana: University of Illinois Press, 2009.

Brandt, Nat. *Harlem at War: The Black Experience in WW II.* New York: Syracuse University Press, 1996.

Brattain, Michelle. "Race, Racism, and Antiracism: UNESCO and the Politics of Presenting Science to the Postwar Public." *American Historical Review* 112 (December 2007): 1386–1413.

Brickman, Celia. *Aboriginal Populations in the Mind: Race and Primitivity in Psychoanalysis.* New York: Columbia University Press, 2003.

Briggs, Laura. *Reproducing Empire: Race, Sex, Science, and U.S. Imperialism in Puerto Rico.* Berkeley: University of California Press, 2002.

Brilliant, Mark. *The Color of America Has Changed: How Racial Diversity Shaped Civil Rights Reform in California, 1941–1978.* New York: Oxford University Press, 2010.

Brinkley, Alan. *The End of Reform: New Deal Liberalism in Recession and War.* New York: Vintage, 1995.

Bromberg, Walter. "Marihuana Intoxication: A Clinical Study of Cannabis Sativa Intoxication." *American Journal of Psychiatry* 91 (September 1934): 303–40.

————. *Psychiatry between the Wars, 1918–1945: A Recollection.* Westport, CT: Greenwood Press, 1982.

————. "Psychotherapy in a Court Clinic." *American Journal of Orthopsychiatry* 11 (October 1941): 770–74.

Brown, Claude. *Manchild in the Promised Land.* New York: MacMillan, 1965.

Brown, Michael K. *Race, Money, and the American Welfare State.* Ithaca, NY: Cornell University Press, 1999.

Brown, Michael K., Martin Camoy, Elliott Currie, and Troy Duster. *Whitewashing Race: The Myth of a Color-Blind Society.* Berkeley: University of California Press, 2005.

Brumberg, Joan Jacobs. *Fasting Girls: The History of Anorexia Nervosa.* New York: Plume, 1989.

Burchell, Graham, Colin Gordon, and Peter Miller, eds. *The Foucault Effect: Studies in Governmentality.* Chicago: University of Chicago Press, 1991.

Butler, Judith. *Bodies That Matter: On the Discursive Limits of Sex.* New York: Routledge, 1993.

——. "Restaging the Universal: Hegemony and the Limits of Formalism." In *Contingency, Hegemony, Universality: Contemporary Dialogues on the Left*, edited by Judith Butler, Ernesto Laclau, and Slavoj Zizek, 11–43. New York: Verso, 2000.

Butts, Hugh F. "Review of William H. Grier and Price M. Cobbs, *Black Rage.*" *Journal of Negro Education* 38 (Spring 1969): 166–68.

——. "Skin Color Perception and Self-Esteem." *Journal of Negro Education* 32 (Spring 1963): 122–28.

Bynum, Cornelius L. *A. Philip Randolph and the Struggle for Civil Rights.* Urbana: University of Illinois Press, 2010.

Byrd, W. Michael, and Linda A. Clayton. *An American Health Dilemma: Race, Medicine, and Health Care in the United States, 1900–2000.* New York: Routledge, 2001.

Calhoon, Claudia Marie. "Tuberculosis, Race, and the Delivery of Health Care in Harlem, 1932–1939." *Radical History Review* 73 (Spring 2001): 101–19.

Cantril, Hadley, and Muzafer Sherif. "The Kingdom of Father Divine." *Journal of Abnormal and Social Psychology* 33 (1938): 147–67.

Capeci, Jr., Dominic J. "Fiorello H. La Guardia and the Harlem 'Crime Wave' of 1941." *The New York Historical Society Quarterly* 64 (January 1980): 7–29.

——. "From Different Liberal Perspectives: Fiorello H. La Guardia, Adam Clayton Powell, Jr., and Civil Rights in New York City, 1941–1943." *Journal of Negro History* 62 (April 1977): 160–73.

——. *The Harlem Riot of 1943.* Philadelphia, PA: Temple University Press, 1977.

Caron, Simone M. "Birth Control and the Black Community in the 1960s: Genocide or Power Politics." *Journal of Social History* 31 (Spring 1998): 545–69.

——. *Who Chooses: American Reproductive History since 1830.* Gainesville: University Press of Florida, 2008.

Carter, Robert T. *The Influence of Race and Racial Identity in Psychotherapy: Towards a Racially Inclusive Model.* New York: John Wiley, 1995.

——, ed. *Theory and Research*, vol. 1 of *Handbook of Racial-Cultural Psychology and Counseling.* Hoboken, NJ: John Wiley & Sons, 2005.

Castel, Robert. "From Dangerous to Risk." In Burchell, Gordon, and Miller, *Foucault Effect*, 281–98.

Castoriadis, Cornelius. *The Imaginary Institution of Society.* Translated by Kathleen Blarney. Cambridge: Massachusetts Institute of Technology Press, 1998.

Chauncey, George, Jr. *Gay New York: Gender, Urban Culture and the Making of the Gay World, 1890–1940.* New York: Basic Books, 1994.

Chen, Anthony S. "'The Hitlerian Rule of Quotas': Conservatism and the Politics of Fair Employment Legislation in New York State, 1941–1945." *Journal of American History* 92 (March 2006): 1238–64.

Chess, Stella, Kenneth D. Clark, and Alexander Thomas. "The Importance of Cultural Evaluation in Psychiatric Diagnosis and Treatment." *Psychiatric Quarterly* 27 (1953): 102–14.

Christmas, June Jackson. "Group Methods in Training and Practice: Nonprofessional Mental Health Personnel in a Deprived Community." *American Journal of Orthopsychiatry* 36 (April 1966): 410–19.

Clark, Kenneth B. "A Conversation with James Baldwin." In Clarke, *Harlem*, 123–30.

——. *Dark Ghetto: Dilemmas of Social Power.* New York: Harper & Row, 1965.

236 ❧ BIBLIOGRAPHY

Clarke, John Henrik, ed. *Harlem: A Community in Transition.* New York: The Citadel Press, 1964.

Coles, Robert. *Children in Crisis: A Study of Courage and Fear.* Boston, MA: Little, Brown, 1967.

Collins, Charles W. "Psychoanalysis of Groups: Critique of a Study of a Small Negro Sample." *Journal of the National Medical Association* 44 (May 1952): 165–71.

Comer, James P., and Alvin F. Poussaint. *Raising Black Children: Two Leading Psychiatrists Confront the Educational, Social, and Emotional Problems Facing Black Children.* New York: Plume, 1992.

Corbould, Clare. *Becoming African Americans: Black Public Life in Harlem, 1919–1939.* Cambridge, MA: Harvard University Press, 2009.

———. "Streets, Sounds and Identity in Interwar Harlem." *Journal of Social History* 40 (Summer 2007): 859–82.

Crenner, Christopher. "Race and Medical Practice in the Kansas City Free Dispensary." *Bulletin of the History of Medicine* 82 (Winter 2008): 820–47.

Dai, Bingham. "Some Problems of Personality Development among Negro Children." In *Personality in Nature, Society, and Culture,* edited by Clyde Kluckholn and Henry A. Murray, 545–66. 2nd ed. New York: Alfred A. Knopf, 1967.

Dain, Norman. *Clifford W. Beers: Advocate for the Insane.* Pittsburgh, PA: University of Pittsburgh Press, 1980.

Dawson, Michael C. *Behind the Mule: Race and Class in African-American Politics.* Princeton, NJ: Princeton University Press, 1995.

Degler, Carl N. *In Search of Human Nature.* New York: Oxford University Press, 1991.

DeJongh, James. *Vicious Modernism: Black Harlem and the Literary Imagination.* New York: Cambridge University Press, 1994.

DeLuzio, Crista. *Female Adolescence in American Scientific Thought, 1830–1930.* Baltimore, MD: Johns Hopkins University Press, 2007.

DeVeaux, Scott. *The Birth of Bebop: A Social and Musical History.* Berkeley: University of California Press, 1997.

Dittmer, John. *The Good Doctors: The Medical Committee for Human Rights and the Struggle for Social Justice in Health Care.* New York: Bloomsbury Press, 2009.

———. *Local People: The Struggle for Civil Rights in Mississippi.* Urbana: University of Illinois Press, 1995.

Donzelot, Jacques. *The Policing of Families.* New York: Random House, 1979.

Doyle, Dennis. "Black Celebrities, Selfhood, and Psychiatry in the Civil Rights Era: The Wiltwyck School for Boys and the Floyd Patterson House." *Social History of Medicine* 28 (May 2015): 330–50.

———. "'A Fine New Child': The Lafargue Mental Hygiene Clinic and Harlem's African American Communities, 1946–1958." *Journal of the History of Medicine and Allied Sciences* 64 (April 2009): 173–212.

———. "'Racial Differences Have to Be Considered': Lauretta Bender, Bellevue Hospital, and the African American Psyche, 1936–1952." *History of Psychiatry* 21 (June 2010): 206–23.

———. "'Where the Need Is Greatest': Social Psychiatry and Race-Blind Universalism in Harlem's Lafargue Clinic, 1946–1958." *Bulletin of the History of Medicine* 83 (Winter 2009): 746–74.

Dreger, Ralph Mason, and Kent S. Miller. "Comparative Psychological Studies of Negroes and Whites in the United States: 1959–1965." Monograph supplement, *Psychological Bulletin* 70, no. 3, pt. 2 (1968): 1–58.

Dudziak, Mary. *Cold War Civil Rights: Race and the Image of American Democracy.* Princeton, NJ: Princeton University Press, 2002.

Dwyer, Ellen. *Homes for the Mad: Life Inside Two Nineteenth-Century Asylums.* New Brunswick, NJ: Rutgers University Press, 1987.

———. "Psychiatry and Race during World War II." *Journal of the History of Medicine and Allied Sciences* 61 (April 2006): 117–43.

Ellison, Ralph. "Harlem Is Nowhere." In *Shadow and Act*, 292–302. New York: Random House, 1964.

Evarts, Arrah B. "Dementia Precox in the Colored Race." *Psychoanalytic Review* 1 (October 1914): 388–403.

Fabian, Johannes. *Out of Our Minds: Reason and Madness in the Exploration of Central Africa.* Berkeley: University of California Press, 2000.

———. *Time and the Other: How Anthropology Makes Its Object.* New York: Columbia University Press, 1983.

Fanon, Frantz. *Black Skin, White Masks.* Translated by Charles Lam Markmann. New York: Grove Press, 1967.

Feldstein, Ruth. *Motherhood in Black and White: Race and Sex in American Liberalism, 1930–1965.* Ithaca, NY: Cornell University Press, 2000.

Fergus, Devin. *Liberalism, Black Power, and the Making of American Politics, 1965–1980.* Athens: University of Georgia Press, 2009.

Fernando, Suman. *Mental Health, Race and Culture.* 2nd ed. New York: Palgrave, 2002.

Fields, Barbara J. *Racecraft: The Soul of Inequality in American Life.* New York: Verso, 2012.

Flynn, Edward J. *You're the Boss.* New York: Viking Press, 1947.

Forman, Seth. *Blacks in the Jewish Mind: A Crisis of Liberalism.* New York: New York University Press, 1998.

Foucault, Michel. *Abnormal: Lectures at the College de France, 1974–1975.* Translated by Graham Burchell. New York: Picador, 2003.

———. *Discipline and Punish: The Birth of the Prison.* Translated by Alan Sheridan. New York: Pantheon, 1977.

Fraser, Nancy, and Linda Gordon. "A Genealogy of *Dependency*: Tracing a Keyword of the U.S. Welfare State." *Signs* 19 (Winter 1994): 309–36.

Fraser, Nancy, and Axel Honneth. *Redistribution or Recognition? A Political-Philosophical Exchange.* New York: Verso, 2003.

Freedman, Estelle. *Maternal Justice: Miriam Van Waters and the Female Reform Tradition.* Chicago: University of Chicago Press, 1996.

Freeman, Joshua. *Working-Class New York: Life and Labor since World War II.* New York: Free Press, 2000.

Freud, Sigmund. *Introductory Lectures on Psychoanalysis.* Translated and edited by James Strachey. New York: Liveright, 1977.

———. *Three Essays on the Theory of Sexuality.* Translated and edited by James Strachey. New York: Basic Books, 1975.

Friedman, Lawrence M. *American Law in the 20th Century.* New Haven, CT: Yale University Press, 2002.

Fuller, Simon. "A Study of Neurofibrils in Dementia Paralytics, Dementia Senilis, Chronic Alcoholism, Cerebral Uses, and Microcephalic Idiocy." *American Journal of Insanity* 63 (1907): 415–68.

Gambino, Matthew. "'These Strangers within our Gates': Race, Psychiatry and Mental Illness among Black Americans at St. Elisabeths Hospital in Washington, DC, 1900–1940." *History of Psychiatry* 19 (2008): 387–408.

Gamble, Vanessa Northington. *The Black Community Hospital: Contemporary Dilemmas in Historical Perspective.* New York: Garland, 1989.

———. *Making a Place for Ourselves: The Black Hospital Movement, 1920–1945.* New York: Oxford University Press, 1995.

Gans, Herbert J. *The Urban Villagers: Group and Class in the Life of Italian Americans.* New York: Free Press, 1965.

Gaonkar, Dilip Paramaesshawar. "Toward New Imaginaries: An Introduction." *Public Culture* 14 (Winter 2002): 1–19.

Garber, Eric. "A Spectacle in Color: The Lesbian and Gay Subculture of Jazz Age Harlem." In *Hidden from History: Reclaiming the Gay and Lesbian Past,* edited by Martin Duberman, Martha Vicinus, and George Chauncey, Jr., 318–31. New York: Meridian, 1989.

Garcia, Jay. *Psychology Comes to Harlem: Rethinking the Race Question in Twentieth-Century America.* Baltimore, MD: Johns Hopkins University Press, 2012.

Garrett, Charles. *The La Guardia Years: Machine and Reform Politics in New York City.* New Brunswick, NJ: Rutgers University Press, 1961.

Gerstle, Gary. "The Crucial Decade: The 1940s and Beyond." *Journal of American History* 92 (March 2006): 1292–99.

———. "The Protean Character of American Liberalism." *American Historical Review* 99 (October 1994): 1043–73.

———. "Race and the Myth of the Liberal Consensus." *Journal of American History* 82 (September 1995): 579–86.

Giddings, Paula. *When and Where I Enter: The Impact of Black Women on Race and Sex in America.* New York: William Morrow, 1984.

Gilbert, James. *A Cycle of Outrage: America's Reaction to the Juvenile Delinquent in the 1950s.* New York: Oxford University Press, 1986.

Gill, Jonathan. *Harlem: The Four Hundred Year History from Dutch Village to Capital of Black America.* New York: Grove, 2011.

Gilman, Sander L. *Difference and Pathology: Stereotypes of Sexuality, Race, and Madness.* Ithaca, NY: Cornell University Press, 1985.

Gilmore, Glenda. *Defying Dixie: The Radical Roots of Civil Rights.* New York: W. W. Norton, 2009.

———. *Gender and Jim Crow: Women and the Politics of White Supremacy in North Carolina, 1896–1920.* Chapel Hill: University of North Carolina Press, 1996.

Gilroy, Paul. *Against Race: Imagining Political Culture beyond the Color Line.* Cambridge, MA: Belknap Press, 2000.

———. "Cosmopolitanism, Blackness, and Utopia." *Transition* 98 (2008): 116–35.

———. *Postcolonial Melancholia.* New York: Columbia University Press, 2005.

Gordon, Colin. "Governmental Rationality: An Introduction." In Burchell, Gordon, and Miller, *Foucault Effect,* 1–51.

Gordon, Linda. *Pitied but Not Entitled: Single Mothers and the History of Welfare.* Cambridge, MA: Harvard University Press, 1994.

Gosling, F. C. *Before Freud: Neurasthenia and the American Medical Community, 1870–1910.* Urbana: University of Illinois Press, 1987.

Gould, Jeffrey L. *To Die in This Way: Nicaraguan Indians and the Myth of Mestizaje, 1880–1965.* Durham, NC: Duke University Press, 1998.

Gould, Stephen Jay. *I Have Landed.* New York: Norton, 2002.

Green, E. M. "Manic-Depressive Psychosis in the Negro." *American Journal of Insanity* 73 (1917): 619–26.

Greenberg, Cheryl. "God and Man in Harlem." *Journal of Urban History* 21 (May 1995): 519–20.

———. *"Or Does It Explode?" Black Harlem in the Great Depression.* New York: Oxford University Press, 1991.

———. "The Politics of Disorder: Reexamining Harlem's Riots of 1935 and 1943." *Journal of Urban History* 18 (August 1992): 395–441.

———. *Troubling the Waters: Black-Jewish Relations in the American Century.* Princeton, NJ: Princeton University Press, 2006.

Gregory, Dick. *From the Back of the Bus.* New York: Avon, 1962.

Gregory, James N. *The Southern Diaspora: How the Great Migrations of Black and White Southerners Changed America.* Chapel Hill: University of North Carolina Press, 2005.

Grier, William H., and Price M. Cobbs, *Black Rage.* Rev. ed. New York: Basic Books, 1992.

Grinspoon, Lester. *Marihuana Reconsidered.* Cambridge, MA: Harvard University Press, 1971.

Grob, Gerald N. *The Mad among Us: A History of the Care of America's Mentally Ill.* New York: Free Press, 1994.

———. *Mental Illness and American Society, 1875–1940.* Princeton, NJ: Princeton University Press, 1987.

———. *Mental Institutions in America: Social Policy to 1875.* New York: Free Press, 1975.

———. "Psychiatry's Holy Grail: The Search for the Mechanisms of Mental Diseases." *Bulletin of the History of Medicine* 72 (1998): 189–219.

Guinier, Lani. "From Racial Liberalism to Racial Literacy: *Brown v. Board of Education* and the Interest-Divergence Dilemma." *Journal of American History* 91 (June 2004): 92–118.

Hacker, Helen Mayer. "Ishmael Complex." *American Journal of Psychotherapy* 6 (July 1952): 494–512.

Hacking, Ian. *Historical Ontology.* Cambridge, MA: Harvard University Press, 2004.

Hale, Grace Elizabeth. *Making Whiteness: The Culture of Segregation in the South, 1890–1940.* New York: Vintage, 1998.

Hale, Nathan G., Jr. *Freud and the Americans: The Beginnings of Psychoanalysis in the United States, 1876–1917.* New York: Oxford University Press, 1971.

———. *The Rise and Crisis of Psychoanalysis in the United States: Freud and the Americans, 1917–1985.* New York: Oxford University Press, 1995.

Hall, Jacquelyn Dowd. "The Long Civil Rights Movement and the Political Uses of the Past." *Journal of American History* 91 (March 2005): 1233–53.

Hambourg, Maria Morris. "Helen Levitt: A Life in Part." In Phillips and Hambourg, *Helen Levitt*, 45–63.

Harlem Project Research Committee. *The Role of the School in Preventing and Correcting Maladjustment and Delinquency; a Study in Three Schools.* New York: New York Foundation, 1949.

Hartigan, John, Jr. "Culture against Race: Reworking the Basis for Racial Analysis." *South Atlantic Quarterly* 104 (Summer 2005): 543–60.

Hauser, Mary E. "Caroline Pratt and the City and Country School." In Semel and Sadovnick, *Founding Mothers and Others*, 77–92.

Healy, William. *Mental Conflicts and Misconduct.* Boston, MA: Little, Brown, 1930.

Healy, William, Augusta F. Bronner, Edith M. H. Baylor, and J. Prentice Murray. *Reconstructing Behavior in Youth: A Study of Problem Children in Foster Families.* New York: Alfred Knopf, 1936.

Hegarty, Marilyn E. *Victory Girls, Khaki-Wackies, and Patriotutes: The Regulation of Female Sexuality during World War II.* New York: New York University Press, 2007.

Henry, Jules. "Environment and Symptom Formation." *American Journal of Orthopsychiatry* 17 (October 1947): 628–51.

Herman, Ellen. *Kinship by Design: A History of Adoption in the Modern United States.* Chicago: University of Chicago Press, 2008.

———. *Romance of American Psychology: Political Culture in the Age of Experts.* Berkeley: University of California Press, 1995.

Herman, Judith. *Trauma and Recovery.* New York: Basic Books, 1997.

Hicks, Cheryl D. "'Bright and Good Looking Colored Girl': Black Women's Sexuality and 'Harmful Intimacy' in Early Twentieth-Century New York." *Journal of the History of Sexuality* 18 (September 2009): 418–56.

———. *Talk with You Like a Woman: African American Women, Justice, and Reform in New York, 1890–1935.* Chapel Hill: University of North Carolina Press, 2010.

Hinitz, Bythe. "Margaret Naumburg and the Walden School." In Semel and Sadovnick, *Founding Mothers and Others*, 37–60.

Hirsch, Arnold. "Massive Resistance in the Urban North: Trumbull Park, Chicago, 1953–1966." *Journal of American History* 82 (September 1995): 522–50.

Hirshbein, Laura D. *American Melancholy: Constructions of Depression in the Twentieth Century.* New Brunswick, NJ: Rutgers University Press, 2009.

———. "Sex and Gender in Psychiatry: A View from History." *Journal of Medical Humanities* 31 (2010): 155–70.

Hollingshead, August de Belmont, and Frederick C. Redlich. "Social Stratification and Psychiatric Disorders." *American Sociological Review* 18 (1953): 163–69.

Holloman, Laynard. "On the Supremacy of the Negro Athlete in White Athletic Competition." *Psychoanalytic Review* 30 (1943): 157–62.

Holt, Thomas. *The Problem of Race in the 21st Century.* Cambridge, MA: Harvard University Press, 2000.

Horn, Margo. *Before It's Too Late: The Child Guidance Movement in the United States, 1922–1945.* Philadelphia, PA: Temple University Press, 1989.

Horwitz, Morton J. *The Transformation of American Law, 1870–1960: The Crisis of Orthodoxy.* New York: Oxford University Press, 1992.

Hoshor, John. *God in a Rolls Royce: The Rise of Father Divine, Madman, Menace, or Messiah.* New York: Hillman-Curl, 1936.

Hunt, Lynn. *Inventing Human Rights: A History.* New York: Norton, 2007.

Hughes, John S. "Labeling and Treating Black Mental Illness in Alabama, 1861–1910." *Journal of Social History* 58 (August 1992): 435–60.

Iton, Richard. *In Search of the Black Fantastic: Politics and Popular Culture in the Post–Civil Rights Era.* New York: Oxford University Press, 2008.

Jackson, Lynette A. *Surfacing Up: Psychiatry and Social Order in Colonial Zimbabwe, 1908–1968.* Ithaca, NY: Cornell University Press, 2005.

Jackson, Thomas. *From Civil Rights to Human Rights: Martin Luther King, Jr. and the Struggle for Economic Justice.* Philadelphia: University of Pennsylvania Press, 2009.

Jackson, Walter A. *Gunnar Myrdal and America's Conscience: Social Engineering and Racial Liberalism, 1938–1987.* Chapel Hill: University of North Carolina Press, 1990.

Jacobson, Matthew Frye. *Whiteness of a Different Color: European Immigrants and the Alchemy of Race.* Cambridge, MA: Harvard University Press, 1999.

Johnson, Laura. "A Generation of Women Activists; African American Female Educators in Harlem, 1930–1950." *Journal of African American History* 89 (Summer 2004): 223–40.

Jones, Jacqueline. *Labor of Love, Labor of Sorrow: Black Women, Work and the Family, from Slavery to the Present.* New York: Vintage, 1995.

Jones, Kathleen W. *Taming the Troublesome Child: American Families, Child Guidance, and the Limits of Psychiatric Authority.* Cambridge, MA: Harvard University Press, 1999.

Jones, Reginald L. *Black Psychology.* 2nd ed. New York: Harper & Row, 1980.

Joseph, Peniel E. "Introduction: Toward a Historiography of the Black Power Movement." In *The Black Power Movement: Rethinking the Civil Rights–Black Power Era,* edited by Peniel E. Joseph, 1–26. New York: Routledge, 2006.

———. *Waiting 'Til the Midnight Hour: A Narrative History of Black Power in America.* New York: Henry Holt, 2006.

Kardiner, Abram. *The Psychological Frontiers of Society.* New York: Columbia University Press, 1945.

Kardiner, Abram, and Lionel Ovesey. *The Mark of Oppression: Explorations in the Personality of the American Negro.* Rev. ed. New York: Meridian, 1962.

Katz, Michael B., Mark J. Stern, and Jamie J. Fader. "The New African American Inequality." *Journal of American History* 92 (June 2005): 75–108.

Katznelson, Ira. *When Affirmative Action Was White: An Untold History of Racial Inequality in Twentieth-Century America.* New York: Norton, 2005.

Kelley, Robin D. G. *Thelonious Monk: The Life and Times of an American Original.* New York: Free Press, 2009.

———. *Yo Mama's Disfunktional! Fighting the Culture Wars in Urban America.* Boston, MA: Beacon Press, 1997.

Kennedy, Janet Alterman. "Problems Posed in the Analysis of Negro Patients." *Psychiatry* 15 (August 1952): 313–27.

Kessner, Thomas. *Fiorello H. LaGuardia and the Making of Modern New York.* New York: McGraw-Hill, 1989.

Kevles, Daniel J. *In the Name of Eugenics: Genetics and the Uses of Human Heredity.* Cambridge, MA: Harvard University Press, 1997.

Klineberg, Otto. *Race Differences.* New York: Harper, 1935.

Kluger, Richard. *Simple Justice: The History of Brown v. Board of Education and Black America's Struggle for Equality.* New York: Alfred A. Knopf, 1976.

Knupfer, Anna Meis. *Reform and Resistance: Gender, Delinquency, and America's First Juvenile Court.* New York: Routledge, 2001.

Kunzel, Regina. *Criminal Intimacy: Prison and the Uneven History of Modern American Sexuality.* Chicago: University of Chicago Press, 2008.

———. *Fallen Women, Problem Girls: Unmarried Mothers and the Professionalization of Social Work, 1890–1945.* New Haven, CT: Yale University Press, 1993.

———. "White Neurosis, Black Pathology: Constructing Out-of-Wedlock Pregnancy in the Wartime and Postwar United States." In *Not Just June Cleaver: Women and Gender in Postwar America, 1945–1960,* edited by Joanne Meyerowitz, 304–34. Philadelphia, PA: Temple University Press, 1994.

Kornbluh, Felicia. *The Battle for Welfare Rights: Politics and Poverty in Modern America.* Philadelphia: University of Pennsylvania Press, 2007.

Kusmer, Kenneth. "African American in the City since World War II: From Industrial to the Post-Industrial Era." *Journal of Urban History* 21 (May 1995): 458–503.

Lagemann, Ellen Condliffe. *An Elusive Science: The Troubling History of Education Research.* Chicago: University of Chicago Press, 2000.

Lait, Jack, and Lee Mortimer. *New York: Confidential!* New York: Dell, 1951.

Lasch-Quinn, Elizabeth. *Race Experts: How Racial Etiquette, Sensitivity Training, and New Age Therapy Hijacked the Civil Rights Revolution.* New York: Norton, 2001.

Lawrence, Sara Lightfoot. *Balm in Gilead: Journey of a Healer.* New York: Merloyd-Lawrence, 1988.

Lears, Jackson. "The Ad Man and the Grand Inquisitor: Intimacy, Publicity, and the Managed Self in America, 1880–1940." In *Constructions of the Self,* edited by George Levine, 107–41. New Brunswick, NJ: Rutgers University Press, 1992.

———. *No Place of Grace: Antimodernism and the Transformation of American Culture.* Chicago: University of Chicago Press, 1994.

———. *Something for Nothing: Luck in America.* New York: Viking, 2003.

Leavitt, Jacqueline, and Susan Seagert. *From Abandonment to Hope: Community-Household in Harlem.* New York: Columbia University Press, 1990.

Lefkowitz, Bonnie. *Community Health Centers: A Movement and the People Who Made It Happen.* New Brunswick, NJ: Rutgers University Press, 2007.

Leighton, Alexander H. "Poverty and Social Change." *Scientific American* 212 (May 1965): 21–27.

Levenson, Jacob. *The Secret Epidemic: The Story of AIDS and Black America.* New York: Anchor, 2004.

Lewis, Carolyn Herbst. *Prescription for Heterosexuality: Sexual Citizenship in the Cold War Era.* Chapel Hill: University of North Carolina Press, 2010.

Lewis, David L. *When Harlem Was in Vogue.* New York: Knopf, 1981.

Lewis, Nolan D. C., and Lewis D. Hubbard. "Epileptic Reactions in the Negro." *American Journal of Psychiatry* 88 (January 1932): 647–77.

———. "Manic Depressive Reactions in Negroes." *Proceedings of the Association of Research in Nervous and Mental Disease* 11 (1931): 779–90.

Lind, John E. "The Dream as Simple Wish-Fulfillment in the Negro." *Psychoanalytic Review* 1 (October 1914): 295–300.

————. "Phylogenetic Elements in the Psychoses of the Negro." *Psychoanalytic Review* 4 (January 1917): 304–32.

Lipsitz, George. *How Racism Takes Place*. Philadelphia, PA: Temple University Press, 2011.

Lipsyte, Robert. *The Contender*. New York: Bantam, 1980.

Livingston, Jane. *The New York School: Photographs, 1936–1963*. New York: Stewart, Tabnori, and Chang, 1992.

Lunbeck, Elizabeth. "American Psychiatrists and the Modern Man, 1900 to 1920." *Men and Masculinities* 1 (July 1998): 58–86.

————. *The Psychiatric Persuasion: Knowledge, Gender, and Power in Modern America*. Princeton, NJ: Princeton University Press, 1994.

Mack, Kenneth W. "Law and Mass Politics in the Making of the Civil Rights Lawyer, 1931–1941." *Journal of American History* 93 (June 2006): 37–62.

Madison, Axel. *The Marshall Fields: The Evolution of an American Business Dynasty*. Hoboken, NJ: John Wiley & Sons, 2002.

Malzberg, Benjamin. "Mental Disease among Negroes in New York State." *Human Biology* 7 (December 1935): 471–513.

————. "Migration and Mental Disease among Negroes in New York State." *American Journal of Physical Anthropology* 21 (January–March 1936): 107–13.

Markowitz, Gerald, and David Rosner. *Children, Race, and Power: Kenneth and Mamie Clark's Northside Center*. Charlottesville: University of Virginia Press, 1996.

————. "Race, Foster Care and the Politics of Abandonment in New York City." *American Journal of Public Health* 87 (November 1997): 1844–49.

Martin, Emily. *Bipolar Expeditions: Mania and Depression in American Culture*. Princeton, NJ: Princeton University Press, 2007.

Martin, Waldo E., Jr. *No Coward Soldiers: Black Cultural Politics and Postwar America*. Cambridge, MA: Harvard University Press, 2005.

Martinez, Daniel HoSang. *Racial Propositions: Ballot Initiatives and the Making of Postwar California*. Berkeley: University of California Press, 2010.

Massey, Douglas, and Nancy A. Denton. *American Apartheid: Segregation and the Making of the Underclass*. Cambridge, MA: Harvard University Press, 1993.

May, Elaine Tyler. *America and the Pill: A History of Promise, Peril, and Liberation*. New York: Basic Books, 2010.

————. *Homeward Bound: American Families in the Cold War Era*. New York: Basic Books, 1988.

Maynard, Aubre de L. *Surgeons to the Poor: The Harlem Hospital Story*. New York: Appleton-Century-Crofts, 1979.

McClintock, Ann. *Imperial Leather: Race, Gender, and Sexuality in the Colonial Conquest*. New York: Routledge, 1991.

————. "No Longer in a Future Heaven: Nationalism, Gender and Race." In *Becoming National: A Reader*, edited by Geoff Eley and Ron Grigor Suny, 259–84. New York: Oxford University Press, 1996.

McKay, Claude. *Harlem: Negro Metropolis*. New York: E. P. Dutton, 1940.

McLean, Helen V. "The Emotional Health of Negroes." *Journal of Negro Education* 18 (1949): 283–90.

————. "Psychodynamic Factors in Race Relation." *Annals of the American Academy of Political and Social Science* 244 (March 1946): 159–66.

———. "Racial Prejudice." *American Journal of Orthopsychiatry* 14 (October 1944): 706–13.

McLeod, Jacqueline A. *Daughter of the Empire State: The Life of Judge Jane Bolin.* Urbana: University of Illinois Press, 2011.

———. "Persona Non-Grata: Judge Jane Matilda Bolin and the NAACP, 1930–1950." *Afro-Americans in New York Life and History* 29 (January 2005): 7–29.

Mehta, Uday S. "Liberal Strategies of Exclusion." In *Tensions of Empire: Colonial Cultures in a Bourgeois World*, edited by Frederick Cooper and Ann Laura Stoler, 59–86. Berkeley: University of California Press, 1997.

Mendes, Gabriel N. "An Underground Extension of Democracy." *Transition* 115 (2014): 4–22.

———. *Under the Strain of Color: Harlem's Lafargue Clinic and the Promise of an Antiracist Psychiatry.* Ithaca, NY: Cornell University Press, 2015.

Mennel, Robert M. *Thorns and Thistles: Juvenile Delinquency in the United States, 1825–1940.* Hanover, NH: University Press of New England, 1973.

Metzl, Jonathan Michel. *The Protest Psychosis: How Schizophrenia Became a Black Disease.* Boston, MA: Beacon Press, 2009.

———. *Prozac on the Couch: Prescribing Gender in the Era of Wonder Drugs.* Durham, NC: Duke University Press, 2003.

Meyerowitz, Joanne. "'How Common Culture Shapes the Separate Lives': Sexuality, Race, and Mid-Twentieth-Century Social Constructivist Thought." *Journal of American History* 96 (March 2010): 1057–84.

———. *How Sex Changed: A History of Transsexuality in the United States.* Cambridge, MA: Harvard University Press, 2002.

Mezzrow, Mezz, and Bernard Wolfe. *Really the Blues.* New York: Random House, 1946.

Miller, William Robert. "The Broadening Horizon: Montgomery, America, and the World." In *Martin Luther King Jr.: A Profile*, edited by C. Eric Lincoln, 40–71. New York: Hill and Wang, 1970.

Mintz, Steven. *Huck's Raft: A History of American Childhood.* Cambridge, MA: Belknap Press, 2006.

Minuchin, Salvador. *Families of the Slums: An Exploration of Their Structure and Treatment.* New York: Basic Books, 1967.

Mio, Jeffrey Scott, and Gayle Y. Iwamesa, eds. *Culturally Diverse Mental Health: The Challenges of Research and Resistance.* New York: Brunner-Routledge, 2003.

Mitchell, Pablo. *Coyote Nation: Sexuality, Race, and Conquest in New Mexico, 1880–1920.* Chicago: University of Chicago Press, 2006.

Mittelstadt, Jennifer. "Philanthropy, Feminism, and Left Liberalism." *Journal of Women's History* 20 (Winter 2008): 105–31.

Monk, Daniel Bertrand. "Hives and Swarms: On the 'Nature' of Neoliberalism and the Rise of the Ecological Insurgent." In *Evil Paradises: Dreamworlds of Neoliberalism*, edited by Mike Davis and Daniel Bertrand Monk, 262–73. New York: Free Press, 2007.

Morantz-Sanchez, Regina Markell. "Physicians." In *Women, Health, and Medicine in America: A Handbook*, edited by Rima Apple, 477–95. New York: Garland, 1990.

———. *Sympathy and Science: Women Physicians in American Medicine.* New York: Oxford University Press, 1985.

Morris, Rosalind C. "The Miner's Ear." *Transition* 98 (2008): 96–115.

Morrison, Toni. *Tar Baby.* New York: Plume, 1982.

Mosse, Hilde. "Is There an Ishmael Complex?" *American Journal of Psychotherapy* 7 (January 1953): 72–79.

Muhammad, Khalil Gibran. *The Condemnation of Blackness: Race, Crime, and the Making of Modern Urban America.* Cambridge, MA: Harvard University Press, 2010.

Mukerji, Chandra. "Space and the Political Pedagogy at the Gardens of Versailles." *Public Culture* 24 (Fall 2012): 509–34.

Muncy, Robin L. *Creating a Female Dominion in American Reform, 1890–1935.* New York: Oxford University Press, 1991.

Nell, Norman W., and John Spiegel. "Social Psychiatry." *Archives in General Psychiatry* 14 (1966): 337–45.

Nelson, Alondra. *Body and Soul: The Black Panther Party and the Fight against Medical Discrimination.* Minneapolis: University of Minnesota Press, 2011.

New York Bureau of Child Guidance. *Five-Year Report, 1932–1937.* New York: Board of Education, 1938.

Ngai, Mae N. "American Immigration Law: A Reexamination of the Immigration Act of 1924." *Journal of American History* 86 (June 1999): 67–92.

Norton, Peter D. *Fighting Traffic: The Dawn of the Motor Age in the American City.* Cambridge, MA: MIT Press, 2008.

Odem, Mary. *Delinquent Daughters: Protecting and Policing Adolescent Female Sexuality in the United States, 1885–1920.* Chapel Hill: University of North Carolina Press, 1995.

O'Malley, Mary. "Psychosis in the Colored Race: A Study in Comparative Psychiatry." *American Journal of Insanity* 71 (October 1914): 309–36.

Orleck, Annelise. *Storming Caesar's Palace: How Black Mothers Fought Their Own War on Poverty.* Boston, MA: Beacon Press, 2005.

Osofsky, Gilbert. *Harlem: The Making of a Ghetto.* New York: Harper, 1966.

Ottley, Roi. *"New World A-Coming": Inside Black America.* New York: Houghton Mifflin, 1945.

Ottley, Roi, and William J. Weatherby. *The Negro in New York: An Informal Social History, 1626–1940.* New York: Praeger, 1967.

Parker, Robert A. *The Incredible Messiah: The Deification of Father Divine.* Boston, MA: Little, Brown, 1937.

Pasamanick, Benjamin. "Some Misconceptions concerning Differences in the Racial Prevalence of Mental Disease." *American Journal of Orthopsychiatry* 33 (January 1963): 72–86.

Patterson, James. *Grand Expectations: The United States, 1945–1975.* New York: Oxford University Press, 1997.

Pearson, Hugh. *When Harlem Nearly Killed King: The 1958 Stabbing of Dr. Martin Luther King Jr.* New York: Seven Stories Press, 2004.

Petry, Ann. *The Street.* 1946. Reprint, Boston, MA: Beacon Press, 1985.

Pfister, Joel, and Nancy Schnog. *Inventing the Psychological: Toward a Cultural History of Emotional Life in America.* New Haven, CT: Yale University Press, 1997.

Phillips, Sandra S. "Helen Levitt's New York." In Phillips and Hambourg, *Helen Levitt,* 15–43.

Phillips, Sandra S., and Maria Morris Hambourg, eds. *Helen Levitt.* San Francisco, CA: San Francisco Museum of Modern Art; New York: Metropolitan Museum of Art, 1991.

Plant, James S. *Personality and the Cultural Pattern.* New York: Commonwealth Fund, 1937.

Pleck, Elizabeth. *Domestic Tyranny: The Making of Social Policy against Family Violence from Colonial Times to the Present.* New York: Oxford University Press, 1987.

Pol, Therese. "Psychiatry in Harlem." *The Protestant* (June–July 1947): 28–30.

Polier, Justine Wise. "Attitudes and Contradictions in Our Culture." *Child Welfare* 39 (November 1960): 1–5.

———. *Everyone's Children, Nobody's Child.* New York: Charles Scribner's Sons, 1941.

———."How I Became Interested in Racial Justice." *Opportunity* 26 (Spring 1948): 63–69.

———. *Juvenile Justice in Double Jeopardy: The Distanced Community and Vengeful Retribution.* Hillsdale, NJ: Lawrence Erlbaum Associates, 1989.

———. "Wartime Needs of Children and Federal Responsibility." *Federal Probation* 8 (April–June 1944): 9–12.

Poussaint, Alvin F. "The Black Child's Image of the Future." In *Learning for Tomorrow: The Role of the Future in Education,* edited by Alfred Toffler, 56–71. New York: Vintage, 1972.

———. "Education and Black Self-Image, No. 4, 1968." In *Freedomways Reader: Prophets in Their Own Country,* edited by Esther Cooper Jackson, 222–28. Boulder, CO: Westview Press, 2000.

Poussaint, Alvin F., and Amy Alexander. *Lay My Burden Down: Unraveling Suicide and the Mental Health Crisis among African-Americans.* Boston, MA: Beacon, 2000.

Pressman, Jack P. *Last Resort: Psychosurgery and the Limits of Medicine.* New York: Cambridge University Press, 1998.

———. "Psychiatry and Its Origins." *Bulletin of the History of Medicine* 71 (1997): 129–39.

Prudhomme, Charles. "The Problem of Suicide in the American Negro." *Psychoanalytic Review* 25 (1938): 187–204.

Prudhomme, Charles, and David F. Musto. "Historical Perspectives on Mental Health and Racism in the United States." In *Racism and Mental Health,* edited by Charles V. Willie, Bernard S. Kramer, and Bertram S. Brown, 25–57. Pittsburgh, PA: University of Pittsburgh Press, 1973.

Quadagno, Jill. *The Color of Welfare: How Racism Undermined the War on Poverty.* New York: Oxford University Press, 1996.

Quen, Jacques M. "Asylum Psychiatry, Neurology, Social Work, and Mental Hygiene: An Explanatory Study in Interprofessional History." *Journal of the History of the Behavioral Sciences* 13 (January 1977): 1–11.

Rai, Amit. *The Rule of Sympathy: Sentiment, Race, and Power, 1750–1850.* New York: Palgrave, 2002.

Rampersad, Arnold. "Afterword." In Richard Wright, *Rite of Passage,* 135–42. New York: Harper Trophy, 1994.

Randolph, Kirby N. "Psychiatry versus the Negro." Paper presented at the New York Academy of Medicine, February 27, 2001, New York.

Ransby, Barbara. *Ella Baker and the Black Freedom Movement: A Radical Democratic Vision.* Chapel Hill: University of North Carolina Press, 2005.

Ravitch, Dianne. *The Great School Wars: A History of the New York City Public Schools.* Rev. ed. Baltimore, MD: Johns Hopkins University Press, 2000.

Raz, Mical. *What's Wrong with the Poor: Psychiatry, Race, and the War on Poverty.* Chapel Hill: University of North Carolina Press, 2013.

Reagan, Leslie J., Nancy Tomes, and Paula Treichler. "Introduction: Medicine, Health, and Bodies in American Film and Television." In *Medicine's Moving Pictures: Medicine, Health, and Bodies in American Film and Television,* edited by Leslie J. Reagan, Nancy Tomes, and Paula Treichler, 1–16. Rochester, NY: University of Rochester Press, 2007.

Reiss, Benjamin. *Theaters of Madness: Insane Asylums and Nineteenth-Century American Culture.* Chicago: University of Chicago Press, 2008.

Reverby, Susan. *Examining Tuskegee: The Infamous Syphilis Study and Its Legacy.* Chapel Hill: University of North Carolina Press, 2009.

Rhodes-Pitts, Sharifa. *Harlem Is Nowhere: A Journey to the Mecca of Black America.* New York: Little, Brown, 2011.

Ripley, Lt. Colonel Herbert S., and Major Stewart Wolf. "Mental Illness among Negro Troops Overseas." *American Journal of Psychiatry* 103 (1947): 499–512.

Risor, Helene. "Twenty Hanging Dolls and a Lynching: Defacing Dangerousness and Enacting Citizenship in El Alto, Bolivia." *Public Culture* 22 (Fall 2010): 465–85.

Roberts, Dorothy. *Killing the Black Body: Race, Reproduction, and the Meaning of Liberty.* New York: Pantheon, 1997.

Roberts, Leigh M., Seymour L. Halleck, and Martin B. Loeb. *Community Psychiatry.* Madison: University of Wisconsin Press, 1966.

Roberts, Samuel Kelton, Jr. *Infectious Fear: Politics, Disease, and the Health Effects of Segregation.* Chapel Hill: University of North Carolina Press, 2009.

Robertson, Stephen. *Crimes against Children: Sexual Violence and Legal Culture in New York City, 1880–1960.* Chapel Hill: University of North Carolina Press, 2005.

Robison, Sophia M. *Juvenile Delinquency: Its Nature and Control.* New York: Holt, 1960.

Roediger, David R. *Colored White: Transcending the Racial Past.* Berkeley: University of California Press, 2003.

Rose, Anne C. *Psychology and Selfhood in the Segregated South.* Chapel Hill: University of North Carolina Press, 2009.

Rose, Nikolas. *Inventing Our Selves: Psychology, Power, and Personhood.* New York: Cambridge University Press, 1998.

———. *The Politics of Life Itself: Biomedicine, Power, and Subjectivity in the Twenty-First Century.* Princeton, NJ: Princeton University Press, 2008.

Rosenthal, Simon P. "Racial Differences in the Mental Diseases." *Journal of Abnormal and Social Psychology* 28 (October–December 1933): 301–18.

Ruiz, Dorothy S., ed. *Handbook of Mental Health and Mental Disorder among Black Americans.* New York: Greenwood Press, 1990.

Russell, Thaddeus. "The Color of Discipline: Civil Rights and Black Sexuality." *American Quarterly* 60 (March 2008): 101–28.

Ryan, Mary P. *Mysteries of Sex: Tracing Women and Men through American History.* Chapel Hill: University of North Carolina Press, 2006.

Ryan, William. *Blaming the Victim.* New York: Vintage, 1972.

Sacco, Lynn. *Unspeakable: Father-Daughter Incest in American History.* Baltimore, MD: Johns Hopkins University Press, 2009.

Sadowsky, Jonathan. *Imperial Bedlam: Institutions of Madness in Colonial Southwest Nigeria.* Berkeley: University of California Press, 1999.

Schilder, Paul, and Sam Parker. "Pupillary Disturbances in Schizophrenic Negroes." *Archives of Neurology and Psychiatry* 25 (March 1931): 838–47.

Schoener, Allon, ed. *Harlem on My Mind: Cultural Capital of Black America, 1900–1968.* New York: New Press, 2007.

Schwartz, Joel. *The New York Approach: Robert Moses, Urban Liberals, and Redevelopment of the Inner City.* Columbus: The Ohio State University Press, 1993.

Schwartz, Robert C., and Kevin P. Feisthamel. "Disproportionate Diagnosis of Mental Disorders among African Americans versus European American Clients: Implications for Counseling Theory, Research, and Practice." *Journal of Counseling & Development* 87 (Summer 2009): 295–301.

Scott, Daryl Michael. *Contempt and Pity: Social Policy and the Image of the Damaged Black Psyche, 1880–1996.* Chapel Hill: University of North Carolina Press, 1997.

———. "Postwar Pluralism, *Brown v. Board of Education,* and the Origins of Multicultural Education." *Journal of American History* 91 (June 2004): 69–82.

Self, Robert O. *All in the Family: The Realignment of American Democracy since the 1960s.* New York: Hill and Wang, 2012.

———. *American Babylon: Race and the Struggle for Postwar Oakland.* Princeton, NJ: Princeton University Press, 2003.

Sellers, Christopher. "Body, Place, and the State: The Making of an 'Environmental' Imaginary in the Post–World War II U.S." *Radical History Review* 74 (Spring 1999): 31–64.

———. "Thoreau's Body: Towards an Embodied Environmental History." Paper presented at 2nd Plenary Session, Annual Meeting of the American Society for Environmental History, March 1997, Baltimore, MD (copy in author's possession).

Semel, Susan, and Alan Sadovnick, eds. *Founding Mothers and Others: Women Educational Leaders during the Progressive Era.* New York: Palgrave, 2002.

Serlin, David. *Replaceable You: Engineering the Body in Postwar America.* Chicago: University of Chicago Press, 2004.

Shah, Nayan. *Contagious Divides: Epidemics and Race in San Francisco's Chinatown.* Berkeley: University of California Press, 2001.

Shepard, Todd. *The Invention of Decolonization: The Algerian War and the Remaking of France.* Ithaca, NY: Cornell University Press, 2008.

Singh, Nikhil Pal. *Black Is a Country: Race and the Unfinished Struggle for Democracy.* Cambridge, MA: Harvard University Press, 2004.

Skinner, B. F. *Beyond Freedom and Dignity.* New York: Bantam, 1972.

Sklaroff, Lauren Rebecca. *Black Culture and the New Deal: The Quest for Civil Rights in the Roosevelt Era.* Chapel Hill: University of North Carolina Press, 2009.

Sloman, Larry. *Reefer Madness: The History of Marijuana in America.* Indianapolis, IN: Bobbs-Merrill, 1979.

Smith, Alan P. "The Availability of Facilities for Negroes Suffering from Mental and Nervous Disease." *Journal of Negro Education* 6 (1937): 450–54.

———. "Mental Hygiene in the American Negro." *Journal of the National Medical Association* 23 (January–March 1931): 1–10.

Smith, Eve P. "Willingness and Resistance to Change: The Case of the Race Discrimination Amendment of 1942." *Social Service Review* 69 (March 1995): 31–56.

Smith, Klytus, et al. *The Harlem Cultural/Political Movements, 1960–1970: From Malcolm X to Black Is Beautiful.* New York: Gumbs & Thomas, 1995.

Solinger, Rickie. *Pregnancy and Power: A Short History of Reproductive Politics in America.* New York: New York University Press, 2005.

————. *Wake Up Little Susie: Single Pregnancy and Race before Roe v. Wade.* New York: Routledge, 1992.

Sommer, Doris. *Foundational Fictions: The National Romances of Latin America.* Berkeley: University of California Press, 1991.

Spiegel, John. "Some Cultural Aspects of Transference and Countertransference." In *Individual and Family Dynamics,* edited by J. H. Masserman, 160–82. New York: Grune and Stratton, 1959.

Srole, Leo. *Mental Health in the Metropolis: The Midtown Manhattan Study.* New York: McGraw-Hill, 1962.

Spurlock, Jeanne, ed. *Black Psychiatrists and American Psychiatry.* Washington, DC: American Psychiatric Association, 1999.

St. Clair, Harvey. "Psychiatric Interview Experiences with Negroes." *American Journal of Psychiatry* 108 (1951): 113–19.

Stearns, Peter N. *Anxious Parents: A History of Modern Childrearing in America.* New York: New York University Press, 2004.

Stevens, Rosemary. *In Sickness and in Wealth: American Hospitals in the Twentieth Century.* Baltimore, MD: Johns Hopkins University Press, 1989.

Stevens, Rutherford B. "Psychoanalysis of Groups." *Journal of the National Medical Association* 6 (November 1952): 457–58.

————. "Racial Aspects of Emotional Problems of Negro Soldiers." *American Journal of Psychiatry* 103 (1947): 493–98.

Stewart, Catherine A. "Crazy for This Democracy": Psychoanalysis, African American Blues Narratives, and the Lafargue Clinic." *American Quarterly* 65 (June 2013): 371–95.

Stoler, Ann Laura. *Along the Archival Grain: Epistemic Anxieties and Colonial Common Sense.* Princeton, NJ: Princeton University Press, 2009.

————. "Interview." Interview by E. Valentine Daniel. *Public Culture* 24 (Fall 2012): 487–508.

————. "Intimations of Empire: Predicaments of the Tactile and Unseen." In *Haunted by Empire: Geographies of Intimacy in North American History,* edited by Ann Laura Stoler, 1–22. Durham, NC: Duke University Press, 2006.

————. *Race and the Education of Desire: Foucault's History of Sexuality and the Colonial Order of Things.* Durham, NC: Duke University Press, 1995.

Sugrue, Thomas J. "Crabgrass-Roots Politics: Race, Rights, and the Reaction against Liberalism in the Urban North." *Journal of American History* 82 (September 1995): 551–77.

————. *The Origins of the Urban Crisis: Race and Inequality in Postwar Detroit.* Princeton, NJ: Princeton University Press, 1996.

————. *Sweet Land of Liberty: The Forgotten Struggle for Civil Rights in the North.* New York: Random House, 2008.

Summers, Martin V. "'Suitable Care of the African When Afflicted with Insanity': Race, Madness, and Social Order in Historical Perspective." *Bulletin of the History of Medicine* 84 (Spring 2010): 58–91.

Susman, Warren I. "'Personality' and the Making of Twentieth-Century Culture." In *Culture as History: The Transformation of American Society in the Twentieth Century,* edited by Warren I. Susman, 274–81. New York: Pantheon, 1984.

Tabili, Laura. "Race Is a Relationship, and Not a Thing." *Journal of Social History* (Fall 2003): 125–30.

Takaki, Ronald. *Double Victory: A Multicultural History of America in World War II.* Boston, MA: Little, Brown, 2000.

Taussig, Michael. *Mimesis and Alterity: A Particular History of the Senses.* New York: Routledge, 1993.

———. *What Color Is the Sacred?* Chicago: University of Chicago Press, 2009.

Taylor, Charles. "Cultures of Democracy and Citizen Efficacy." *Public Culture* 19 (Winter 2007): 117–50.

———. *Modern Social Imaginaries.* Durham, NC: Duke University Press, 2004.

———. "Modernity and Difference." In *Without Guarantees: In Honor of Stuart Hall,* edited by Paul Gilroy, Lawrence Grossberg, and Angela McRobbie, 364–74. London: Verso, 2000.

Taylor, Clarence, ed. *Civil Rights in New York City: From World War II to the Giuliani Era.* New York: Fordham University Press, 2011.

———. "Conservative and Liberal Opposition to the New York City School-Integration Campaign." In Taylor, *Civil Rights in New York City,* 95–117.

———. *Knocking at Our Own Door: Milton A. Galamison and the Struggle to Integrate New York City Schools.* Lanham, MD: Lexington, 2001.

Thomas, Alexander, and Samuel Sillen. *Racism and Psychiatry.* New York: Brunner/Mazel, 1972.

Thomas, Karen Kruse. *Deluxe Jim Crow: Civil Rights and American Health Policy, 1935–1954.* Athens: University of Georgia Press, 2011.

———. "The Hill-Burton Act and Civil Rights: Expanding Hospital Care for Black Southerners, 1939–1960." *Journal of Southern History* 72 (November 2006): 823–70.

Thomas, Lorrin. *Puerto Rican Citizen: History and Political Identity in Twentieth-Century New York City.* Chicago: University of Chicago Press, 2010.

Thurston, Henry W. *The Dependent Child: A Story of Changing Aims and Methods in the Care of Dependent Children.* New York: Columbia University Press, 1930.

Tice, Karen W. *Tales of Wayward Girls and Immoral Women: Case Records and the Professionalization of Social Work.* Urbana: University of Illinois Press, 1998.

Tomes, Nancy. *The Art of Asylum-Keeping: Thomas Story Kirkbride and the Origins of American Psychiatry.* 1984. Reprint, Philadelphia: University of Pennsylvania Press, 1994.

———. "Merchants of Health: Medicine and Consumer Culture in the United States, 1900–1940." *Journal of American History* 88 (2001): 519–47.

Torgovnick, Marianna. *Gone Primitive: Savage Intellects, Modern Lives.* Chicago: University of Chicago Press, 1990.

Tyson, Timothy. *Radio Free Dixie: Robert F. Williams and the Roots of Black Power.* Chapel Hill: University of North Carolina Press, 1999.

Urofsky, Melvin I. *A Voice That Spoke for Justice: The Life and Time of Stephen S. Wise.* Albany: State University of New York Press, 1982.

Vaughan, Megan. *Curing Their Ills: Colonial Power and African Illness.* Stanford, CA: Stanford University Press, 1992.

Vitullo-Martin, Julio, ed. *Breaking Away, the Future of Cities: Essays in Honor of Robert F. Wagner, Jr.* New York: Twentieth Century Fund, 1996.

Von Eschen, Penny. *Race against Empire: Black Americans and Anticolonialism, 1937–1957.* Ithaca, NY: Cornell University Press, 1997.

Wagner, Philip Sigmund. "A Comparative Study of Negro and White Admissions to the Psychiatric Pavilion of the Cincinnati General Hospital." *American Journal of Psychiatry* 95 (July 1938): 167–83.

Wailoo, Keith. *Dying in the City of the Blues: Sickle Cell Anemia and the Politics of Race and Health.* Chapel Hill: University of North Carolina, 2001.

———. *How Cancer Crossed the Color Line.* New York: Oxford University Press, 2011.

Waldinger, Roger. *Still the Promised City? African Americans and New Immigrants in Postindustrial New York.* Cambridge, MA: Harvard University Press, 1999.

Walker, Margaret. *Richard Wright, Daemonic Genius: A Portrait of the Man, a Critical Look at His Work.* New York: Warner, 1988.

Walter, John C. *The Harlem Fox: J. Raymond Jones and Tammany, 1920–1970.* Albany: State University of New York Press, 1989.

Waquant, Loic. *Punishing the Poor: The Neoliberal Government of Social Insecurity.* Durham, NC: Duke University Press, 2009.

Ward, Jason Morgan. *Defending White Democracy: The Making of a Segregationist Movement and the Remaking of Racial Politics, 1936–1965.* Chapel Hill: University of North Carolina Press, 2011.

Warner, W. Lloyd, Buford H. Junker, and Walter A. Adams. *Color and Human Nature: Negro Personality Development in a Northern City.* Washington, DC: American Council of Education, 1941.

Watkins-Owens, Irma. *Blood Relations: Caribbean Immigrants and the Harlem Community, 1900–1930.* Bloomington: University of Indiana Press, 1994.

Watkins, Rychetta. *Black Power, Yellow Power, and the Making of Revolutionary Identities.* Jackson: University of Mississippi Press, 2014.

Watson, Maud E. *Children and Their Parents.* New York: F. S. Crofts, 1932.

Watts, Jill. *God, Harlem, U.S.A.: The Father Divine Story.* Berkeley: University of California Press, 1992.

Weinstein, Deborah. *The Pathological Family: Postwar America and the Rise of Family Therapy.* Ithaca, NY: Cornell University Press, 2013.

Welsing, Frances Cress. *The Isis Papers: The Keys to Color.* Chicago: Third World Press, 1991.

Weisbord, Robert. *Genocide? Birth Control and the Black American.* New York: Greenwood Press, 1975.

Weisbrot, Robert. *Father Divine and the Struggle for Racial Equality.* Urbana: University of Illinois Press, 1983.

Wertham, Fredric. "Psychological Effects of School Segregation." *American Journal of Psychotherapy* 6 (January 1952): 94–103.

———. "An Unconscious Determinant in *Native Son.*" *Journal of Clinical Psychopathology* 6 (July 1944): 111–15.

White, Joseph L. *The Psychology of Blacks: An Afro-American Perspective.* Englewood Cliffs, NJ: Prentice-Hall, 1984.

White, Walter. *A Man Called White: The Autobiography of Walter White.* 1948. Reprint, Athens: University of Georgia Press, 1995.

Wickberg, Daniel. "What Is the History of Sensibilities? On Cultural Histories, Old and New." *American Historical Review* 112 (June 2007): 661–84.

Wiggins, E. J., and R. S. Lyman. "Manic Psychosis in a Negro: With Special Reference to the Role of the Psychogenic and Sociogenic Factors." *American Journal of Psychiatry* 100 (May 1944): 781–87.

Wilcox, Roger, ed. *The Psychological Consequences of Being a Black American: A Sourcebook of Research by Black Psychologists.* New York: Wiley & Sons, 1971.

Williams, Ernest Y. "The Incidence of Mental Disease in the Negro." *Journal of Negro Education Quarterly* 6 (1937): 377–92.

————. "Some Observations on the Psychological Aspects of Suicide." *Journal of Social and Abnormal Psychology* 31 (October–November 1936): 260–65.

————. "Thieves and Punishment." *Journal of Criminal Law and Criminology* 26 (May 1935): 52–60.

Williams, Mason B. *City of Ambition: FDR, La Guardia, and the Making of Modern New York.* New York: Norton, 2013.

Winant, Howard. *Racial Conditions: Politics, Theory, Comparisons.* Minneapolis: University of Minnesota Press, 1994.

Winsor, Charlotte. "Introduction." In *Experimental Schools Revisited: Bulletins of the Bureau of Educational Experiments,* edited by Charlotte Winsor, 7–19. New York: Agathon Press, 1973.

Winsor, Max. "Children in Need." *Atlantic Monthly,* July 1943, 59–60.

————. "Delinquency in Wartime." *American Journal of Orthopsychiatry* 13 (July 1943): 510–13.

Wittenberg, Rudolph M. "Rethinking the Clinic Function in a Public School Setting." *American Journal of Orthopsychiatry* 14 (October 1944): 722–30.

Wolcott, Victoria W. "The Culture of the Informal Economy: Numbers Runners in Inter-War Detroit." *Radical History Review* 69 (Fall 1997): 46–75.

Wray, Matt. *Not Quite White: White Trash and the Boundaries of Whiteness.* Durham, NC: Duke University Press, 2006.

Wright, Richard. "Psychiatry Comes to Harlem." *Free World* 12 (September 1946): 45–51.

Yamamoto, Joe, and Marcia Kraft Coin. "On the Treatment of the Poor." *American Journal of Psychiatry* 122 (September 1965): 267–71.

Young, Cynthia. *Soul Power: Culture, Radicalism, and the Making of a U.S. Third World Left.* Durham, NC: Duke University Press, 2006.

Yuval-Davis, Nira. *Gender and Nation.* Thousand Oaks, CA: Sage, 1997.

Zunz, Oliver. *Philanthropy in America: A History.* Princeton, NJ: Princeton University Press, 2012.

Index

Printed in the United States
By Bookmasters